BARRON'S

NURSING SCHOOL ENTRANCE EXAMS

5TH EDITION

Sandra Swick, R.N.

Rita Callahan, R.N., B.S.N., M.A., Ph.D.

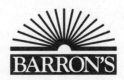

BARRON'S

12-9-16
Roc

Copyright © 2016, 2011, 2007, by Barron's Educational Series, Inc. Originally published under the title *How to Prepare for the Nursing School Entrance Exams*, Copyright © 2004, 1998 by Barron's Educational Series, Inc.

All inquiries should be addressed to:
Barron's Educational Series, Inc.
250 Wireless Boulevard
Hauppauge, New York 11788
www.barronseduc.com

ISBN: 978-1-4380-0627-7

Library of Congress Catalog Card No. 2015945202

Printed in the United States of America

9 8 7 6 5 4 3 2 1

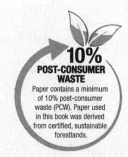

10%
POST-CONSUMER
WASTE
Paper contains a minimum
of 10% post-consumer
waste (PCW). Paper used
in this book was derived
from certified, sustainable
forestlands.

CONTENTS

Introduction

1

IS THIS BOOK FOR YOU?

Are you wondering what might be included on a nursing school entrance exam, or does the nursing program you've applied to require an entrance exam? If you answered yes to either of these questions, then *Nursing School Entrance Exams* is the reference you need.

Nursing school entrance examinations provide associate, diploma, and baccalaureate nursing programs with specific information relating to an applicant's or newly admitted individual's abilities in content areas that provide the foundation for nursing courses such as verbal ability, reading comprehension, numerical or mathematical ability, and life and/or physical sciences. Nursing school entrance examinations generally use a multiple-choice format.

Verbal ability includes elements such as vocabulary, antonyms, synonyms, verbal reasoning, and the use of analogy. Included in verbal ability are English usage and grammar, spelling, prefixes, suffixes, and root words.

Reading comprehension involves reading sentences, paragraphs, or short articles and answering questions, interpreting, and/or making inferences about the literary material. Prior knowledge of the topic is not requisite for reading comprehension because the examination is asking you to think logically and make decisions based on the information presented.

Topics for verbal ability and reading comprehension may address technical or scientific knowledge and/or general, everyday knowledge. Information may come from discipline-specific vocabulary, English grammar, history, geography, literature, art and architecture, humanities, general information, natural sciences, social sciences, and mathematics.

Numerical ability encompasses arithmetic, algebra, and geometry. Computation and interpretation of word problems, charts, ratios and proportions, decimals, percentages, and fractions may also be included. Word problems, drawn from common life events, may address such areas as sales, taxation, insurance, distance or travel, geometry, age, mixtures, investments, interest, and averages.

Life and/or physical sciences sections focus on basic premises of biology, chemistry, human anatomy and physiology. Life sciences specifically addresses human structure and functioning, development, and genetics.

This book is intended to assist you to prepare or review for a nursing school entrance examination. This book is not intended to provide sufficient instruction on any topic in which you have little or no previous experience. For example, if you have never taken algebra or geometry, it is doubtful that the algebra and geometry sections found in this book will provide a background that will enable you to be successful on similar sections of a nursing school entrance examination.

Nursing School Entrance Exams is not intended to address a specific nursing school entrance examination. Nursing programs using entrance exams have a number of examinations from which to choose. These standardized exams are used nationwide. A brief overview of selected nursing school entrance examinations is presented in the following table:

Overview of Selected Nursing School Entrance Examinations

Test	Content Areas	Number of Questions	Time Allowed (in minutes)
HESI A²	Anatomy and Physiology	25	50
	Grammar	50	50
	Biology	25	25
	Chemistry	25	25
	Mathematics	50	50
	Reading Comprehension	47	60
	Vocabulary & General Knowledge	50	50
NET	Reading Comprehension	33	30
	Mathematics	60	60
	*(Reading Rate, Test-Taking Skills, Stress Level Profile, Social Interaction Profile, Learning Style)		
NLN PAX-RN	Mathematics	40	60
	Science	60	60
	Verbal Skills	60	60
PSB-RN	Part I: Vocabulary, Arithmetic, and Form Relationships (minitests)	30, 30, 30	30/minitest
	Part II: Spelling	50	
	Part III: Reading Comprehension	40	
	Part IV: Natural Science	90	
	Part V: Vocational Adjustment Index	90	
RNEE	Life Science	40	
	Numerical Ability	40	
	Physical Science	40	
	Reading Skill	45	
	Verbal Skill	50	
TEAS	English	55	65
	Mathematics	45	56
	Reading	40	50
	Science	30	38

*Does not count toward score

NURSES AND WHAT THEY DO

So you think you want to be a nurse. Nursing is one of the most gratifying careers you'll ever find. But nursing is not what you've seen on television or read about in books. Nursing is hard work, and learning to become a nurse requires dedication and long hours of study and preparation.

Unlike many disciplines in which the academic curricula has foundation courses with many related subjected areas, nursing courses usually build on one another. Prerequisite courses, such as anatomy and physiology, chemistry, microbiology, and biology, are the foundation for what you will learn in your nursing courses, such as medical-surgical nursing, pharmacology, obstetric nursing, and mental health nursing.

When enrolling in prerequisite courses, it should be with the intention of seriously learning information for use as your basic foundation in your nursing courses. Weaknesses in your prerequisite courses may cause problems not only in your nursing coursework, but also on your nursing entrance exam. Remember, nursing courses depend heavily on knowledge learned in prerequisites.

Today's nurses work in numerous roles and settings, and opportunities are virtually unlimited. The following list includes settings in which nurses may practice:

Hospitals	Cruise ships
Clinics	Retirement/nursing homes
Doctors' offices	Volunteer organizations
Business/industry	Occupational health programs
Community agencies	Ambulatory care agencies
Schools	Hospices
Nursing schools	Federal/state agencies
Military	
Resorts and summer camps	

What a nurse actually does depends upon the scope of the practice setting. In the majority of institutional or home health settings, nurses provide care to individuals with chronic, acute physical, and/or mental conditions. What a nurse does also depends upon the needs of the individual patient. The nurse may assume total care of a patient who is unable to meet any of his or her needs or may help only in areas where assistance is needed.

When working with patients, nurses assume a number of roles. In many cases, these roles overlap and are interdependent in nature. They include:

Caregiver	Role model
Comforter	Decision maker
Patient advocate	Case manager
Teacher	Communicator
Counselor	Researcher

When practicing in these various roles, the nurse works to meet, or helps the patient meet, hygiene, elimination, safety, nutritional, spiritual, comfort, activity, sensory, adaptation, and/or mental health needs. The nurse focuses on assessing, analyzing, planning, and resolving actual or potential health problems and evaluates the effectiveness of nursing interventions based on the patient's responses.

Most people think of nurses as working with individuals on a one-to-one basis. In the community setting, however, the patient may not be an individual but a family or group of families, a group of individuals, or an entire community.

Educational preparation plays an important role in career planning in nursing. Career opportunities run hand in hand with a nurse's educational preparation. Simply put, opportunities for advancement increase as education increases. For some levels of practice, an associate degree in nursing is acceptable. For others, a bachelor's degree, a master's degree, or a doctoral degree in nursing or education is required. Career opportunities include:

Staff nurse	Nurse educator
Home health nurse	Nurse researcher
Clinical nurse specialist	Nurse consultant
Nurse midwife	Nurse anesthetist
Nurse administrator	Nurse practitioner
Hospice nurse	Public health nurse

Successful completion and graduation from a nursing program does not allow you to practice or work as a registered nurse. You must be licensed by the state you live in to practice as a *registered* nurse. You will be issued a temporary permit by the state board of nursing. It will allow you to work as a graduate nurse for a specified time. The state board of nursing grants you licensure after you successfully complete the NCLEX-RN examination.

IS NURSING RIGHT FOR ME?

Nursing is not for everyone, and it takes more than "desire" and a "big heart" to be a good nurse. Nursing requires intelligence, self-discipline, critical thinking, communication skills, compassion, dedication, high moral and ethical standards, endurance, as well as respect and concern for the welfare of others regardless of race, creed, culture, religion, or gender orientation.

When considering nursing as a career, think about the following questions.

❏ Is nursing a job or a career?

There is a difference between a job and a career. A job is something you do in exchange for something else, usually money. A career, on the other hand, is something you are dedicated to. A career is an endeavor in which you constantly strive to be the best at your craft and in which life-long learning is not only a necessity but a consuming desire.

❏ Am I a good team player?

In the majority of instances, nursing is a team effort focusing on an identified patient. No one person or specialty is more important than the other. The entire team works together for the patient's welfare.

Broadly speaking, nurses are part of a team that includes a physician and other health care professionals. Depending upon the patient's needs, the team may also include case managers; physical, occupational, respiratory, enterostomal, and speech therapists; nutritionists; social workers; pharmacists; psychologists; and spiritual advisors. Narrowly speaking, the team is the group of health care individuals the nurse works with on a daily basis.

❏ Am I honest, dependable, responsible, and accountable?

These qualities are the hallmarks of a good nurse. Nurses must be honest in their relationships with patients and their families, physicians, and other health care workers. Nurses must also be honest with themselves and be able to seek appropriate assistance in situations in which they are uncomfortable, unsure, or incompetent. Nurses must be dependable and come to work as scheduled and correctly perform responsibilities that are within their scope of practice. Nurses must also be responsible and accountable for their own behavior and actions. The patient, physician, or other health care workers cannot be blamed when nurses make mistakes.

❏ Do I engage in behaviors that have the potential to bring harm to myself, a patient, or others?

When addressing behaviors that have the potential to bring harm to others, as well as oneself, it is impossible to find an individual who has not engaged in potentially harmful behaviors. *Almost* everyone's done it—from running a yellow light because we're going too fast to safely stop, to drinking too much alcohol (being over the legal limit), to inappropriately using cell phones while driving.

Alcohol, prescription medications, over-the-counter medications, and illegal drugs are all chemicals that have the ability to alter behavior, judgment, motor skills, perceptions, physiology, and more. Cemeteries are full of individuals who swore they'd never drive while under the influence. Cemeteries are also full of their victims.

It's essential to remember that behaviors or activities that have the potential to bring harm to yourself or others often violate the law or bring about circumstances where the law is broken. A criminal record can prevent you from being admitted to a nursing program, lead you to dismissal from a nursing program, prevent you from taking the NCLEX-RN after successfully completing your nursing studies, or cause your nursing license to be revoked.

❏ Can past behaviors influence my admission to a nursing program?

Simply put, yes they can. If you have had legal issues or problems in the past, contact the nursing programs you've applied to, as well as the state board of nursing. They can give you the advice you need.

Do not make decisions based on what friends or family tell you. Information that the board of nursing considers is viewed on an individual basis and not based on what might have been done in another case. While cases may look the same, they are not.

❏ Do I follow directions?

There is little nurses do that does not involve following directions of some sort. All health care agencies have policies and procedures that dictate proper behavior or actions to be taken with virtually any responsibility occurring within the institution. Nurses who take shortcuts or ignore institutional policies and procedures when performing patient-related tasks place themselves, patients, and others at risk for injury or even death.

❑ Do I care for others?

Nurses do not selectively determine who they will care for. Nurses provide care to all regardless of gender, race, creed, culture, or religion. Nurses also do not selectively determine the quality of care that a patient receives. All patients deserve the highest standard of care possible.

❑ Am I comfortable with decisions others make even when I disagree with decisions they have made?

Individuals do not forfeit their constitutional rights or their ability to make decisions when they enter the health care system. Competent patients have the right to refuse any and all treatments without fear of reproach or retaliation, even if the end result will ultimately be death.

❑ How do I manage stress or crisis?

Nursing is a profession laden with stressful situations and ever-impending crises, be it patient or institution related. A patient's condition may suddenly worsen, or a nursing unit may have to work short staffed because of absenteeism. Nurses must have the ability to remain calm and collected during stressful or crisis situations in order to focus on the patient.

❑ How do I feel about death and dying?

Human life is fragile, and individuals entering the health care system sometimes die. The process of dying as well as death itself are normal parts of the human existence. An ancient Chinese proverb states "a child born is a child dying" because every minute of life is one minute closer to death. Death is a visitor to those too ill to recover, and death intervenes when all else fails. In order for nurses to work effectively with death and dying, they must understand and accept their own mortality.

❑ How do I handle frustration?

Caring for individuals in any health care setting can be frustrating. Working with others can be frustrating as well. Patients may not be compliant with their medications or keep needed appointments. During a crisis, an institution may have difficulty in obtaining necessary resources. Nurses must be able to control their frustrations. Losing focus could bring harm to all involved.

❑ How do I respond to abusive behaviors?

Patients and their families are under great stress as a result of a serious illness and the possible need for hospitalization. As such, they may not always respond in an appropriate fashion. When patients are verbally abusive, they are usually striking out in frustration, grief, fear, pain, or anxiety. Often times the nurse just happens to be the one to catch their wrath. For the nurse to be verbally abusive in return would be inappropriate and would make an already difficult situation even worse.

Physicians may be verbally abusive to nurses and other health care workers, or health care workers may vent their anger on each other. In all such cases, verbal abuse should not be tolerated.

Physical abuse should also not be tolerated and should be addressed according to institutional policy.

SELECTING A NURSING PROGRAM

If you are seriously considering a career in nursing, you should realize that there is a difference in the types of nursing programs that can lead to a registered nurse designation. Each meets the needs of different types of students.

When selecting a school of nursing, it is important to consider the following questions:

❏ **What is the pass rate for the past five years of the school?**

The pass rate is the percentage of graduates that have successfully completed the NCLEX-RN examination. Schools with consistently low pass rates over a number of years may have inadequately prepared faculty, new or outdated curriculum, or poor instructional methods. Some may have lowered their admission standards and therefore are graduating lower caliber students.

❏ **Is the school of nursing nationally accredited by a volunteer nursing agency or agency of higher education such as the National League for Nursing (NLN), American Nurses Association (ANA), the Commission on Collegiate Nursing Education (CCNE), or one of the associations of colleges and universities?**

Accreditation from a national nursing agency is essential for admission to many graduate programs in nursing. Health care institutions are also interested in the credentials of a nursing program. They may not hire graduates or nurses from nonaccredited programs.

❏ **Is the school of nursing recognized by the state's Board of Nursing?**

The board extends licensure to graduates who successfully write the NCLEX-RN and regulates the practice for registered nurses in a given state. The purpose of a state's Board of Nursing is to protect the public. It may suspend or remove an individual's license to practice nursing if that person is unable to meet the standards of practice for a given state.

❏ **How good a fit would you be at a particular school of nursing or institution of higher education in which the school of nursing is located?**

Do you prefer large educational institutions with a sizeable student population and numerous social and work opportunities, or do you prefer a smaller educational institution with a modest student population and fewer social and work opportunities? Larger institutions may offer more from a nonacademic standpoint. Smaller institutions may provide a close-knit community atmosphere and offer more personalized relationships with faculty and one-to-one assistance when necessary.

❏ **Do you need your own transportation to get to and from classes or clinical experience?**

Schools of nursing typically do not furnish transportation to or from learning experiences on or off campus. Didactic or lecture courses are normally offered on campus. Clinical experience, that is, taking care of patients or clients in various health care settings, is usually conducted off campus, and may be many miles away. There is also no guarantee that clinical sites will be within walking distance.

There are currently three avenues or programs to become a registered nurse in the United States. Each program has its specific educational foundation, type of curriculum, accrediting agencies, educational location, and professional organizations.

Associate degree programs are the shortest in length and usually require two years of nursing course work in addition to non-nursing subjects. Associate degree programs are often referred to as ADN programs and are usually found in community or junior colleges.

Students enrolled in ADN programs are required to take the general education courses all states require of college graduates. These include courses in English, history, psychology, literature or humanities, math, and general sciences. Required non-nursing courses may include anatomy and physiology, chemistry, nutrition, algebra, and microbiology. Associate degree nursing courses usually include nursing fundamentals, medical surgical nursing, mental health nursing, pediatric nursing, obstetric nursing, and history and issues in nursing. Critical thinking, ethical decision making, and problem solving are integrated into all nursing courses.

The second type of nursing program, *diploma programs*, are affiliated with hospitals and are usually three years in length. Diploma programs do not lead to an associate or baccalaureate degree so general education courses may not be required. Diploma programs do, however, require prerequisite courses. These may include anatomy and physiology, microbiology, nutrition, pharmacology, and psychology.

Nursing programs leading to a *baccalaureate degree*, the last type of program, are at least four years in length. These programs are located in four-year colleges, universities, university-affiliated medical centers, and health sciences centers. Like associate degree students, baccalaureate students are required to take the college's or university's general education requirements. Non-nursing or prerequisite courses may include anatomy and physiology, microbiology, chemistry, literature, fine arts, nutrition, ethics, mathematics, logic, statistics, sociology, and psychology.

Nursing courses in baccalaureate programs typically include fundamentals of nursing; health and physical assessment; nursing care of adults, children, and the child-bearing family; perioperative nursing; mental health nursing; community health nursing; nursing management and leadership; nursing theory; nursing research; nursing history and philosophy; and professional nursing concepts, issues, and development. As with ADN programs, critical thinking, ethical decision making, and problem solving are integrated into nursing courses.

Graduates of ADN and diploma programs may, as registered nurses, enter completion or mobility programs found within baccalaureate nursing programs. These types of programs build on the nursing experiences their students have, and students complete the educational requirements for the baccalaureate degree.

Graduates of all three nursing programs take the same licensure examination—the NCLEX-RN. Individuals passing this examination may use the initials R.N. after their name and are allowed to practice or work as a registered nurse in the state that issued the license. This is usually in the state in which the NCLEX-RN is successfully written. Registered nurses may hold multiple licenses to practice in multiple states.

TECHNICIANS VERSUS GENERALISTS

Even though graduates of all three types of nursing programs take the same licensure examination, there is a difference in the focus of each program and in the overall abilities of the graduate. Associate degree and diploma programs prepare graduates for technical nursing practice. These graduates are viewed as care givers in structured care settings. The focus of their care is the individual patient or client.

Baccalaureate programs prepare graduates for professional nursing practice. These nurses are considered generalists because of their ability to perform diverse roles in various health care settings. Baccalaureate programs ask the most of their students, and society expects the most of its graduates. Baccalaureate graduates, in addition to being care givers, also serve as educators in vocational or practical nursing programs, researchers, case managers, client advocates, leaders, and consultants. Generalists deal with the individual patient or client, an individual family or group of families, groups of individuals, populations within communities, or entire communities. Generalists practice in both structured and unstructured health care settings.

GRADUATE EDUCATION

The baccalaureate degree in nursing is the stepping stone to graduate education. Many jobs require advanced education at the master's level and/or doctoral level.

Master's level programs prepare nurses for roles as educators in ADN, diploma, or baccalaureate nursing programs; researchers; managers or administrators in institutional or health care settings; or nurse practitioners. Master's programs in nursing are usually two years in length, providing the individual attends full time.

Doctoral programs offer professional degrees such as the Doctor of Education (Ed.D.), Doctor of Nursing Science (D.N.Sc.), and Doctor of Nursing Practice (DNP), and research degrees such as the Doctor of Philosophy (Ph.D.). Doctoral programs prepare master's educated nurses to practice as nurse educators in undergraduate and graduate nursing programs, administrators in health care or nonhealth care related settings, advanced clinical researchers, consultants, and practitioners.

GETTING INTO NURSING SCHOOL

Entry into a nursing program is dependent upon many factors—grade point average, SAT/ACT scores, references, interviews, writing ability, community or public service, and entrance examinations.

Admission is competitive and schools of nursing may accept only those individuals who, according to the school's standardized criteria, have the greatest chance of success. Nursing schools typically have set standards for the number of admissions each academic year. For this reason, it is a good idea to apply to more than one nursing program.

High school or community college grades are extremely important, and the higher the grade point average, the better. Many schools of nursing require a specific grade point average for consideration for entry into their programs. Most schools require a "B" or "C" average.

It is important to remember that having the required grade point average does not guarantee admission. For example, if the applicant pool for a particular academic year has an average grade point of 3.1 on a 4.0 scale, an individual with a grade point average of 2.0 who meets admission standards may not be granted admission. This is not because this individual could not succeed, but that other more qualified individuals were admitted.

ACT or SAT scores are utilized as admission criteria for many schools of nursing. Again, the higher your score, the better.

Most programs require a number of references. Your references should speak to your critical thinking and problem solving skills, your ability to master difficult and challenging content and material, and your ability to stick with and complete a project with or without difficult circumstances. You should be selective when asking for references and seek them from qualified, appropriate individuals, such as science or math teachers, professors, or better yet, from teachers whose honors or college prep courses you took. Employers may be good references if they are acquainted with your abilities to think logically, solve problems, and work responsibly.

Family, personal friends, clergy, and neighbors are inappropriate references. These individuals know you too well and are probably biased. If you are seeking admission to a religiously affiliated college or university, however, reference from clergy may be required.

Always contact individuals you may use as references before writing their names down. Do not assume because an individual is nice to you that he or she will give you a good reference. When approaching an individual, you might say, "I am applying to the university nursing program. Would you feel comfortable giving me a reference?" His or her enthusiasm or tentativeness may be a good indicator of whether or not that person would make a good reference.

Many nursing programs require a personal interview as part of the admission process. If you interview, make sure that you arrive 15 to 20 minutes early and look your best. Wear business-oriented clothing, not what is fashionable at the moment. Remove visible body piercings. Visible tattoos should be covered. Look and act professionally. Don't chew gum or suck on hard candy during your interview. Remember, the interviewers not only will be listening to what you have to say and how you say it but also will be critiquing how you look and present yourself.

A handwritten essay on a selected topic may be required. Reviewers are interested in your writing and reasoning abilities as well as your proficiency to discuss on paper a topic either known or unknown to you.

Some programs may be interested in the types of public or community service you've done. Performance of such service demonstrates an interest in society as a whole and indicates a well-rounded individual.

SPECIAL TESTING CONSIDERATIONS

The Americans with Disabilities Act (ADA) of 1990 and Section 504 of the Rehabilitation Act of 1973 mandate equal opportunities for individuals with disabilities in all public activities, facilities, programs, services, and benefits derived from them. If you have, or suspect that you have, a disability, it is imperative for you to notify the nursing program (whose nursing entrance test you are preparing to take) as soon as possible.

You simply cannot announce that you have a disability on the day of the test and expect accommodation. Educational institutions have strict policies and procedures for establishing reasonable accommodations for qualified disabled students. The nursing program can advise you on what you need to do and who you need to contact.

FINANCIAL ASSISTANCE

Cost is an important factor when considering a school of nursing. Baccalaureate programs, by their very nature, will be more expensive than diploma or ADN programs because of the length of time required to complete course work.

The decision to work or not while attending school is an important one. Nursing education at any level is expensive. Many students have no choice but to work in order to pay for their education. Ideally, a student who does not have to work can devote all of the time necessary for study, preparation, class attendance, and clinical experiences.

The majority of individuals coming into a nursing program do not realize the time and effort required to be successful. Nursing students typically spend many more hours in daily study and preparation for classes and clinicals than do students in nonhealth-related disciplines. Clinicals may be scheduled for 6 to 12 hours a day for two to three days a week. Students who work 10+ hours a week rarely have adequate time to prepare the required work or care for themselves.

The ideal situation is not to work unless there is no other option available to cover the cost of your education. If you must work, try to get a job in the health care field.

CONSIDER ALL COSTS

When considering the cost of a nursing education, allow for the following expenses each semester or quarter:

1. Tuition and fees
2. Room and board, if any, including money for meals at clinical sites
3. Books and other supplementary materials. Nursing books are expensive and should be kept, not sold, because they serve as reference material for subsequent courses.
4. Uniforms, lab coat, and shoes
5. Malpractice insurance, purchased through the nursing program
6. Stethoscope, bandage scissors, a watch with a second hand, a laptop computer, and other required equipment. Some items are bought only once and others need to be replaced periodically.
7. Transportation and/or vehicle upkeep costs
8. Personal health screening
9. Miscellaneous, hidden, or unexpected expenses
10. Money for entertainment, recreation, and relaxation. All study and no fun can lead to burnout and failure.

Whatever the cost of a nursing education, financial assistance is available in many forms and in various amounts. The institution or the school of nursing you attend can provide specific information.

Prior to accepting any financial assistance, make sure you understand the terms of the contract. Educational loans typically have low interest rates and must be repaid after graduation. Failure to repay can negatively affect your credit rating and may, at some point in time, result in forfeiture of your nursing license. Although this issue is currently being debated, keep in mind that you cannot practice as a nurse without a valid license.

Scholarships and grants may be available that do not require repayment. These sources may not be based upon financial need but may be intended for individuals with certain interests or other needs. Numerous scholarships and grants are provided by private individuals or groups, nursing associations, and the business sector.

Continued financial assistance is often contingent upon grade point average and the number of credit hours taken each semester. Grade point averages falling below stated levels or failure to complete the required number of credit hours may cancel financial assistance, or require repayment.

For any additional questions about preparing for your nursing school entrance exam, you may contact the author at: *picket31644@mypacks.net*

Testing and Test-Taking Strategies

2

Testing is a thread that runs through the tapestry of our lives. Virtually everywhere we turn, there is something that requires testing. Most people develop some measure of anxiety when it comes to test taking. This anxiety is not necessarily bad as long as it does not paralyze your thinking. A little anxiety is normal and can actually be beneficial. If you have anxiety that causes problems with testing, and you haven't sought help already, you should do so now.

There are many different types of tests and test questions. Many tests are offered on computers, and some provide almost immediate feedback. Individuals working on advanced degrees (masters level and higher) may be required to complete both a written and oral exam at the end of their program. There are also many different kinds of test questions. Having passed through the K–12 public or private school system, and having had to take a number of college courses, has introduced you to most of them.

PREPARING FOR YOUR ENTRANCE EXAM

If you're reading this book, you probably have a nursing entrance test ahead of you. What can you do to help yourself prepare for such an important exam? Start by asking yourself the answers to these important questions:

❑ What does your nursing entrance test require?

In order to review and prepare for the entrance test, you need to know what topics will be covered. The nursing program you are interested in can provide this information, and may also have suggestions for preparation.

❑ How did you do in your prerequisite courses?

Most nursing programs require some college work to demonstrate how well you handle topics dealing with post-public school knowledge. Courses such as biology, anatomy and physiology, pharmacology, chemistry, algebra, geometry, or statistics may be required as prerequisites. Too many students tend to think of prerequisites as something they have to get through in order to take the courses required for their major—in your case, nursing. Nothing could be farther from the truth. Look at the word *prerequisite*. What does it mean? Get your dictionary and look the word up if you do not know.

Prerequisite courses set the foundation for more advanced courses in a discipline. If you have a weakness in your prerequisite courses, you have already increased your risk of academic problems in your nursing program. This is not the time to learn what you don't know.

Think of yourself sitting in a nursing lecture class. The topic is oral medications and patients with liver dysfunction. The lecturer starts to talk about the physiologic changes that occur with liver dysfunction and then begins to specifically talk about the "first pass" that all oral medications must go through before the body can use them. If you do not know that "first pass" occurs in the liver, and you do not understand normal liver physiology (from your prerequisite anatomy and physiology course), how will you understand "first pass" and patients with a dysfunctional liver?

To do well on your entrance exam, you need to understand that the writers of the exam assume you bring the necessary knowledge about the topics the exam will cover.

❑ How do you prepare for a test?

There is no one guaranteed method to prepare for a test. You need to develop a system that works for you, and you alone.

There are a number of considerations that can help make a suitable learning environment. Think about the following.

■ *How's your attitude?*

Attitude and education go hand in hand. If you are excited and interested in learning, you will find it easier to prepare for class, go to class, and prepare for exams. Most importantly, you will learn more and perform better. Remember, reviewing for the nursing entrance exam is the first step toward attaining your goal of becoming a nurse.

It is unlikely that you will be successful with your review, or with taking the entrance exam, if you have a poor attitude and find that preparing for class, attending class, and preparing for exams is bothersome.

■ *Where do you study?*

This area should be used only for studying, and supplies for studying should be kept here. There should be no distractions—no music, no cell phones, no interruptions. You will not have any of these things when you take your entrance test, so get used to not having them now.

■ *Do you have dedicated study times?*

Study times should be regular and consistent. Make a schedule you can follow with ease. These should be peak times during your day. Your friends and family need to know when these times are, so that they do not interrupt you while you study. You need an uninterrupted period that is yours. If those who care for you truly want you to be successful on your entrance test, they will give you the uninterrupted time you need to prepare for the exam.

■ *How long do you study?*

Studying for prolonged periods of time without breaks and cramming for exams can be a waste of time. Get into the habit of studying for approximately 50 minutes and then break for 10 minutes (50/10). This gives you time to clear your head, and a chance to stretch and move around. Use your break time constructively—leave your study area and exercise, meditate, or do another activity you enjoy for ten minutes. Using the 50/10 study method allows you to study longer without tiring.

Cramming is for the foolish and does not contribute to long-term memory. The majority of information learned when cramming is short term and rarely remembered over time.

Remember, do not take any over-the-counter medications to keep yourself awake or alert. These preparations may hinder your learning.

■ *What do you have with you when you study?*

Your study area should have everything you need for your study session. Having to constantly get up and find study aids wastes your time and is a distraction. Use this review book with your own books and class notes, plus any other materials you have that may aid your review.

■ *How do you determine that you have mastered content?*

Reviewing does little good if you have no way to determine that you have learned or know what you have been reviewing. Identify a section, such as mitosis, and study it. When you have finished, take a sheet of paper and write out or draw all of the steps of mitosis and what each step means. If you can do this successfully, then you most likely have a good handle on the content. As an extra measure, when you begin a new study session, write out everything you learned from your previous session. Retesting yourself reinforces your learning for the long term.

■ *What do you do the day before the exam?*

Drive to the testing site if you have not been there before. Identify the building or business. If the testing site is in a large multistory building, park and go into the building so that you can locate where you will take your exam. Determine where the parking area is—will you have a long walk from the parking lot to the testing site? Will you have to pay for parking? You probably will not be able to take the test if you arrive late. Make sure you know where you're going and arrive early.

Your preparation for your entrance exam should be complete. Review areas that are still difficult, or test yourself for mastery.

Make sure you have everything you need for the next day's test. Having to search for something the morning of the test can be distracting and unsettling. What clothes and shoes will you wear? What identification materials do you need? Do you need money? Plan on getting around 8 hours of sleep the night before. You need to be well rested and alert for your exam.

■ *What to do the morning/day of the exam?*

Set your alarm if necessary, get up early, and give yourself plenty of time to get ready. Eat a moderate breakfast and don't stuff yourself. You need to be alert and at your best, not drowsy from eating too much. Double-check and make sure you have everything you need. Make a list if you have to. Take a sweater or light jacket with you. Testing areas are sometimes kept cooler. Leave an extra thirty minutes to an hour earlier than you need to. It won't hurt to arrive early. Many events could delay your arrival at the testing center—you could have a flat tire or car trouble, or you could be involved in or come upon an accident with backed-up traffic. Arrive at the testing check-in area early. Locate the nearest bathroom and go there ahead of time—you may not be able to leave the testing area once the exam starts. Get a drink of water if you need to. You may have many more things you want to include when preparing for your entrance exam. What you've just read are suggestions.

The word

CHALLENGE

appears before those practice questions in this book that represent the higher level questions you may encounter on an actual exam.

MULTIPLE-CHOICE TEST QUESTIONS

By this time in your education, you have, in all likelihood, experienced the majority of different types of test questions. The type of questions you will see on your entrance exam will be multiple-choice questions—the name means exactly what it says, you will have more than one choice to choose from on each question. Your job is to select the correct, or most correct, answer.

When you look at a question, the stem presents a definite problem and focuses on a learning outcome. The stem can also be an incomplete sentence. The list of possible choices in multiple-choice questions contains one correct answer choice and a number of distracters or incorrect choices. Table 2.1 presents the different types of multiple-choice questions you may see on your entrance exam.

Table 2.1. Multiple-Choice Question Types

True/False	Most Accurate
There are 51 states in the United States of America. (A) True (B) False**	The large vessel that pumps blood from the left ventricle to the body is (A) a blood vessel. (B) an artery. (C) the aorta.** (D) the largest vessel in the body.
Odd One Out	**Completion**
Select the option that is different from the others. (A) 15, 45, 72 (B) 4, 32, 88** (C) 70, 42, 14 (D) 63, 90, 117	Two angles whose sum is 90° are called (A) adjacent angles. (B) complementary angles.** (C) right angles. (D) supplementary angles.
Grid	
The shopping list included selecting three different kinds of fruit. Which of the following should be selected? 1. Apples 4. Oranges 2. Broccoli 5. Potatoes 3. Kiwi 6. Squash (A) 1, 2, 5 (B) 1, 3, 4** (C) 2, 5, 6 (D) 3, 4, 6	

**Correct answer

TEST-TAKING STRATEGIES
General Strategies

- Pay attention to the instructions! Listen carefully to verbal instructions. Read printed instructions carefully and thoroughly. If the test is computerized, can you leave an unanswered question and go back to it later? If not, and you're unsure of the answer, make your best choice.
- Keep your mind open when reading stems and possible answers. Do not make assumptions. Do not argue with the question. Do not read into the question. Remember, the stem will give you all of the information you need!
- Be careful when changing answers unless you know you mismarked an answer. If you do change an answer, make sure you know why the originally selected answer is incorrect *and* why the new answer is correct. Do not guess!
- Take your time, within reason, on an untimed test.
- Monitor yourself on a timed test. If you're spending much more than one minute per question, or more than two minutes per question on numerical tests, you may run out of time.
- Know the number of questions on your test. If you are taking a paper-and-pencil test, look in the back of the booklet for the number of questions. The information you were given on the entrance test should also provide the number of questions on each section of the test. Knowing the number of questions will help you manage your time.

Understand the Stem of the Question

- Read the stem carefully and determine what you need to do.
- Cover the possible answer choices and do not look at them until you understand the stem.
- Circle important words in the stem if you are taking a paper-and-pencil test.
- Quickly answer the question before looking at the possible answer choices.

Review Every Answer Choice

- Read all of the possible choices before making a decision. One choice may be 90% correct, but another choice is 100% correct. Rapidly selecting the first choice that "sounds good" may be incorrect.
- Reread each possible choice. If you believe a choice is incorrect, you should be able to justify why it is incorrect. If you cannot justify your reasoning, the choice may be correct.
- Eliminate and forget any answer choice you've deemed as incorrect. Using this strategy, you may be able to eliminate all but one choice, the correct answer.
- Just as you justified why some answer choices were incorrect, you need to be able to justify why your selected "correct" answer is the appropriate choice.
- If you're having problems determining a correct answer to a test question, treat the options as true/false statements. You can eliminate the false or incorrect options until only the true, correct answer choice remains.

There are myths that students sometimes use when trying to determine correct answers on multiple-choice tests. It is important to remember the test writers are also aware of these myths. The longest answer option is not always the correct one, and "C" is not necessarily the option to choose if you are guessing.

- Try to break down words that you are not familiar with. Identify prefixes, root words, and suffixes in an effort to define the word.
- Pay attention to words used in the answer choices. Be careful when choosing options that contain: all, always, more, never, none, not, or only.

Choose the Correct Answer

- If you are still uncertain of the correct answer, make an **educated** guess after using the process of elimination.
- Look for possible wording in the stem or answer choices that may give a clue to the correct answer. Do not read into the question or make assumptions during this process.
- Eliminate answer choices that do not represent what the stem requests.

Review Your Work

- If possible, review your test before submitting it. This is not the time to frantically change answers, but rather it is the time to make sure that you did not skip any questions or fill in the answer bubble for choice B when you meant to select choice C.
- If you are taking a paper-and-pencil test, make sure all erasures are complete and do not leave smudges that could cause your answer to be mismarked.
- Hand in your test and be confident that you did your best.

EXAMPLE QUESTIONS

Practice the strategies that you just learned. Read the following questions and attempt to determine the correct answer.

1. Upon learning that you have completed your first year of nursing school, your 55-year-old neighbor, who lives with her family, asks if giving up cigarette smoking would be beneficial at her age. Which of the following statements could you say in response that would most likely encourage the neighbor to stop smoking cigarettes?

    (A) "Cigarettes are expensive and the cost is constantly going up."
    (B) "Second-hand smoke has been associated with a number of serious illnesses. Does your family have any health problems?"
    (C) "As sad as it is to say, it doesn't matter because the damage is irreversible after twenty or thirty years of cigarette smoking. Your present health won't improve."
    (D) "Stopping smoking at any age reduces the risk of heart disease, stroke, and peripheral vascular disease."

The correct answer is choice D. Research has shown that stopping smoking at any age can be beneficial. Based on information given in the question, choice D is the only logical statement.

Choice A is incorrect because the stem gives no indication that the cost of cigarettes is an issue for the neighbor, even though it is true that cigarettes are expensive with the cost continually going up.

Choice B is a true statement, but again, it doesn't apply because the question does not suggest that second-hand smoke is an issue for your neighbor. Also, no additional information is provided as to what is meant by "family." How many members are in this family? What are their ages? Do they also smoke cigarettes?

Choice C is also incorrect because it is a false statement.

Did you miss this question? What led you to select an incorrect answer? Go back and reread the question. Look specifically at the information that the question provides, namely the neighbor's age, the fact that she lives with others, the fact that she is a smoker, and that she wants to know if quitting smoking would be beneficial at her age. **Beneficial** is a key word. Synonyms of beneficial are helpful, advantageous, and gainful. The neighbor wants to know if quitting smoking will help her. This is basically all that you need to know to answer the question. Do not select an answer choice that has nothing to do with the information provided in the question.

2. Which of the following temperatures is required to bring water to a boil at sea level?

(A) 0° Fahrenheit
(B) 100° Fahrenheit
(C) 0° Celsius
(D) 100° Celsius

The correct answer is choice D. Read the answer choices carefully. If you know that water boils at 212° Fahrenheit, or 100° Celsius, this question may be easy for you. Be careful. You may have selected choice B if you remembered 100° and chose the first answer that contained that number without reading all of the choices closely.

3. Select the risk factor that is *most closely identified* with cardiovascular disease.

(A) diabetes
(B) family history of heart disease
(C) hypertension
(D) obesity

The correct answer is choice B. Family history of heart disease is the correct answer because, of the choices given, it is the only one that cannot be modified or changed. Diabetes, hypertension, and obesity are risk factors for cardiovascular disease, but they can be treated or changed.

The question asks for you to decipher the best answer choice out of all the options. Obviously, all are correct to some degree, but one choice must be more correct than all the others. How are the options different? The difference is that three choices, A, C, and D, are all modifiable, while choice B is nonmodifiable.

4. According to the Centers for Disease Control (CDC) and Prevention, the leading cause of mortality among adolescents aged 15–19 is

(A) homicide.
(B) suicide.
(C) unintentional injury.
(D) adolescent cancer.

The correct answer is choice C. Like the previous question, all of the answer choices are leading causes of death in adolescents. This question can be reasoned out if you stop and consider each choice separately.

Choice A is not the best answer. Homicide, from the perspective of the CDC, refers to all adolescent homicide in the United States, regardless of gender or ethnic group.

Choice B is a possibility. The news frequently reports the suicide of individuals as young as six or seven years of age to nineteen-year-olds. Suicide unfortunately seems more and more common, but is it the leading cause?

Choice C is the best answer. Stop and consider what the word *unintentional* means. Synonyms are accidental, unplanned, involuntary, unpremeditated, or not deliberate. Homicide and suicide are normally considered intentional or premeditated. Take a minute and consider all of the ways 15–19-year-olds could suffer an accidental injury leading to death—the list is virtually endless.

Choice D would require an expert to determine the answer. How many types of cancer are considered solely adolescent cancers? Cancers are commonly referred to as "childhood," not adolescent. Therefore, this choice is not the answer.

DIAGNOSTIC TEST

The remainder of this chapter includes a diagnostic test to take before you begin preparing for your entrance exam. While this test contains all sections covered in this book, it is important to remember that it is not all-inclusive. Its purpose is to test what you know, and what you need to review further. When you look at the number of questions missed in each section, a good rule of thumb is that the more questions you missed on a section, the more time you should spend reviewing that material.

ANSWER SHEET
Diagnostic Test

Section 1: Verbal Ability

1. Ⓐ Ⓑ Ⓒ Ⓓ
2. Ⓐ Ⓑ Ⓒ Ⓓ
3. Ⓐ Ⓑ Ⓒ Ⓓ
4. Ⓐ Ⓑ Ⓒ Ⓓ

5. Ⓐ Ⓑ Ⓒ Ⓓ
6. Ⓐ Ⓑ Ⓒ Ⓓ
7. Ⓐ Ⓑ Ⓒ Ⓓ
8. Ⓐ Ⓑ Ⓒ Ⓓ

9. Ⓐ Ⓑ Ⓒ Ⓓ
10. Ⓐ Ⓑ Ⓒ Ⓓ

Section 2: Reading Comprehension

1. Ⓐ Ⓑ Ⓒ Ⓓ
2. Ⓐ Ⓑ Ⓒ Ⓓ

3. Ⓐ Ⓑ Ⓒ Ⓓ
4. Ⓐ Ⓑ Ⓒ Ⓓ

Section 3: Numerical Ability

1. Ⓐ Ⓑ Ⓒ Ⓓ
2. Ⓐ Ⓑ Ⓒ Ⓓ
3. Ⓐ Ⓑ Ⓒ Ⓓ
4. Ⓐ Ⓑ Ⓒ Ⓓ

5. Ⓐ Ⓑ Ⓒ Ⓓ
6. Ⓐ Ⓑ Ⓒ Ⓓ
7. Ⓐ Ⓑ Ⓒ Ⓓ
8. Ⓐ Ⓑ Ⓒ Ⓓ

9. Ⓐ Ⓑ Ⓒ Ⓓ
10. Ⓐ Ⓑ Ⓒ Ⓓ

Section 4: Biology/Chemistry

1. Ⓐ Ⓑ Ⓒ Ⓓ
2. Ⓐ Ⓑ Ⓒ Ⓓ
3. Ⓐ Ⓑ Ⓒ Ⓓ
4. Ⓐ Ⓑ Ⓒ Ⓓ

5. Ⓐ Ⓑ Ⓒ Ⓓ
6. Ⓐ Ⓑ Ⓒ Ⓓ
7. Ⓐ Ⓑ Ⓒ Ⓓ
8. Ⓐ Ⓑ Ⓒ Ⓓ

9. Ⓐ Ⓑ Ⓒ Ⓓ
10. Ⓐ Ⓑ Ⓒ Ⓓ

Section 5: Anatomy & Physiology

1. Ⓐ Ⓑ Ⓒ Ⓓ
2. Ⓐ Ⓑ Ⓒ Ⓓ
3. Ⓐ Ⓑ Ⓒ Ⓓ
4. Ⓐ Ⓑ Ⓒ Ⓓ
5. Ⓐ Ⓑ Ⓒ Ⓓ
6. Ⓐ Ⓑ Ⓒ Ⓓ
7. Ⓐ Ⓑ Ⓒ Ⓓ

8. Ⓐ Ⓑ Ⓒ Ⓓ
9. Ⓐ Ⓑ Ⓒ Ⓓ
10. Ⓐ Ⓑ Ⓒ Ⓓ
11. Ⓐ Ⓑ Ⓒ Ⓓ
12. Ⓐ Ⓑ Ⓒ Ⓓ
13. Ⓐ Ⓑ Ⓒ Ⓓ
14. Ⓐ Ⓑ Ⓒ Ⓓ

15. Ⓐ Ⓑ Ⓒ Ⓓ
16. Ⓐ Ⓑ Ⓒ Ⓓ
17. Ⓐ Ⓑ Ⓒ Ⓓ
18. Ⓐ Ⓑ Ⓒ Ⓓ
19. Ⓐ Ⓑ Ⓒ Ⓓ
20. Ⓐ Ⓑ Ⓒ Ⓓ

SECTION 1: VERBAL ABILITY

For Questions 1–6, select the letter (A, B, C, or D) that best matches the paired words. Record your answers in Section 1 of the Diagnostic Answer Sheet on page 21.

1. ALTERCATE : STRIFE : : ALTRUISM : _____

   (A) GENTLENESS
   (B) GOODWILL
   (C) SELFISHNESS
   (D) TRANQUIL

2. COVETOUS : GUILTY : : _____ : CULPABLE

   (A) JEALOUS
   (B) INDIFFERENT
   (C) INNOCENT
   (D) LIBERAL

3. IGNOBLE : _____ : : IMPRECATION : BLESSING

   (A) BASE
   (B) CURSE
   (C) HONORABLE
   (D) MALEDICTION

4. OSTENTATIOUS : MODEST : : OSTENSIBLE : _____

   (A) APPARENT
   (B) IMPROBABLE
   (C) PRESUME
   (D) SEEMING

5. $3 + 5 = 5 + 3$: COMMUTATIVE PROPERTY OF ADDITION : : $(3 + 4) + 8 = 3 + (4 + 8)$: _____

   (A) ADDITIVE INVERSE
   (B) ASSOCIATIVE PROPERTY OF ADDITION
   (C) CLOSURE
   (D) IDENTITY ELEMENT

6. $A(B + C + D) = (AB) + (AC) + (AD)$: TRUE STATEMENT : : $A(B + C + D) = (AB)(AC)(AD)$: _____

   (A) CANNOT BE DETERMINED
   (B) CANNOT BE DETERMINED UNLESS NUMBERS ARE USED INSTEAD OF LETTERS
   (C) FALSE STATEMENT
   (D) TRUE STATEMENT

For Questions 7–10, select the letter (A, B, C, or D) that best represents the definition of the word in the question. Record your answers in Section 1 of the Diagnostic Answer Sheet on page 21.

7. The old man had an *assemblage* of foreign coins from the early 19th century. The suffix *–age* in the word *assemblage* means

(A) characteristic of
(B) collection of
(C) inclination for
(D) knowledge

8. The root word *fract* means

(A) break
(B) design
(C) joint
(D) part

9. The suffix *–osis* means

(A) acquire
(B) condition
(C) cut
(D) turn

10. *Bounty* means

(A) abundance
(B) bombast
(C) limit
(D) roll

SECTION 2: READING COMPREHENSION

> For Questions 1–4, select the letter (A, B, C, or D) that best answers the question. Record your answers in Section 2 of the Diagnostic Answer Sheet on page 21.

I Heard a Fly Buzz When I Died

I heard a fly buzz – when I died –
The stillness round my form
Was like the stillness in the air –
Between the heaves of storm –

Line

(5) The eyes around – had wrung them dry –
And breaths were gathering firm
For that last onset – when the King
Be witnessed – in the room –

I willed my keepsakes – signed away
(10)   What portion of me be
Assignable – and then it was
There interposed a fly –

With blue – uncertain stumbling buzz,
Between the light – and me –
(15)   And then the windows failed –
And then I could not see to see

1. A conclusion that one can draw from this poem is
   - (A) an individual is dreaming that he is dying, and the buzzing fly is a part of the dream.
   - (B) the dying individual's last thoughts are stopped by a fly in the room.
   - (C) odd occurrences may happen at the moment of death.
   - (D) the speaker of this poem is dead and talking about the fly from beyond the grave.

2. What does "interposed" in line 12 suggest?
   - (A) The fly came between two things.
   - (B) The fly became part of the situation.
   - (C) The fly delayed the death of the person.
   - (D) The fly probably isn't real. It's a hallucination.

3. In the second stanza (lines 5–8), who is the King that comes into the room?
   - (A) Death
   - (B) God
   - (C) The husband of the dying woman
   - (D) The King of the country

4. What is happening in the last two lines (15 and 16) of the poem?
   - (A) Darkness comes and no light is shining through the window.
   - (B) Death comes, and the individual's eyes close.
   - (C) The individual is speaking from the other side.
   - (D) The window curtains were closed by someone.

SECTION 3: NUMERICAL ABILITY

> For Questions 1–10, solve for the unknown on a separate sheet of paper, if necessary. Then, select the letter (A, B, C, or D) that represents your answer. Record your answers in Section 3 of the Diagnostic Answer Sheet on page 21.

1. $\dfrac{4}{x} = \dfrac{2}{5} =$

   (A) 10
   (B) 20
   (C) 30
   (D) 40

2. $\dfrac{3}{4} \div \left(-\dfrac{4}{8} \right) =$

   (A) $\dfrac{3}{8}$

   (B) $-\dfrac{3}{8}$

   (C) $1\dfrac{1}{2}$

   (D) $-1\dfrac{1}{2}$

3. Solve for k if b is to k as d is to a. $\left(\dfrac{b}{k} = \dfrac{d}{a} \right)$

   (A) $k = \dfrac{da}{b}$

   (B) $k = \dfrac{ba}{d}$

   (C) $k = \dfrac{bd}{a}$

   (D) Not enough information is given to solve for k.

4. Penicillin 250 mg/tablet is ordered 4 times a day for 12 days. Each tablet costs $2.38. What is the total cost of the prescription?

   (A) $28.56
   (B) $49.55
   (C) $114.24
   (D) $207.65

5. A plane flies from Point A to Point B, a distance of 1,500 miles at 500 mph. On the return trip from Point B to Point A, it encounters a storm and averages 375 mph. How many total hours was the plane in the air for the entire trip?

   (A) 3.4 hours
   (B) 7.0 hours
   (C) 8.0 hours
   (D) 8.6 hours

6. A jacket that normally sells for $245.99 is on sale with a 30% markdown. The sales tax is 6.88%. What is the markdown, in dollars, for the jacket?

   (A) $73.80
   (B) $172.19
   (C) $184.04
   (D) $215.99

7. One number exceeds another number by 15. Find the smaller number if the sum of the two numbers is 83.

   (A) 5.18
   (B) 34
   (C) 49
   (D) 53

8. Sarah and Abigail are sisters. Sarah is 7 years older than Abigail. In 2 years, Sarah will be twice as old as Abigail. How old is Abigail now?

   (A) 2-years-old
   (B) 3-years-old
   (C) 4-years-old
   (D) 5-years-old

9. Tickets for the fair are $10.00 for adults and $6.00 for seniors. Over a two-week period, 10,000 tickets were sold. The total income from both sets of tickets was $94,988. How many of each type of ticket were sold?

(A) 5,649 adult tickets and 4,351 senior tickets
(B) 6,000 adult tickets and 4,000 senior tickets
(C) 8,747 adult tickets and 1,253 senior tickets
(D) 9,156 adult tickets and 844 senior tickets

10. What is the volume of a cube whose side is 8.35 inches?

(A) 200.00 inches
(B) 269.34 inches
(C) 448.13 cubic inches
(D) 582.18 cubic inches

SECTION 4: BIOLOGY/CHEMISTRY

For Questions 1–10, select the letter (A, B, C, or D) that best answers the question. Record your answers in Section 4 of the Diagnostic Answer Sheet on page 21.

1. Basic biological concepts include all of the following EXCEPT

   (A) adaptation.
   (B) homeostasis.
   (C) metabolism.
   (D) nutrition.

2. Life is best defined in terms

   (A) of breathing and respiration.
   (B) of functions performed by all living things.
   (C) of movement of fluid and other materials throughout the organism.
   (D) of processes included with ingestion and digestion.

3. _____ is defined as the production of a substance by the coming together of chemical elements, groups, of simpler compounds or by the degradation of a complex compound where simple molecules are built larger and more complex.

   (A) Excretion
   (B) Regulation
   (C) Respiration
   (D) Synthesis

4. Types of reproduction are

   1. Asexual requiring a single parent
   2. Asexual requiring two parents
   3. Sexual requiring two parents
   4. Sexual requiring one parent

   (A) 1 and 2
   (B) 3 and 4
   (C) 1 and 3
   (D) 2 and 4

5. Which of the following is TRUE regarding cellular organization?

   (A) Living matter is always divided into small units known as cells.
   (B) Cells vary in size, shape, and function, yet all have important characteristics in common.
   (C) Cell response time and duration varies slowly over time.
   (D) All members of one species of cell in one region of the body have similar characteristics.

6. Anything that has weight and occupies space is considered (a)

   (A) antimatter.
   (B) compound.
   (C) matter.
   (D) suspension.

7. _____ is an example/are examples of a solution.

   (A) Alcohol and water
   (B) Fog
   (C) Italian salad dressing
   (D) White of an egg

8. Acids and bases _____.

   (A) are almost the same
   (B) are opposites
   (C) are separated by filtration
   (D) release hydrogen ions in water suspensions

9. During embryonic/fetal development, all of the following are derived from the ectoderm EXCEPT the
   (A) circulatory system.
   (B) epidermis.
   (C) nervous system.
   (D) pituitary gland.

10. Which of Mendel's laws of heredity is the following statement based on?

   Genes for different traits are sorted separately from one another so that the inheritance of one trait is not dependent on the inheritance of another.

   (A) Dominance
   (B) Genes
   (C) Independent assortment
   (D) Segregation

SECTION 5: ANATOMY AND PHYSIOLOGY

For Questions 1–20, select the letter (A, B, C, or D) that best answers the question. Record your answers in Section 5 of the Diagnostic Answer Sheet on page 21.

1. The position of the _____ is located in the mediastinum of the thorax, approximately between the second and fifth ribs. It rests on the diaphragm, lies posterior to the sternum, is bordered by the lungs that overlie it, and lies anterior to the vertebral column.

    (A) heart
    (B) kidneys
    (C) liver
    (D) spleen

2. Which of the following has the ability to adjust blood flow by dilation or constriction, and pumps high-pressure blood to the body?

    (A) arteries
    (B) arterioles
    (C) capillaries
    (D) veins

3. A man has a blood pressure of 142/78. The 142 is indicative of

    (A) peak pressure applied against artery walls during contraction of the heart.
    (B) the contraction phase brought on by depolarization and contraction of the ventricles.
    (C) remaining pressure within the arterial system during cardiac relaxation.
    (D) the volume of blood pumped out of the right and left ventricles.

4. _____ regulate(s) fluid and electrolyte balance, reproduction, growth and development, adaptation to stress, and metabolism.

    (A) Glands
    (B) Gonads
    (C) Hormones
    (D) Vasopressin

5. Which of the following glands produces the adrenocorticotropic hormone (ACTH)?

    (A) adrenal gland
    (B) anterior lobe of the pituitary
    (C) hypothalamus
    (D) thyroid gland

6. Mineralocorticoids

    (A) control sodium and mineral balance.
    (B) influence secondary sex hormones.
    (C) regulate blood pressure, respiration, and temperature.
    (D) regulate sugar and protein metabolism.

7. Homeostasis is a state of equilibrium

    (A) where fluid balance exists when water in equals water out.
    (B) when all solutes in the body are dissolved or suspended in water.
    (C) when distribution of body fluids among body fluid compartments is regulated.
    (D) within the body when all body systems are balanced.

8. Body fluid is primarily

    (A) blood.
    (B) electrolytes.
    (C) oxygen.
    (D) water.

9. The _____ is a hollow tube or passageway that extends from the pharynx to the stomach.

    (A) duodenum
    (B) esophagus
    (C) oral cavity
    (D) pyloric sphincter

10. Which of the following is essential for absorption of vitamin B_{12} in the small intestine?

  (A) amylase
  (B) chyme
  (C) hydrochloric acid
  (D) intrinsic factor

11. Hematopoiesis is the

  (A) formation of blood or blood cells in the living body.
  (B) liquid portion of whole blood with clotting factors.
  (C) number of blood cells in the body.
  (D) synthesis of plasma factors including albumin and clotting factors.

12. The function of red blood cells (RBCs) is to

  (A) carry hemoglobin via circulation to cells and carbon dioxide to the lungs.
  (B) circulate self-renewing cells from the bone marrow.
  (C) disseminate folic acid, vitamin D, and iron.
  (D) synthesize coagulation factors VII, IX, and X.

13. The thymus gland, areas of the spleen, tonsils, and Peyer's patches

  (A) are found primarily in the inguinal and axillary areas.
  (B) are organs of the lymph system.
  (C) produce antibodies.
  (D) secrete monocytes that transform into macrophages.

14. _____ is an example of passive acquired immunity.

  (A) Acquired from having the disease
  (B) Gamma globulin injection
  (C) Opsonization
  (D) Vaccination

15. Neurons

  (A) contain no special structures.
  (B) have a nucleus that contains genes.
  (C) have no cell membrane.
  (D) speed conduction time along nerve fibers.

16. Which of the following regulates activity of smooth muscles?

  (A) acetylcholine reflexes
  (B) autonomic reflexes
  (C) neuropeptide reflexes
  (D) somatic reflexes

17. The risk of aspiration is greater in the right main stem bronchus because

  (A) of the difference in pressure gradients between the left and right stem bronchi.
  (B) it does not participate in gas exchange.
  (C) it is shorter, wider, and more vertical.
  (D) of its association with the trachea.

18. The pneumotaxic area of respiration is located in the

  (A) brain stem.
  (B) medulla.
  (C) pons.
  (D) stretch receptors.

19. Renal system nerve fibers regulate blood flow. Sympathetic fibers _____ and parasympathetic fibers _____.

  (A) constrict arterioles, dilate arterioles
  (B) dilate arterioles, constrict arterioles
  (C) constrict venules, dilate venules
  (D) dilate venules, constrict venules

20. Urine is expelled from the body via the

  (A) collecting duct.
  (B) tubules.
  (C) ureters.
  (D) urethra.

ANSWER KEY
Diagnostic Test

Section 1: Verbal Ability

1. **B**		3. **C**		5. **B**		7. **B**		9. **B**	
2. **A**		4. **B**		6. **C**		8. **A**		10. **A**	

Section 2: Reading Comprehension

1. **D**		3. **A**
2. **A**		4. **B**

Section 3: Numerical Ability

1. **A**	3. **B**	5. **B**	7. **B**	9. **C**
2. **D**	4. **C**	6. **A**	8. **D**	10. **D**

Section 4: Biology/Chemistry

1. **D**	3. **D**	5. **B**	7. **A**	9. **A**
2. **B**	4. **C**	6. **C**	8. **B**	10. **C**

Section 5: Anatomy & Physiology

1. **A**	5. **B**	9. **B**	13. **B**	17. **C**
2. **A**	6. **A**	10. **D**	14. **B**	18. **C**
3. **A**	7. **D**	11. **A**	15. **B**	19. **A**
4. **C**	8. **D**	12. **A**	16. **B**	20. **D**

ANSWERS EXPLAINED

Section 1: Verbal Ability

1. **(B)** Altruism and goodwill are synonyms, as are altercate and strife.

2. **(A)** Covetous and jealous are synonyms, as are guilty and culpable.

3. **(C)** Ignoble and honorable are antonyms, as are imprecation and blessing.

4. **(B)** Ostentatious and modest are antonyms, as are ostensible and improbable.

5. **(B)** The commutative property of addition means that the order of numbers does not make any difference. The associative property of addition means that the grouping of numbers does not make any difference.

6. **(C)** Use real numbers for A, B, C, and D to determine your answer.

$$A = 2, B = 4, C = 6, D = 8$$

$$A(B + C + D) = (AB) + (AC) + (AD)$$
$$2(4 + 6 + 8) = (2 \times 4) + (2 \times 6) + (2 \times 8)$$
$$2(4 + 6 + 8) = (8) + (12) + (16)$$
$$2(18) = 36$$
$$36 = 36$$

$$A(B + C + D) = (AB)(AC)(AD)$$
$$2(4 + 6 + 8) = (2 \times 4)(2 \times 6)(2 \times 8)$$
$$2(4 + 6 + 8) = (8)(12)(16)$$
$$2(18) = 1,536$$
$$36 \neq 1,536$$

7. **(B)** The suffix *–age* in the word *assemblage* means *collection of*. In this sentence, the man has a collection of coins.

8. **(A)** The root word *fract* means *break* as in a *fracture* or a *break*.

9. **(B)** The suffix *–osis* means *condition* as in *hypnosis* or the *condition* or state of being hypnotized.

10. **(A)** The word *bounty* means *abundance* as in a *bounty* of apples collected from apple picking.

Section 2: Reading Comprehension

1. **(D)** The first line of the poem provides the answer, "I heard a fly buzz—when I died." The remaining responses are incorrect. There is nothing in the poem to suggest that the individual is dreaming about death, so choice A is incorrect. Choice B is wrong because the fly in the room did not stop the last thought of the dying individual. The fly is merely an interruption, but it did not stop his thoughts. Choice C is a general statement for when all individuals die. This response is not specific to the dying individual in the poem.

2. **(A)** The buzzing fly comes between the light and the dying person. The remaining responses are incorrect. The fly never becomes a part of the situation, so choice B is wrong, nor does it delay the individual's death, so choice C is incorrect. There is also nothing to suggest hallucinations as choice D incorrectly states.

3. **(A)** Death has been personified, and there is the notion that death is present when an individual dies. The remaining responses are incorrect. God is not personified and may not be present during a person's death, as choice B suggests. There is nothing in the poem that implies that the dying individual has a husband or lives in a country that has a King, making choices C and D both incorrect.

4. **(B)** The eyes are often referred to as the "windows to the soul" and would "fail" at the moment of death when the soul theoretically leaves the body. The remaining responses are incorrect. There is nothing to suggest that darkness has come and no light is shining through the window, so choice A is wrong. It is possible to select choice C and assume that the individual is speaking from the other side. This choice, however, does not address what the question is asking, which is to answer what is happening in lines 15 and 16 specifically. Choice D is incorrect as well. Although the poem uses the word "windows," it does not mean windows in the literal sense, which have curtains that can be opened or closed, nor is there a "someone" described in the poem who might be closing these windows.

Section 3: Numerical Ability

1. **(A)** $\dfrac{4}{x} = \dfrac{2}{5}$

   $2x = 20$

   $x = 10$

2. **(D)** $\dfrac{3}{4} \div \left(-\dfrac{4}{8}\right)$

   $\dfrac{3}{4} \times \left(-\dfrac{8}{4}\right)$

   $\dfrac{3}{4} \times -\dfrac{2}{1} = -\dfrac{6}{4} = -1\dfrac{1}{2}$

3. **(B)** $\dfrac{b}{k} = \dfrac{d}{a}$

   $kd = ba$

   $k = \dfrac{ba}{d}$

4. **(C)** 4 tablets a day × 12 days = 48 tablets over the course of 12 days

   48 tablets × $2.38 per tablet = $114.24

5. **(B)** Note that distance = rate × time ($d = r \times t$)

Distance to = 1,500 miles	Distance back = 1,500 miles
Rate = 500 mph	Rate = 375 mph
$d = r \times t$	$d = r \times t$
$1,500 = 500(t)$	$1,500 = 375(t)$
$t = 3$ hours	$t = 4$ hours

Total time = $3 + 4 = 7.0$ hours

6. **(A)** Jacket = \$245.99   Discount = 30%

$245.99 \times 0.30 = \$73.80$

7. **(B)** $x = 15$ (first number) $x + 15$ (second number)

$x + (x + 15) = 83$	$x + (x + 15) = 83$
$x + x + 15 = 83$	$34 + 34 + 15 = 83$
$2x = 68$	$34 + 49 = 83$
$x = 34$	$83 = 83$

8. **(D)**

	Age Now	Age +2 Years
Abigail	x	$x + 2$
Sarah	$x + 7$	$x + 9$

In two years, Sarah	will be	twice	as old as	Abigail
$x + 9$	=	2	×	$x + 2$

$$x + 9 = 2x + 4$$
$$9 = x + 4$$
$$5 = x$$

Abigail is currently 5-years-old, and Sarah is 12-years-old ($5 + 7 = 12$). In 2 years, Abigail will be 7-years-old ($5 + 2 = 7$) and Sarah will be 14-years-old ($5 + 9 = 14$), which will be twice Abigail's age.

9. **(C)**

	Number of Tickets	Cost per Ticket	Income
Adult	x	\$10.00	$10(x)$
Senior	$10,000 - x$	\$6.00	$6(10,000 - x)$

Income from Adult tickets	+	Income from Senior tickets	=	Total Income
$10x$	+	$6(10,000x)$	=	\$94,988

First, solve for x to find the number of adult tickets sold.

$$10x + 6(10,000 - x) = 94,988$$
$$10x + 60,000 - 6x = 94,988$$
$$4x + 60,000 = 94,988$$
$$4x = 34,988$$
$$x = 8,747$$

Then, plug in 8,747 for x in the equation to check your answer.

$$10(8,747) + 6(10,000 - 8,747) = 94,988$$
$$87,470 + 7,518 = 94,988$$
$$94,988 = 94,988$$

Finally, subtract 8,747 from 10,000 to find the number of senior tickets sold.
$10,000 - x = 10,000 - 8,747 = 1,253$ senior tickets.
Therefore, there were 8,747 adult tickets and 1,253 senior tickets sold.

10. **(D)** Volume = $(s)(s)(s)$ Side(s) = 8.35
$V = s^3$
$V = 8.35 \times 8.35 \times 8.35$
$V = 582.18$ cubic inches

Section 4: Biology/Chemistry

1. **(D)** Nutrition is not a biologic concept because it supports adaptation, homeostasis, and metabolism. These things cannot occur without nutrition.

2. **(B)** Life is best defined in terms of its various functions, which are growth, cellular organization, cell respiration, favorable response to the environment, adaptation to the environment through natural selection, and reproduction. Choices A, C, and D are each one function only.

3. **(D)** "Synthesis" best completes this statement.

4. **(C)** The two types of reproduction are asexual reproduction, which requires a single parent (1) and sexual reproduction, which requires two parents (3).

5. **(B)** Choice B is the only true statement about cellular organization. None of the other choices are correct.

6. **(C)** Matter both has weight and occupies space.

7. **(A)** Solutions are formed when a mixture is homogenous, the solute does not separate from the solvent by itself, and the solution passes completely through filter paper leaving no residue. Water is the solvent with alcohol (the solute) dissolved in it.

8. **(B)** Acids release hydrogen (H^+) in solutions. The greater the number of hydrogen ions released, the stronger the acid. Acidity ranges from 0–6 on the pH scale. Acids attract hydroxyl ions in solution. Bases release hydroxyl (OH^-). The greater number of hydroxyl released, the stronger the base. Bases range from 8–14 on the pH scale. Bases attract hydrogen ions in solution.

9. **(A)** The circulatory system derives from the mesoderm.

10. **(C)** This statement best describes independent assortment.

Section 5: Anatomy and Physiology

1. **(A)** This statement best describes the position of the heart.

2. **(A)** The phrase "pumps high-pressure blood to the body" is the key to selecting choice A as the correct answer as opposed to choosing choices C or D. Capillaries and veins do not pump blood to the body.

3. **(A)** The beating of the heart contracts and pushes blood through the arteries to the rest of the body. This creates the systolic pressure in the arteries.

4. **(C)** Hormones, produced by the endocrine system, are instrumental in maintaining homeostasis and regulating production and development.

5. **(B)** The anterior lobe of the pituitary gland produces the adrenocorticotropic hormone (ACTH).

6. **(A)** Mineralocorticoids regulate minerals and inorganic molecules such as sodium, potassium, and hydrogen. For the most part, these hormones balance mineral levels to maintain water balance in and around cells.

7. **(D)** This is a basic concept of biology, and it is characteristic of all living systems. Homeostasis is the upkeep or maintenance of steady, internal conditions within specific limits.

8. **(D)** The major fluid within the human body is water.

9. **(B)** The esophagus is the passageway described by this statement.

10. **(D)** Intrinsic factor is an important protein that helps the body absorb vitamin B_{12}. Vitamin B_{12} is needed for red blood cells to form and grow. The stomach produces intrinsic factor.

11. **(A)** Hematopoiesis best describes the formation of blood or blood cells, choice A. None of the other choices accurately describe hematopoiesis.

12. **(A)** The primary function of RBCs is carrying hemoglobin via circulation to cells and carbon dioxide to the lungs.

13. **(B)** The question notes organs that are specific to the lymph system. Choice A does not accurately describe where these organs are located, while choices C and D do not represent what these organs do.

14. **(B)** Passive immunity refers to the process of providing IgG antibodies to protect against infection. It gives immediate, but short-lived protection lasting from several weeks to 3 or 4 months. Passive acquired immunity refers to the process of obtaining serum from immune individuals, concentrating the immunoglobulin fraction, and then injecting it into a vulnerable person for protection. Injections of gamma globulin are used to produce a rapid, but short-term immunity in individuals who have been exposed to certain diseases.

15. **(B)** It is true that neurons have a nucleus that contains genes. None of the other choices describe the correct contents of a neuron or the function of a neuron.

16. **(B)** Autonomic reflexes control/regulate smooth muscle cells, cardiac muscle cells, and glands. In general, these reflexes have the same basic components as somatic reflexes. A crucial difference is that autonomic reflexes have the ability to either stimulate or inhibit the smooth muscle/gland.

17. **(C)** The right main stem bronchus can best be described as shorter, wider, and more vertical, as stated in choice C.

18. **(C)** Pons are the source of the pneumotaxic area of respiration. None of the other answer choices describe the correct location.

19. **(A)** Sympathetic fibers and parasympathetic fibers neither constrict nor dilate venules, so choices C and D can easily be eliminated first. The function of sympathetic fibers is to constrict arterioles, while the function of parasympathetic fibers is to dilate arterioles. This makes choice A the correct answer.

20. **(D)** The urethra controls the release of urine from the human body.

Verbal Ability

3

One of the most important skills that a registered nurse can have is the ability to communicate effectively with patients, families, and other health care workers. Verbal ability, or the capacity to use and comprehend spoken language competently, forms the basis of effective communication and is necessary for success in everyday life.

Communication based on weak verbal ability places all involved at risk. For example, someone may misunderstand what was said and feel offended. A nurse may misinterpret a physician's verbal order and give a patient an incorrect treatment. Effective communication may cease between nurse and patient or between nurse and other health care workers if the nurse cannot listen carefully and speak concisely.

ENHANCE WHAT YOU ALREADY HAVE

There are many techniques to increase your verbal ability. Start with increasing your vocabulary. Make this activity a part of your everyday learning and conversation.

There are a number of strategies that you might employ to increase your vocabulary:

1. Write new or undefinable words you hear or see in a notebook and look them up in a dictionary. Write out all the definitions because words frequently have a number of different meanings and can be used in many different ways. Consider the word *pass*:

   The highway sign said, "Do not *pass*."
   The quarterback threw a long *pass* to a receiver.
   The child asked his mother to *pass* the green beans.
   The teacher hoped all the students would *pass* the test.
   Everyone thought the man would *pass* away since his condition had worsened.
   The mountain *pass* contained many obstacles for the climbers.
   The student requested a library *pass*.

2. Practice using new words in conversations with others to incorporate them into your vocabulary. Merely knowing how to define words strengthens your vocabulary only slightly. You must actively use the words to strengthen your vocabulary.

3. Read different types of materials to expose yourself to new words. Most public libraries subscribe to numerous newspapers, magazines, and trade journals. Find time each week to read articles with information unfamiliar to you. Take a dictionary with you and define new words as you encounter them. Remember to use these words in your daily conversations. British and Canadian spelling of some words is different than some American spellings. If you are planning to take entrance examinations for American schools of nursing, make sure that you learn the American spelling of words.

4. Attend lectures and speeches to hear others speak. Most public speakers have excellent vocabularies. Again, write down the new words, define them, and use them in your daily conversations with others.

5. Review self-help books on verbal ability. Such information may be contained in books dealing with vocabulary, grammar, and spelling.

6. Engage in activities that require you to spell correctly and know the meanings of words. Practice working crossword puzzles or playing board games such as Scrabble.

7. After you've defined and incorporated new words into your active vocabulary, consult a thesaurus or synonym-antonym finder to learn antonyms and synonyms of the words.

ETYMOLOGY

Simply defined, etymology is the study of the origin or formation of words. All the words used in our daily speech and writing have come from other sources. Our words are a hodge-podge of words or word pieces from languages and times all over the world. Some words have existed for so long that they are considered as old as time, whereas other words can be traced back to a specific era in world history.

Words are often formed by putting together what might be considered word pieces or groups of letters. These pieces are prefixes, roots, and suffixes. If you understand these pieces, you can break down a specific word into its individual pieces or parts in order to define the word.

Prefixes

A prefix is a word, syllable, or group of letters that comes before a root word and alters the meaning of the word. Many prefixes come from Old English, Greek, Latin, and French. Prefixes have comprehensive, commonplace meanings like with, through, among, and beyond.

Consider the use of the prefix *dis* and the root word *obedient*. The prefix *dis* means not or the opposite of. *Obedient* means dutiful or obeying. An obedient child is one who is dutiful or obeys, whereas a disobedient child is one who does not behave or does not do what he is supposed to do. Our language contains hundreds of prefixes. Many are in common use and some are rarely used.

When adding a prefix to a root word, the spelling of the word remains the same. Consider the following examples using the prefixes *peri*, *hemi*, *co*, and *ultra*:

EXAMPLES

peri + scope = periscope
hemi + sphere = hemisphere
co + exist = coexist
ultra + modern = ultramodern

A partial list of common prefixes is provided in Table 3.1. To learn more prefixes, consult a dictionary or other source containing prefixes.

Table 3.1. Common Prefixes

Prefix	Meaning	Example
a	not; without	The article described the man as *amoral*.
ab	away from	The couple would *abstain* from sex until they were married.
ad	toward; to	All children looked forward to the *adventure*.
ante	before	Our telephone was in the *anteroom*.
anti	against	The woman supported the *antidemocracy* movement.
be	by; near	The child sat *beside* her mother.
bene	good; well	The man was *benevolent*.
bi	two	Many older adults wear *bifocals*.
circum	around; about	The planets in our solar system have a *circumsolar* orbit.
co	with; together	The man and woman were *coanchors* on the evening news.
com	together	The recipe said to *combine* the dry ingredients.
contra	against	The couple went to their doctor to discuss methods of *contraception*.
counter	opposite	During the debate, the woman made a *counter-proposal*.
de	from; down; away	The guard instructed the group to *descend* the stairs and turn right.
equi	equal	The river is *equidistant* between the two cities.
ex	out of; former	A woman was *excommunicated* from the church when she divorced her husband.
extra	beyond	The man was sure he saw an *extraterrestrial* being.
infra	below; beneath	The *infrastructure* of the building was damaged in the earthquake.
inter	between	Group *interaction* was better than expected.
intra	within	*Intramural* sports were offered in public schools.
macro	large	The scientist said proteins are *macromolecular*.
mal	bad	The infant was *malformed*.
mega	large	Nuclear explosions in heavily populated areas would cause *megadeath*.
micro	small	A student used a *microscope* to examine the fly's wing.
mid	middle	The family decided on a *midday* picnic.
mini	small	Our *minivan* was too small for family needs.
mis	wrong	There were many *misspellings* in the paper.
multi	many	The SAT is a *multiple*-choice exam.
non	not	The country was *nonaligned* during the war.
ob	against	No one on the committee would *object* to the rule changes.
over	excessive	The owner *overcharged* for the computer repair.

Table 3.1. Common Prefixes (*Continued*)

Prefix	Meaning	Example
peri	around	The pregnant woman was entering the *perinatal* period.
poly	many	*Polygamy* is against the law in the United States.
post	after; later	A *posttest* was administered at the end of the seminar.
pre	before	The couple enrolled in *premarital* counseling courses.
pro	supporting	The man lived in a *procommunist* country.
pseudo	false	The woman published her books using a *pseudonym*.
re	again	Smart students *review* their notes the night before the exam.
retro	backward	Pay raises are *retroactive*.
semi	half	The recipe called for *semisweet* chocolate.
socio	social; society	*Sociology* class met three times a week.
sub	under	The building contractor offered four *subcontracts*.
super	above	Farmers had a *superabundant* harvest.
supra	above	The football player sustained a *supraorbital* injury.
trans	across	His goal was to enter a *transcountry* race.
ultra	beyond	The man was known as an *ultraconservative* politician.
un	not	Many of the group's activities were considered *un-American*.
under	beneath	The migrants were *underpaid* for their work.
vice	in place of; next to in rank	The woman listed her occupation as *vice president* of the company.
with	against; back	The family asked the doctor to *withhold* medical treatment.

Suffixes

Suffixes are the opposite of prefixes and are found at the end of a root word instead of at the beginning. Suffixes do one of two things. They may create a new word, as when adding the suffix *dom* to the word *free* to make a new word *freedom*. Suffixes may also alter the original word in some fashion but not change the meaning of the word. Consider the suffix *ed* and the root word *edit*. The suffix *ed* changes a word from the present tense to the past tense. *Edit* means to correct or change. An edited paper is one that has been corrected or changed. The editing of the paper took place in the past instead of the present. The suffix *ed* does not tell when the editing took place, only that it occurred.

A number of mechanical rules apply to adding suffixes to root words.

1. When the suffix begins with a vowel, double the final consonant of the root word before the suffix—provided that the root word has only one syllable or the accent is on the last syllable.

   brag + g + art = braggart
   rob + b + ery = robbery
   regret + t + ing = regretting
   profit + able = profitable

2. When the suffix *less*, *ness*, *ly*, or *en* is added to a root word, the spelling of the root word does not change.

   heart + less = heartless
   fond + ness = fondness
   late + ly = lately
   wood + en = wooden

   Exceptions to this rule are when the root word ends in *y* and the *y* changes to an *i* before the suffixes *ness* and *ly*.

   dingy + ness = dingi + ness = dinginess
   swarthy + ness = swarthi + ness = swarthiness

3. When the suffix begins with a vowel, drop the final *e* in the root words ending in *e*.

   write + ing = writ + ing = writing
   deflate + ing = deflat + ing = deflating
   desire + able = desir + able = desirable

4. When the suffix begins with a consonant, keep the final *e* of root words ending with *e*.

   lone + some = lonesome
   hope + less = hopeless
   state + hood = statehood

   Exceptions to this rule are words such as *judgment*, *acknowledgment*, and *argument*.

5. When root words end in *y* preceded by a consonant, change the *y* to *i* before adding the suffix. This applies to suffixes not starting with *i*.

   beauty + ful = beauti + ful = beautiful
   lazy + ness = lazi + ness = laziness

A partial list of common suffixes is found in Table 3.2. Consult a dictionary or other appropriate source for more suffixes.

Table 3.2. Common Suffixes

Suffix	Meaning	Example
ability	inclination for	The first lesson he learned at the academy was *respectability*.
able	worthy of an act	The woman was a *capable* leader.
ac	pertaining to	A *cardiac* muscle had ruptured.
acy	having the quality of	The team's target practice had an *accuracy* rate of 90 percent.
age	collection, connection	The museum was an *assemblage* of antique cars.
al	related to; process of	His *approval* rating was the lowest ever obtained.
ance	condition of	The building was not in *compliance* with city codes.
ate	having	Church members would *alienate* divorced couples.
ation	process of; action	The *publication* date was set for the end of the month.
cy	condition of; state of	*Vagrancy* was a problem for the city.
ed	past tense of a verb	The child *walked* five miles to go fishing.
en	to cause to be	The father carved a *wooden* horse for his daughter's birthday present.
ence	state of; condition of	People should value their *independence*.
er	one who performs	Everyone said she should be a *teacher*.
ery	state of; place	The nurse worked in *surgery*.
ese	quality of	The restaurant served *Chinese* food.
ia, ial	pertaining to	The student read the *tutorial* for the program.
ian	related to; belonging to	Her secretary was the *historian* for the city.
ing	action	*Running* the mile in less than six minutes was her goal.
ist	one who performs an action	The orchestra had a violin *soloist*.
ious	full of; having	The deacon was a *religious* man.
ish	characteristic of	Children often act *foolish*.
ism	action; quality of	*Alcoholism* is a serious problem in some segments of society.
ity	action; process of	There was one *abnormality* in the test results.
ive	performing an action	The couple had an *abusive* relationship.
ize	to cause to be	Instructions said to *sterilize* the instruments.
less	without	The procedure was advertised as a *bloodless* surgery.
logy	study of	*Biology* is required for a high school diploma.
ment	action; process of	The coat was a *replacement* for the one he lost.
meter	measurement of	The *thermometer* indicated the patient's temperature was above normal.
ness	quality; condition	Male pattern *baldness* is a problem for some men.
oid	resembling	The being had *humanoid* qualities.
or	state of	Her child's *behavior* was offensive.
ory	characterized by	The church's *advisory* committee voted against a raise in pay for the minister.

Table 3.2. Common Suffixes (*Continued*)

Suffix	Meaning	Example
ose	full of; possessing	After being hit on the head, the man was *comatose*.
osis	condition	*Osmosis* is the dispersion of fluid through a semipermeable membrane.
s, es	plural of a noun; more than one	Ten *drivers* registered for the race.
ship	state of; quality of	Their *friendship* had lasted for years.
some	full of	The police made a *gruesome* discovery.
tion	action; condition of	The minister gave the *benediction*.
ty	quality; condition of	Singing is an *activity* enjoyed by children.

Root Words

Root words are words that communicate the fundamental meaning of a particular word. Root words form the nucleus of a word and are the basis for words in a language. Prefixes and suffixes are combined with or attached to these words to create other words or to change the meaning of the root words. Some words are combinations of more than one root word and are used to create another word that may have a similar or completely opposite meaning.

A partial list of root words follows in Table 3.3. Consult a dictionary for more root words.

Table 3.3. Common Root Words

Root	Meaning	Example
ac	to do	No *action* was taken against the trespassers.
ag	to do	The secretary read the *agenda* to the committee members.
agri	farm	Her college major was *agribusiness*.
anthropo	man	*Anthropology* is the study of man.
aqua	water	The new swimming pool was called the *aquatic* center.
aud	hearing	*Audiovisuals* enhanced the student's difficult presentation.
auto	self	The car had an *automatic* transmission.
biblio	book	A *bibliography* or reference section is at the end of the paper.
bio	life	The actor completed his *autobiography* two weeks ago.
cad	fall	The drum *cadence* could be heard for blocks.
capit	head	Austin is the *capital* of Texas.
cede	go	The parents *interceded* when their children were fighting.
celer	speed	He pushed the car's *accelerator* to the floor.
chron	time	A *chronograph* recorded the duration of the event.
cide	kill; cut	The gardener sprayed an *insecticide* on the trees.
clude	close	Adults did not want to *include* the children.
cog	know; knowledge	Our psychologist tested the child's *cognitive* abilities.
ded	give	The *dedication* for the monument was scheduled for next week.
dent	tooth	The child needed a *dental* appointment.
duc	lead	The adult could not *induce* the child to take the money.

Table 3.3. Common Root Words (*Continued*)

Root	Meaning	Example
fac	make; do	Our company *manufactured* leather shoes.
fer	carry	The nurse *transferred* to another floor.
fract	break	The child *fractured* his arm when he fell.
frater	brother	He wanted to join a *fraternity*.
gen	produce	The job would *generate* money for the family.
geo	earth	Children learn about different countries in *geography* class.
graph	picture; writing	The couple bought software containing computer *graphics*.
hemo	blood	The woman's *hemoglobin* was lower than normal.
homo	man	The police investigated the *homicide*.
hydr	water	The dam produced *hydroelectricity*.
ject	throw	A child was *rejected* by his friends.
jud	right	The *judge* suspended the sentence and freed the man.
junct	join	A *conjunction* is a part of speech.
juris	justice; law	This crime occurred outside of the police department's *jurisdiction*.
lect	read	The *lecture* lasted for an hour.
logue	speech	Her *dialogue* confused the students who had not read the material.
loq	speak	The author was an *eloquent* speaker.
lude	play	The *interlude* lasted for fifteen minutes.
manu	hand	The old *manuscript* was written by Aristotle.
mand	order	The major was the *commander* of the unit.
mater	mother	The woman was his *maternal* grandmother.
mort	death	A *mortician* prepared the body for the funeral.
mute	change	A judge *commuted* the sentence.
naut	sailor; ship	The islands were ten *nautical* miles apart.
nounce	declare	The judge *announced* the winners of the games.
ped	foot	The teenager thought her feet would look better after a *pedicure*.
philo	love	A student studied *philosophy* as an undergraduate.
port	carry	The woman took her *portable* radio to the park.
psych	mind	He studied to be a clinical *psychologist*.
reg	rule	The company had many *regulations*.
rupt	break	Children *disrupted* the game.
sect	cut	Students taking gross anatomy *dissect* cadavers.
sert	bind	The missing pages were *inserted* into the manuscript.
scend	climb	The man fell while *descending* the ladder.
scribe	write	The jeweler *inscribed*, "To my husband of fifty wonderful years," on the plaque.
spect	look at	The man was a *spectator* at all of his son's football games.
spir	breath	The *respiratory* rate of an infant is faster than that of an adult.

Table 3.3. Common Root Words (*Continued*)

Root	Meaning	Example
strict	tighten	There were no *restrictions* on travel.
tain	hold	The woman asked for a one-quart *container*.
term	end	His business *terminated* the contract.
tract	draw	The car's tires had little *traction* on the ice.
typ	print	Most students would rather use a computer than a *typewriter*.
ven	come	The meeting *convened* at dusk.
vict	conquer	The football team had a *victorious* season.
vis	see	The child needed a *visual* exam because he was seeing double.
volt	turn	Soldiers *revolted* against the king.

Medical Terminology

Numerous disciplines have their own terminology. Nursing draws its terminology from medicine and the sciences. You will be learning terminology throughout your nursing program. A good place to begin learning this new terminology is with anatomical directional terms in Table 3.4.

Table 3.4. Anatomical Directional Terms

Term	Definition	Example
Anterior	Near the front of the body	The navel is on the *anterior* body.
Contralateral	Opposite of the body	The liver and spleen are *contralateral* to each other.
Deep	Away from body surface	The heart is *deep* to the ribs of the chest.
Distal	Farther away from the point of attachment	The hand is *distal* to the elbow.
Inferior	Away from the head (usually applies to the trunk of the body)	The breasts are *inferior* to the brain.
Intermediate	Between structures	The heart is *intermediate* to the lungs.
Ipsilateral	Same side of the body	The ascending colon and the appendix are *ipsilateral*.
Lateral	Away from the midline of the body	The kidneys are *lateral* to the aorta.
Medial	Nearer the midline of the body	The bladder is *medial* to the liver.
Posterior	Near to the back of the body	The spinal column is *posterior* to the sternum.
Proximal	Closer to the point of attachment	The hip is *proximal* to the knee.
Superficial	Toward the surface of the body	The ribs of the chest wall are *superficial* to the viscera of the chest cavity.
Superior	Toward the head (usually applies to the trunk of the body)	The lungs are *superior* to the small intestines.

ANTONYMS AND SYNONYMS

Words are more than their parts—prefixes, roots, and suffixes. They have meanings. Numerous words have almost the same or identical meanings, and many other words are opposite in meaning. These are the synonyms and antonyms.

Using antonyms and synonyms can enhance your written and verbal communication with others. Listening to or writing the same word or words again and again is repetitive, and suggests that your vocabulary may be limited. Your reader or listener may lose interest when you use the same word or words repeatedly.

Antonyms are words that are opposite in meaning. Words such as hot and cold, happy and sad, young and old, good and bad, and inside and outside are antonyms. Antonyms do not reveal the degree or condition of the word. Take hot and cold water for example; the words *hot* and *cold* do not tell us how hot or how cold the water actually is. They only tell us the relative temperature of the water.

Synonyms are often thought of as being the opposite of antonyms; they are words that are identical or almost the same in meaning. Words such as audacity and boldness, bondage and slavery, nomad and wanderer, hazard and danger, and ingenious and clever are synonyms. Like antonyms, synonyms do not indicate the degree or amount. The words *hazard* and *danger* suggest a potential for injury in a given situation, but how hazardous or how dangerous a situation is cannot be determined from the words alone.

Antonym and synonym sample tests with answer sheets and answer keys follow. You will learn more if you take the test before looking at the answer key. When selecting answers using a multiple-choice format, make sure that you determine why each response is right or wrong. Good test takers know why a response is right as well as why the remaining responses are wrong.

ANSWER SHEET
Antonyms Sample Test One

1. Ⓐ Ⓑ Ⓒ Ⓓ
2. Ⓐ Ⓑ Ⓒ Ⓓ
3. Ⓐ Ⓑ Ⓒ Ⓓ
4. Ⓐ Ⓑ Ⓒ Ⓓ
5. Ⓐ Ⓑ Ⓒ Ⓓ
6. Ⓐ Ⓑ Ⓒ Ⓓ
7. Ⓐ Ⓑ Ⓒ Ⓓ
8. Ⓐ Ⓑ Ⓒ Ⓓ
9. Ⓐ Ⓑ Ⓒ Ⓓ

10. Ⓐ Ⓑ Ⓒ Ⓓ
11. Ⓐ Ⓑ Ⓒ Ⓓ
12. Ⓐ Ⓑ Ⓒ Ⓓ
13. Ⓐ Ⓑ Ⓒ Ⓓ
14. Ⓐ Ⓑ Ⓒ Ⓓ
15. Ⓐ Ⓑ Ⓒ Ⓓ
16. Ⓐ Ⓑ Ⓒ Ⓓ
17. Ⓐ Ⓑ Ⓒ Ⓓ
18. Ⓐ Ⓑ Ⓒ Ⓓ

19. Ⓐ Ⓑ Ⓒ Ⓓ
20. Ⓐ Ⓑ Ⓒ Ⓓ
21. Ⓐ Ⓑ Ⓒ Ⓓ
22. Ⓐ Ⓑ Ⓒ Ⓓ
23. Ⓐ Ⓑ Ⓒ Ⓓ
24. Ⓐ Ⓑ Ⓒ Ⓓ
25. Ⓐ Ⓑ Ⓒ Ⓓ

Directions: For each of the numbered pairs of words, select the letter (A, B, C, or D) in which the paired words are *opposite* in meaning. Record your answers on the answer sheet on page 49.

1. (A) Teach—Learn
   (B) Counter—Workbench
   (C) Conceal—Camouflage
   (D) Offensive—Distasteful

2. (A) Obesity—Adiposity
   (B) Nag—Nuisance
   (C) Specific—Indefinite
   (D) Adherence—Association

3. (A) Deceptive—Misleading
   (B) Vulnerable—Susceptible
   (C) Durable—Impermanent
   (D) Solitude—Seclusion

4. (A) Frugal—Spartan
   (B) Recant—Take back
   (C) Turgid—Swollen
   (D) Wicked—Innocent

   CHALLENGE

5. (A) Secret—Open
   (B) Indictment—Charge
   (C) Hollow—Vacuous
   (D) Hectic—Chaotic

6. (A) Laudable—Praiseworthy
   (B) Deplete—Hoard
   (C) Prior—Former
   (D) Ability—Aptitude

7. (A) Include—Exclude
   (B) Later—Subsequent
   (C) Eager—Ardent
   (D) Discipline—Correction

8. (A) Private—Known
   (B) Diligent—Industrious
   (C) Prolific—Fruitful
   (D) Replete—Full

9. (A) Absolve—Pardon
   (B) Inept—Adroit
   (C) Compliant—Submissive
   (D) Affinity—Rapport

10. (A) Nullify—Abolish
    (B) Acrimony—Irascibility
    (C) Concur—Agree
    (D) Abstinent—Insatiable

    CHALLENGE

11. (A) Ardor—Fervor
    (B) Blunt—Sharp
    (C) Cauterize—Burn
    (D) Bovine—Cowlike

12. (A) Posterior—Dorsal
    (B) Ipsilateral—Lateral
    (C) Medial—Intermediate
    (D) Anterior—Ventral

13. (A) Indubitable—Inconclusive
    (B) Germane—Relevant
    (C) Solemn—Grave
    (D) Appraise—Estimate

14. (A) Scorn—Mock
    (B) Silent—Loquacious
    (C) Pretend—Concoct
    (D) Fetish—Amulet

15. (A) Candid—Frank
    (B) Happy—Merry
    (C) Avoid—Shun
    (D) Impudent—Courteous

16. (A) Flagon—Flask
    (B) Precipitous—Steep
    (C) Humble—Pompous
    (D) Peruse—Study

17. (A) Sequester—Set apart
    (B) Tepid—Lukewarm
    (C) Stringent—Lax
    (D) Wan—Sickly

    CHALLENGE

18. (A) Homogeneous—Uniform
    (B) Proscribe—Outlaw
    (C) Venial—Forgivable
    (D) Morbid—Wholesome

19. (A) False—Forged
    (B) Boorish—Urbane
    (C) Surmise—Imagine
    (D) Temerity—Audacity

20. (A) Flux—Change
    (B) Perfidy—Fidelity
    (C) Stealthy—Shifty
    (D) Gregarious—Sociable

21. (A) Alms—Charity
    (B) Dauntless—Fearless
    (C) Hood—Cowl
    (D) Impromptu—Planned

22. (A) Judicious—Imprudent
    (B) Flaccid—Limp
    (C) Hirsute—Hairy
    (D) Gulch—Ravine

23. (A) Pariah—Outcast
    (B) Tawdry—Cheap
    (C) Inept—Dexterous
    (D) Terse—Concise

24. (A) Tacit—Explicit
    (B) Flaunt—Exhibit
    (C) Illicit—Unlawful
    (D) Flammable—Combustible

25. (A) Windward—Leeward
    (B) Harsh—Grating
    (C) Revile—Scold
    (D) Quell—Suppress

Antonyms Sample Test One Answer Key

1. **A**	6. **B**	11. **B**	16. **C**	21. **D**
2. **C**	7. **A**	12. **B**	17. **C**	22. **A**
3. **C**	8. **A**	13. **A**	18. **D**	23. **C**
4. **D**	9. **B**	14. **B**	19. **B**	24. **A**
5. **A**	10. **D**	15. **D**	20. **B**	25. **A**

ANSWER SHEET
Antonyms Sample Test Two

1. Ⓐ Ⓑ Ⓒ Ⓓ
2. Ⓐ Ⓑ Ⓒ Ⓓ
3. Ⓐ Ⓑ Ⓒ Ⓓ
4. Ⓐ Ⓑ Ⓒ Ⓓ
5. Ⓐ Ⓑ Ⓒ Ⓓ
6. Ⓐ Ⓑ Ⓒ Ⓓ
7. Ⓐ Ⓑ Ⓒ Ⓓ
8. Ⓐ Ⓑ Ⓒ Ⓓ
9. Ⓐ Ⓑ Ⓒ Ⓓ

10. Ⓐ Ⓑ Ⓒ Ⓓ
11. Ⓐ Ⓑ Ⓒ Ⓓ
12. Ⓐ Ⓑ Ⓒ Ⓓ
13. Ⓐ Ⓑ Ⓒ Ⓓ
14. Ⓐ Ⓑ Ⓒ Ⓓ
15. Ⓐ Ⓑ Ⓒ Ⓓ
16. Ⓐ Ⓑ Ⓒ Ⓓ
17. Ⓐ Ⓑ Ⓒ Ⓓ
18. Ⓐ Ⓑ Ⓒ Ⓓ

19. Ⓐ Ⓑ Ⓒ Ⓓ
20. Ⓐ Ⓑ Ⓒ Ⓓ
21. Ⓐ Ⓑ Ⓒ Ⓓ
22. Ⓐ Ⓑ Ⓒ Ⓓ
23. Ⓐ Ⓑ Ⓒ Ⓓ
24. Ⓐ Ⓑ Ⓒ Ⓓ
25. Ⓐ Ⓑ Ⓒ Ⓓ

Directions: For each of the numbered words, select the letter (A, B, C, or D) in which the paired words are *opposite* in meaning. Record your answers on the answer sheet on page 53.

1. Rigid
   - (A) Format
   - (B) Right
   - (C) Yielding
   - (D) Rickety

2. Modern
   - (A) Avant-garde
   - (B) Antiquated
   - (C) Impact
   - (D) Kind

3. Archaic
   - (A) Arch
   - (B) Medieval
   - (C) Lightning
   - (D) Young

4. Refuse
   - (A) Accept
   - (B) Spurn
   - (C) Garbage
   - (D) Regain

5. Announce
   - (A) Forswear
   - (B) Dovetail
   - (C) Conceal
   - (D) Drive

6. Cunning
   - (A) Naive
   - (B) Exact
   - (C) Smart
   - (D) Trustworthy

7. Unforeseen
   - (A) Predictable
   - (B) Umbrage
   - (C) Undulate
   - (D) Marginal

8. Shape
   - (A) Round
   - (B) Tighten
   - (C) Destroy
   - (D) Empower

9. Deep
   - (A) Extending down
   - (B) Ocean
   - (C) Involved
   - (D) Superficial

10. Flexible
    - (A) Reflex
    - (B) Tight
    - (C) Weight
    - (D) Extend

11. Boil
    - (A) Anger
    - (B) Material
    - (C) Enrapture
    - (D) Assuage

12. Defective
    - (A) Faultless
    - (B) Police
    - (C) Reject
    - (D) Rejoin

13. Inhospitable

    (A) Corrupt

    (B) Askew

    (C) Genial

    (D) Independence

14. Sever

    (A) Cut

    (B) Unify

    (C) Hard

    (D) Nourish

15. Charge

    (A) Rent

    (B) Rotate

    (C) Chemical

    (D) Absolve

16. Rehabilitate

    (A) Walk

    (B) Investigate

    (C) Destroy

    (D) Comprehensive

17. Manifest   **CHALLENGE**

    (A) Invaluable

    (B) Unclear

    (C) Natural

    (D) Developing

18. Fertile

    (A) Crescent

    (B) Soil

    (C) Gestation

    (D) Unproductive

19. Felicitous

    (A) Improper

    (B) Catlike

    (C) Mourning

    (D) Defeat

20. Cordial

    (A) Party

    (B) Unsociable

    (C) Headstrong

    (D) Enjoyable

21. Rupture

    (A) Heaven

    (B) Torn

    (C) Mend

    (D) Elastic

22. Strong   **CHALLENGE**

    (A) Chary

    (B) Irresolute

    (C) Overwrought

    (D) Incline

23. Impasse

    (A) Parch

    (B) Destroy

    (C) Flow

    (D) Agreement

24. Torpid   **CHALLENGE**

    (A) Kidnap

    (B) Compliant

    (C) Essential

    (D) Energetic

25. Crude

    (A) Polished

    (B) Rough

    (C) Gasoline

    (D) Graded

Antonyms Sample Test Two Answer Key

1. **C**	6. **A**	11. **D**	16. **C**	21. **C**
2. **B**	7. **A**	12. **A**	17. **B**	22. **B**
3. **D**	8. **C**	13. **C**	18. **D**	23. **D**
4. **A**	9. **D**	14. **B**	19. **A**	24. **D**
5. **C**	10. **B**	15. **D**	20. **B**	25. **A**

ANSWER SHEET
Synonyms Sample Test One

1. Ⓐ Ⓑ Ⓒ Ⓓ
2. Ⓐ Ⓑ Ⓒ Ⓓ
3. Ⓐ Ⓑ Ⓒ Ⓓ
4. Ⓐ Ⓑ Ⓒ Ⓓ
5. Ⓐ Ⓑ Ⓒ Ⓓ
6. Ⓐ Ⓑ Ⓒ Ⓓ
7. Ⓐ Ⓑ Ⓒ Ⓓ
8. Ⓐ Ⓑ Ⓒ Ⓓ
9. Ⓐ Ⓑ Ⓒ Ⓓ

10. Ⓐ Ⓑ Ⓒ Ⓓ
11. Ⓐ Ⓑ Ⓒ Ⓓ
12. Ⓐ Ⓑ Ⓒ Ⓓ
13. Ⓐ Ⓑ Ⓒ Ⓓ
14. Ⓐ Ⓑ Ⓒ Ⓓ
15. Ⓐ Ⓑ Ⓒ Ⓓ
16. Ⓐ Ⓑ Ⓒ Ⓓ
17. Ⓐ Ⓑ Ⓒ Ⓓ
18. Ⓐ Ⓑ Ⓒ Ⓓ

19. Ⓐ Ⓑ Ⓒ Ⓓ
20. Ⓐ Ⓑ Ⓒ Ⓓ
21. Ⓐ Ⓑ Ⓒ Ⓓ
22. Ⓐ Ⓑ Ⓒ Ⓓ
23. Ⓐ Ⓑ Ⓒ Ⓓ
24. Ⓐ Ⓑ Ⓒ Ⓓ
25. Ⓐ Ⓑ Ⓒ Ⓓ

Directions: For each of the numbered words, select the letter (A, B, C, or D) in which the words are the *same* or *almost the same* in meaning. Record your answers on the answer sheet on page 57.

1. (A) Defend—Abandon
   (B) Phenomenon—Marvel
   (C) Applaud—Decry
   (D) Reflect—Dismiss

2. (A) Ubiquitous—Everywhere   `CHALLENGE`
   (B) Curl—Straighten
   (C) Odious—Kind
   (D) Bizarre—Conventional

3. (A) Incomplete—Fully
   (B) Umbrage—Anger
   (C) Estranged—Friendly
   (D) Following—Ahead

4. (A) Blighted—Blessed
   (B) Attach—Unconfined
   (C) Sweet—Biting
   (D) Posterity—Children

5. (A) Barbarous—Civilized
   (B) Whimper—Howl
   (C) Impeach—Accuse
   (D) Whet—Dull

6. (A) Twilight—Daybreak
   (B) Vacant—Overflowing
   (C) Forsake—Abandon
   (D) Valiant—Timid

7. (A) Yearn—Ache
   (B) Blur—Clear
   (C) Bloom—Shrink
   (D) Harebrained—Wise

8. (A) Dour—Bright
   (B) Attest—Deny
   (C) Tenacious—Sticky
   (D) Intuitive—Calculate

9. (A) Posterior—Dorsal
   (B) Ventral—Distal
   (C) Lateral—Ipsilateral
   (D) Anterior—Deep

10. (A) Pout—Grin
    (B) Mar—Heal
    (C) Sweet—Rancid
    (D) Allege—Adduce

11. (A) Roll—Steady
    (B) Malign—Blacken
    (C) Like—Diverse
    (D) Dolt—Brain

12. (A) Paraphrase—Restate
    (B) Smooth—Wrinkle
    (C) Enormous—Minute
    (D) Complicated—Easy

13. (A) Think—Disbelieve
    (B) Maritime—Aquatic
    (C) Struggle—Idle
    (D) Stint—Spend

14. (A) Sore—Happy
    (B) Spare—Condemn
    (C) Douse—Deluge
    (D) Abscond—Offer

15. (A) Robust—Flabby
    (B) Calm—Rouse
    (C) Quack—Genuine
    (D) Cooperative—Obliging

16. (A) Puzzle—Clarify   `CHALLENGE`
    (B) Cosmetic—Corrective
    (C) Promiscuous—Temperate
    (D) Downsize—Augment

17. (A) Verdant—Flourishing
    (B) Flaccid—Firm
    (C) Lavish—Economize
    (D) Admonish—Laud

18. (A) Abide—Vacate
    (B) Theological—Secular
    (C) Vibration—Beating
    (D) Dramatic—Straight

19. (A) Oaf—Sage
    (B) August—Common
    (C) Spawn—Create
    (D) Executive—Underling

20. (A) Ghastly—Pleasing
    (B) Reflect—Absorb
    (C) Rough—Nice
    (D) Boisterous—Clamorous

21. (A) Consummate—Begin
    (B) Burrow—Cover
    (C) Flighty—Steady
    (D) Catholic—Broad

22. (A) Censure—Berate
    (B) Ace—Inept
    (C) Flux—Stability
    (D) Impertinent—Civil

23. (A) Covet—Abjure
    (B) Deep—Abysmal
    (C) Defeat—Give up
    (D) Fine—Award

24. (A) Curtail—Extend
    (B) Limber—Tense
    (C) Drudge—Dig
    (D) Desecrate—Honor

25. (A) Immune—Subject
    (B) Mollify—Abate
    (C) Ludicrous—Logical
    (D) Rank—Scatter

Synonyms Sample Test One Answer Key

1. **B**	6. **C**	11. **B**	16. **B**	21. **D**
2. **A**	7. **A**	12. **A**	17. **A**	22. **A**
3. **B**	8. **C**	13. **B**	18. **C**	23. **B**
4. **D**	9. **A**	14. **C**	19. **C**	24. **C**
5. **C**	10. **D**	15. **D**	20. **D**	25. **B**

ANSWER SHEET
Synonyms Sample Test Two

1. Ⓐ Ⓑ Ⓒ Ⓓ

2. Ⓐ Ⓑ Ⓒ Ⓓ

3. Ⓐ Ⓑ Ⓒ Ⓓ

4. Ⓐ Ⓑ Ⓒ Ⓓ

5. Ⓐ Ⓑ Ⓒ Ⓓ

6. Ⓐ Ⓑ Ⓒ Ⓓ

7. Ⓐ Ⓑ Ⓒ Ⓓ

8. Ⓐ Ⓑ Ⓒ Ⓓ

9. Ⓐ Ⓑ Ⓒ Ⓓ

10. Ⓐ Ⓑ Ⓒ Ⓓ

11. Ⓐ Ⓑ Ⓒ Ⓓ

12. Ⓐ Ⓑ Ⓒ Ⓓ

13. Ⓐ Ⓑ Ⓒ Ⓓ

14. Ⓐ Ⓑ Ⓒ Ⓓ

15. Ⓐ Ⓑ Ⓒ Ⓓ

16. Ⓐ Ⓑ Ⓒ Ⓓ

17. Ⓐ Ⓑ Ⓒ Ⓓ

18. Ⓐ Ⓑ Ⓒ Ⓓ

19. Ⓐ Ⓑ Ⓒ Ⓓ

20. Ⓐ Ⓑ Ⓒ Ⓓ

21. Ⓐ Ⓑ Ⓒ Ⓓ

22. Ⓐ Ⓑ Ⓒ Ⓓ

23. Ⓐ Ⓑ Ⓒ Ⓓ

24. Ⓐ Ⓑ Ⓒ Ⓓ

25. Ⓐ Ⓑ Ⓒ Ⓓ

Directions: For each of the numbered words, select the letter (A, B, C, or D) in which the words are the *same* or *almost the same* in meaning. Record your answers on the answer sheet on page 61.

1. Abstruse   CHALLENGE

    (A) Instruct
    (B) Obscure
    (C) Obtuse
    (D) Rigging

2. Nimble

    (A) Skillful
    (B) Simple
    (C) Personal
    (D) Historical

3. Adversary

    (A) Averse
    (B) Caution
    (C) Opponent
    (D) Zeal

4. Oblivion

    (A) Forgetfulness
    (B) Avarice
    (C) Profess
    (D) Fatal

5. Opulence

    (A) Inane
    (B) Chandelier
    (C) Sagacious
    (D) Luxuriousness

6. Muted

    (A) Initiate
    (B) Silent
    (C) Oversight
    (D) Enrage

7. Plight

    (A) Condition
    (B) Hinder
    (C) Imprison
    (D) Minor

8. Disputatious   CHALLENGE

    (A) Polemical
    (B) Immutable
    (C) Iconoclast
    (D) Motive

9. Combativeness

    (A) Malign
    (B) Bungling
    (C) Pugnacity
    (D) Obedient

10. Reticent

    (A) Disfigured
    (B) Reserved
    (C) Lucid
    (D) Graphic

11. Rudimentary

    (A) Offensive
    (B) Peripheral
    (C) Tedium
    (D) Elementary

12. Tyranny

    (A) Suspend
    (B) Dinosaur
    (C) Turbulence
    (D) Oppression

13. Virulent

   (A) Defective

   (B) Violent

   (C) Hostile

   (D) Fallacious

14. Magnanimous

   (A) Exuberance

   (B) Generous

   (C) Comprehensive

   (D) Vanishing

15. Ventral

   (A) Intermediate

   (B) Inferior

   (C) Anterior

   (D) Dorsal

16. Lassitude

   (A) Embitter

   (B) Adopt

   (C) Robust

   (D) Languor

17. Indubitable   **CHALLENGE**

   (A) Unquestionable

   (B) Irreverence

   (C) Threatening

   (D) Stupid

18. Hone

   (A) Dark

   (B) Sharpen

   (C) Dwelling

   (D) Nebulous

19. Blessed

   (A) Naiveté

   (B) Wicked

   (C) Worldly

   (D) Hallowed

20. Germane

   (A) Pertinent

   (B) Foreign

   (C) Stubborn

   (D) Trite

21. Founder

   (A) Vertebrate

   (B) Condition

   (C) Sink

   (D) Insightful

22. Garbled

   (A) Biased

   (B) Marginal

   (C) Jumbled

   (D) Pliant

23. Innocuous

   (A) Commonplace

   (B) Harmless

   (C) Hedonist

   (D) Sneaky

24. Dull

   (A) Obstruct

   (B) Disoriented

   (C) Duplicity

   (D) Insipid

25. Ephemeral   **CHALLENGE**

   (A) Arrogance

   (B) Fruitless

   (C) Encourage

   (D) Fleeting

Synonyms Sample Test Two Answer Key

1. **B**	6. **B**	11. **D**	16. **D**	21. **C**
2. **A**	7. **A**	12. **D**	17. **A**	22. **C**
3. **C**	8. **A**	13. **C**	18. **B**	23. **B**
4. **A**	9. **C**	14. **B**	19. **D**	24. **D**
5. **D**	10. **B**	15. **C**	20. **A**	25. **D**

ANALOGIES

Verbal analogies are word problems based on logical assumptions and are an indicator of an individual's ability to analyze, think, and reason critically. The capacity to perform these higher-level tasks is related to intelligence.

Verbal Analogy Format

Verbal analogies are presented like proportion problems commonly found in math or algebra. Analogies may be presented in one of five different formats. In each format, a missing term or terms must be furnished.

EXAMPLE OF FORMAT ONE

BIG : LITTLE :: _____

(A) GREEN : APPLE
(B) ROAD : CAR
(C) FISH : FISHERMAN
(D) FAT : SKINNY

The correct answer is FAT : SKINNY, choice D. The problem can be solved utilizing two different approaches. By looking at the relationships between the words, you can see that BIG and LITTLE are antonyms as are FAT and SKINNY. You can also see that BIG and FAT are synonyms as are LITTLE and SKINNY.

EXAMPLE OF FORMAT TWO

_____ : LITTLE :: FAT : SKINNY

(A) ROMANCE
(B) LARGE
(C) BIG
(D) PILLOW

The correct answer is BIG, choice C. The same reasoning used to solve Format One is used to solve Format Two.

EXAMPLE OF FORMAT THREE

BIG : _____ :: FAT : SKINNY

(A) MOUNTAIN
(B) BIGGER
(C) PAPER
(D) LITTLE

The correct answer is LITTLE, choice D.

BIG : LITTLE :: _____ : SKINNY

(A) FAT
(B) THIN
(C) MONDO
(D) FISH

The correct answer is FAT, choice A.

BIG : LITTLE :: FAT : _____

(A) OBESE
(B) OBSESSIVE
(C) IMPORTANT
(D) SKINNY

The correct answer is SKINNY, choice D.

Verbal Analogy Content

Verbal analogies are grouped according to subject matter or content. Content areas include the social and natural sciences, mathematics, humanities, commonplace information, and English grammar, usage, and vocabulary. Here is an example of each.

DEMOCRACY : BY THE PEOPLE :: _____ : STATE RULE

(A) FRANCHISE
(B) JUNTA
(C) CHECKS AND BALANCES
(D) DICTATORSHIP

The correct answer is DICTATORSHIP, choice D. Both democracy and dictatorship are forms of government. In a democracy, the government is by the people. In a dictatorship, the government is state ruled by an individual with strict power and authority.

DARWIN : EVOLUTION :: _____ : RELATIVITY

(A) GALILEO
(B) MENDEL
(C) EINSTEIN
(D) SALK

The correct answer is EINSTEIN, choice C. Darwin developed the theory of evolution; Einstein developed the theory of relativity.

MATHEMATICS EXAMPLE

_____ : 10, 14, 18 :: 2, 14, 26 : 6, 12, 18

(A) 11, 13, 15
(B) –2, 2, 6
(C) 7, 15, 23
(D) 3, 13, 23

The correct answer is choice C, 7, 15, and 23. Complete the statement by putting the correct answer on the blank line and look for the relationships. There is a relationship that includes the entire statement, as well as a relationship on each side of the double colons (::).

The first statement to the left of the double colon is 7, 15, 23 : 10, 14, 18.

$$7 + 8 = 15, 15 + 8 = 23 \qquad 10 + 4 = 14, 14 + 4 = 18$$
An increase of 8   An increase of 4

The increase of 8 decreases by half (from 8 to 4).
The second statement to the right of the double colon is 2, 14, 26 : 6, 12, 18.

$$2 + 12 = 14, 14 + 12 = 26 \qquad 6 + 6 = 12, 12 + 6 = 18$$
An increase of 12   An increase of 6

The increase of 12 decreased by half (from 12 to 6).

HUMANITIES EXAMPLE

PARABLE : MORAL TRUTH :: PARODY : _____

(A) RIDICULE
(B) ROMANTICIZE
(C) TRILOGY
(D) POLITICAL INSIGHT

The correct answer is RIDICULE, choice A. A parable is a story that portrays a moral truth or teaching. A parody is an amusing literary composition that makes fun of a serious literary work.

COMMONPLACE INFORMATION EXAMPLE

SHEEP : _____ ::.SWAN : CYGNET

(A) VIXEN
(B) COB
(C) LAMB
(D) CALF

The correct answer is LAMB, choice C. The offspring of a ewe, a female sheep, is a lamb. The offspring of a swan is a cygnet.

ENGLISH GRAMMAR AND USAGE EXAMPLE

CONCRETE NOUN : CINNAMON :: _____ : FREEDOM

(A) COLLECTIVE NOUN
(B) COMMON NOUN
(C) PROPER NOUN
(D) ABSTRACT NOUN

The correct answer is ABSTRACT NOUN, chioce D. A concrete noun is one that can be perceived by the senses. Cinnamon has a distinctive aroma. An abstract noun is one that cannot be pictured or reasoned by the senses. Freedom is an abstract concept.

Verbal Analogy Relationship Patterns

Verbal analogies fall into a number of basic relationship patterns that require the test taker to recognize relationships between pairs of abstractions or ideas. Recognizing these relationships requires higher levels of reasoning and thinking. Here are some examples of the various types of relationship patterns.

PART TO WHOLE EXAMPLE

LEAD : PENCIL :: _____ : EYE

(A) SKULL
(B) REACTION
(C) IRIS
(D) SKIN

The correct answer is IRIS, choice C. Lead is a part of a pencil. The iris is a part of the eye.

WHOLE TO PART EXAMPLE

ENGINE : _____ :: FOOT : TOE

(A) CAR
(B) GASOLINE
(C) SPARK PLUG
(D) TIRE

The correct answer is SPARK PLUG, choice C. One of the parts of an engine is a spark plug. One of the parts of the foot is the toe.

PROCLIVITY : INCLINATION :: BARBAROUS : _____

(A) UNCOUTH
(B) REFINED
(C) TYPICAL
(D) VOLATILE

The correct answer is UNCOUTH, choice A. Barbarous and uncouth are synonyms, as are proclivity and inclination.

ATTENUATE : INTENSIFY :: _____ : _____

(A) EFFETE : EXHAUSTED
(B) POLTROON : COWARD
(C) RUMINATE : PONDER
(D) VERBOSE : LACONIC

The correct answer is VERBOSE : LACONIC, choice D. Verbose means wordy or long-winded; laconic means brief or to the point. The words are antonyms.

RAIN : FLOOD :: _____ : DEATH

(A) TRUMP
(B) HEMORRHAGE
(C) NIGHT
(D) WINTER

The correct answer is HEMORRHAGE, choice B. Too much rain can cause a flood. Too much hemorrhage, or uncontrolled bleeding, can cause death.

DECIBEL : SOUND :: _____ : EARTHQUAKE

(A) RIPPLES
(B) METRONOME
(C) MAGNITUDE
(D) QUIVER

The correct answer is MAGNITUDE, choice C. Decibels are units used to express differences in loudness or softness of sound. Earthquakes are measured in terms of their magnitude.

DEFINING CHARACTERISTIC EXAMPLE

CLAWS : CAT :: _____ : HORSE

(A) FOOT
(B) HOOVES
(C) STAG
(D) SPINE

The correct answer is HOOVES, choice B. A cat by definition has claws; horses have hooves.

SEQUENCE EXAMPLE

_____ : BIRTH :: BUD : FLOWER

(A) DEATH
(B) ABSTINENCE
(C) CONCEPTION
(D) LEAF

The correct answer is CONCEPTION, choice C. Conception takes place before birth can occur, and a bud develops before a flower blooms.

GENDER EXAMPLE

BULL : _____ :: ROOSTER : CAPON

(A) GELDING
(B) BUCK
(C) STEER
(D) COW

The correct answer is STEER, choice C. A castrated bull is referred to as a steer. A castrated rooster is referred to as a capon.

Analogy sample tests with answer sheets and answer keys follow. As with the previous tests, you will learn more if you answer the questions before looking at the answer key. Make sure that you determine why each response is right or wrong. Remember that good test takers know why a response is right as well as why the remaining responses are wrong.

ANSWER SHEET
Analogies Sample Test One

1. Ⓐ Ⓑ Ⓒ Ⓓ
2. Ⓐ Ⓑ Ⓒ Ⓓ
3. Ⓐ Ⓑ Ⓒ Ⓓ
4. Ⓐ Ⓑ Ⓒ Ⓓ
5. Ⓐ Ⓑ Ⓒ Ⓓ
6. Ⓐ Ⓑ Ⓒ Ⓓ
7. Ⓐ Ⓑ Ⓒ Ⓓ
8. Ⓐ Ⓑ Ⓒ Ⓓ
9. Ⓐ Ⓑ Ⓒ Ⓓ

10. Ⓐ Ⓑ Ⓒ Ⓓ
11. Ⓐ Ⓑ Ⓒ Ⓓ
12. Ⓐ Ⓑ Ⓒ Ⓓ
13. Ⓐ Ⓑ Ⓒ Ⓓ
14. Ⓐ Ⓑ Ⓒ Ⓓ
15. Ⓐ Ⓑ Ⓒ Ⓓ
16. Ⓐ Ⓑ Ⓒ Ⓓ
17. Ⓐ Ⓑ Ⓒ Ⓓ
18. Ⓐ Ⓑ Ⓒ Ⓓ

19. Ⓐ Ⓑ Ⓒ Ⓓ
20. Ⓐ Ⓑ Ⓒ Ⓓ
21. Ⓐ Ⓑ Ⓒ Ⓓ
22. Ⓐ Ⓑ Ⓒ Ⓓ
23. Ⓐ Ⓑ Ⓒ Ⓓ
24. Ⓐ Ⓑ Ⓒ Ⓓ
25. Ⓐ Ⓑ Ⓒ Ⓓ

Directions: For each of the questions, select the letter (A, B, C, or D) that makes the best match with the remaining analogous terms. Record your answers on the answer sheet on page 71.

1. RADISH : GARDEN :: _____ : ORCHARD

   (A) TULIP
   (B) GREEN BEAN
   (C) ROSE
   (D) APPLE

2. WE : PERSONAL PRONOUN :: MYSELF :
   _____

   (A) RELATIVE PRONOUN
   (B) INTERROGATIVE PRONOUN
   (C) INDEFINITE PRONOUN
   (D) REFLEXIVE PRONOUN

3. _____ : _____ :: 4, 6, 8, 10 :
   COMPOSITE NUMBERS

   (A) 2, 3, 5, 7 : PRIME   **CHALLENGE**
       NUMBERS
   (B) 1, 4, 6, 7 : RATIONAL NUMBERS
   (C) −3, −2, −1, 0 : NEGATIVE NUMBERS
   (D) 2, 2, 2, 2 : SQUARE NUMBERS

4. SHAKESPEARE : _____ :: HOMER : *THE ODYSSEY*

   (A) *STOPPING BY WOODS ON A SNOWY EVENING*
   (B) *GREAT EXPECTATIONS*
   (C) *HAMLET*
   (D) *THE RANSOM OF RED CHIEF*

5. 4 : 12 :: _____ : _____

   (A) 10 : 16
   (B) 9 : 27
   (C) 3 : 4
   (D) 12 : 6

6. FAMILY : _____ :: GENUS : HOMO

   (A) SAPIENS
   (B) CHORDATA
   (C) ANIMALIA
   (D) HOMINIDAE

7. ANTIETAM : SHILOH :: BUNKER HILL :
   _____

   (A) VALLEY FORGE
   (B) GETTYSBURG
   (C) VERDUN
   (D) DUNKIRK

8. GAGGLE : _____ :: SWARM : BEES

   (A) SWANS
   (B) PUPPIES
   (C) SNAILS
   (D) GEESE

9. SURNAME : FAMILY NAME :: _____ : PEN NAME

   (A) ANCESTOR
   (B) PSEUDONYM
   (C) PHILISTINE
   (D) BANAL

10. FLOUR : BREAD :: _____ : _____

    (A) IRIS : FRUIT
    (B) RUBBER : STRETCH
    (C) EGG : OMELET
    (D) THEATER : ARTS

11. ABIDE : _____ :: SLINK : SLUNK

    (A) ABODE
    (B) ABIDES
    (C) ABODEN
    (D) ABUDEN

12. ELECTRICAL SYSTEM : WIRES :: FLOWER :
    _____

    (A) SOIL
    (B) PETAL
    (C) ROSE
    (D) WATER

13. RUNNING : EXHAUSTION :: INFECTION :
_____

    (A) WELLNESS
    (B) WOUND
    (C) VIRUS
    (D) FEVER

14. _____ : SLOW :: ALLEGRO : LIVELY

    (A) FUGUE
    (B) CODA
    (C) ADAGIO
    (D) FORTISSIMO

15. SUN : HEAT :: SKUNK : _____

    (A) NOCTURNAL
    (B) ODOR
    (C) ANIMAL
    (D) INVERTEBRATE

16. ENGAGED : MARRIAGE : _____ :
DIVORCE

    (A) SEPARATION
    (B) ANNULMENT
    (C) AVAILABLE
    (D) REPULSIVE

17. DONNE : "DEATH BE NOT PROUD" ::
_____ : "BECAUSE I COULD NOT STOP
FOR DEATH"

    (A) DICKINSON
    (B) EMERSON
    (C) FROST
    (D) CLEMENS

18. PALEOZOIC ERA : _____ :: MESOZOIC
ERA : MAMMALS

    (A) HUMANKIND   CHALLENGE
    (B) DINOSAURS
    (C) SPORES
    (D) FISH

19. _____ : JUPITER :: HADES : PLUTO

    (A) VENUS
    (B) HERMES
    (C) ZEUS
    (D) APOLLO

20. ABSTRUSE : RUDIMENTARY :: ESOTERIC :
_____

    (A) VORACIOUS   CHALLENGE
    (B) ELEMENTARY
    (C) RECONDITE
    (D) DEVOTION

21. AURORA BOREALIS : NORTHERN LIGHTS ::
_____ : SOUTHERN LIGHTS

    (A) AURORA AUSTRALIS
    (B) AURORA ENNUE
    (C) AURORA GLISSANDO
    (D) AURORA GEOTROPISM

22. 100 METERS : HECTOMETER :: _____ :
DECAMETER

    (A) 10,000 METERS   CHALLENGE
    (B) 1,000 METERS
    (C) 10 METERS
    (D) 1 METER

23. HEART : CIRCULATION :: LUNGS : _____

    (A) GESTATION
    (B) DIGESTION
    (C) DECEREBRATION
    (D) OXYGENATION

24. PIAGET : INTELLECTUAL DEVELOPMENT ::
_____ : MORAL DEVELOPMENT

    (A) JUNG
    (B) KOHLBERG
    (C) FREUD
    (D) PAVLOV

25. DECLARATION OF INDEPENDENCE :
_____ :: THE U. S. CONSTITUTION :
JAMES MADISON

    (A) ROGER WILLIAMS
    (B) THOMAS JEFFERSON
    (C) BRIGHAM YOUNG
    (D) ALEXANDER HAMILTON

Analogies Sample Test One Answer Key

1. **D**	6. **D**	11. **A**	16. **A**	21. **A**
2. **D**	7. **A**	12. **B**	17. **A**	22. **C**
3. **A**	8. **D**	13. **D**	18. **D**	23. **D**
4. **C**	9. **B**	14. **C**	19. **C**	24. **B**
5. **B**	10. **C**	15. **B**	20. **B**	25. **B**

ANALOGIES SAMPLE TEST ONE ANSWERS EXPLAINED

1. **(D)** A radish is a vegetable, and vegetables are typically grown in a garden. An apple is a fruit, and fruits are typically grown in an orchard.

2. **(D)** We is a personal pronoun; myself is a reflexive pronoun. Pronouns are words used in place of one or more nouns.

3. **(A)** Prime numbers are numbers that can only be divided by themselves and 1. The numbers 2, 3, 5, and 7 are prime numbers. For example, 13 is a prime number that can evenly be divided by 13 and by 1 only. Composite numbers are divisible by more than 1 and themselves. Four, six, eight, and ten are composite numbers. For example, 24 is a composite number that is divisible by 1, 2, 3, 4, 6, 8, 12, and 24.

4. **(C)** Shakespeare, an English dramatist, wrote the play *Hamlet*. Homer, a Greek writer, wrote the epic *The Odyssey*.

5. **(B)** $4 \times 3 = 12.$ $9 \times 3 = 27.$

6. **(D)** Living organisms are classified or grouped by scientific names. Members of the classification, Family, include Hominidae. Members of the classification, Genus, include Homo.

7. **(A)** Antietam and Shiloh were battles in the American Civil War. Bunker Hill and Valley Forge were battles in the American Revolutionary War.

8. **(D)** A gaggle is a group of geese. A swarm is a group of bees.

9. **(B)** Surnames are family names such as Jones, Walker, or Barlett. Pseudonyms are pen names or false names assumed by a writer.

10. **(C)** One of the components or ingredients of bread is flour. One of the components or ingredients of an omelet is eggs.

11. **(A)** Abide and abode are verbs. Abide is present tense and abode is past tense. The same is true for slink and slunk. Both are verbs with slink indicating present tense and slunk indicating past tense.

12. **(B)** One part or component of an electrical system is wires. One part or component of a flower is a petal.

13. **(D)** The end result of running can be exhaustion, or running can cause exhaustion. An indicator of an infection is a fever, or an infection can cause a fever.

14. **(C)** The musical term adagio means slow or a slow movement or piece of music. The musical term allegro means lively or a lively movement. The paired terms are synonyms.

15. **(B)** One of the defining characteristics of the sun is that it gives off heat. One of the defining characteristics of a skunk is its distinctive odor.

16. **(A)** A period of engagement usually precedes, or goes before, a marriage. A period or time of separation usually precedes a divorce.

17. **(A)** John Donne, an English poet, wrote "Death Be Not Proud." Emily Dickinson, an American poet, wrote "Because I Could Not Stop For Death."

18. **(D)** Paleozoic and Mesozoic are eras in geological time. Fish, as life forms, appeared during the Paleozoic era; mammals, as life forms, appeared during the Mesozoic era.

19. **(C)** Zeus was the king of the Greek gods. Jupiter was king of the Roman gods, or his Roman counterpart. Hades was the Greek god of the underworld; Pluto was his Roman counterpart.

20. **(B)** Abstruse and rudimentary are antonyms, as are esoteric and elementary. Abstruse and esoteric are synonyms, as are rudimentary and elementary.

21. **(A)** The northern lights are the common, everyday name for the Aurora Borealis. The southern lights are the common name for the Aurora Australis. The word aurora is defined as polar lights. Austral means southern, and boreal means northern.

22. **(C)** The measurements are based on the metric system. One hundred meters is the same as a hectometer. Ten meters is the same as a decameter. The prefix "hecto" means one hundred, and the prefix "deca" means ten.

23. **(D)** The heart is responsible for the pumping or circulation of the blood. The lungs are responsible for the oxygenation of the blood.

24. **(B)** Piaget was a Swiss psychologist who formulated the stage theory of intellectual development. Kohlberg was an American psychologist who formulated the stages of moral development.

25. **(B)** The Declaration of Independence was authored by Thomas Jefferson. The Constitution of the United States was authored by many men, including James Madison. The Declaration of Independence and the Constitution of the United States are both documents that deal with the growth of democracy and establishment of the American nation. Both Jefferson and Madison were presidents of the United States.

ANSWER SHEET
Analogies Sample Test Two

1. Ⓐ Ⓑ Ⓒ Ⓓ
2. Ⓐ Ⓑ Ⓒ Ⓓ
3. Ⓐ Ⓑ Ⓒ Ⓓ
4. Ⓐ Ⓑ Ⓒ Ⓓ
5. Ⓐ Ⓑ Ⓒ Ⓓ
6. Ⓐ Ⓑ Ⓒ Ⓓ
7. Ⓐ Ⓑ Ⓒ Ⓓ
8. Ⓐ Ⓑ Ⓒ Ⓓ
9. Ⓐ Ⓑ Ⓒ Ⓓ

10. Ⓐ Ⓑ Ⓒ Ⓓ
11. Ⓐ Ⓑ Ⓒ Ⓓ
12. Ⓐ Ⓑ Ⓒ Ⓓ
13. Ⓐ Ⓑ Ⓒ Ⓓ
14. Ⓐ Ⓑ Ⓒ Ⓓ
15. Ⓐ Ⓑ Ⓒ Ⓓ
16. Ⓐ Ⓑ Ⓒ Ⓓ
17. Ⓐ Ⓑ Ⓒ Ⓓ
18. Ⓐ Ⓑ Ⓒ Ⓓ

19. Ⓐ Ⓑ Ⓒ Ⓓ
20. Ⓐ Ⓑ Ⓒ Ⓓ
21. Ⓐ Ⓑ Ⓒ Ⓓ
22. Ⓐ Ⓑ Ⓒ Ⓓ
23. Ⓐ Ⓑ Ⓒ Ⓓ
24. Ⓐ Ⓑ Ⓒ Ⓓ
25. Ⓐ Ⓑ Ⓒ Ⓓ

Directions: For each of the questions, select the letter (A, B, C, or D) that makes the best match with the remaining analogous terms. Record your answers on the answer sheet on page 77.

1. FEMALE : OVARY :: _____ : _____

   (A) MALE : TESTIS
   (B) MALE : MEIOSIS
   (C) MALE : PENUMBRA
   (D) MALE : ORGAN

2. CAN : ABILITY :: MAY : _____

   (A) JUNE
   (B) CAPABILITY
   (C) PERMISSION
   (D) MOVEMENT

3. STALLION : HORSE :: ROOSTER : _____

   (A) SHAM
   (B) CHICKEN
   (C) HEN
   (D) SPUR

4. BUTTE : _____ :: CANYON : NARROW
   DEEP VALLEY

   (A) FAN-SHAPED AREA
   (B) BARREN LAND
   (C) ROUND-TOPPED HILL
   (D) MESA

   CHALLENGE

5. ILLUSTRATION : FOR EXAMPLE ::
   ADDITIONAL ITEMS : _____

   (A) IN SUCH CASES
   (B) ACCORDINGLY
   (C) NEVERTHELESS
   (D) AS WELL AS

6. ALLEGORY : _____ :: COMEDY : *ALL'S
   WELL THAT ENDS WELL*

   (A) *PILGRIM'S PROGRESS*
   (B) *THE RIME OF THE
       ANCIENT MARINER*
   (C) *CHICAGO*
   (D) *GULLIVER'S TRAVELS*

   CHALLENGE

7. 24/36 : 2/3 :: 12/64 : _____

   (A) 1/3
   (B) 3/16
   (C) 3/8
   (D) 6/32

8. PRINCIPLE : PRINCIPAL :: MEAT : _____

   (A) MEET
   (B) MET
   (C) MAT
   (D) MATE

9. PHARMACOLOGY : DRUGS :: CARDIOLOGY :
   _____

   (A) KIDNEYS
   (B) BODY MOVEMENT
   (C) HEART
   (D) DEATH

10. FARMER : HOE :: FISHERMAN : _____

    (A) BOAT
    (B) FISH
    (C) ROD
    (D) RIVER

11. _____ : MIXED :: HOMOGENEOUS :
    UNIFORM

    (A) INGENIOUS
    (B) HETEROGENEOUS
    (C) MERETRICIOUS
    (D) LIGNEOUS

12. PERSONA NON GRATA : UNWELCOME ::
    _____ : ACTING AS PARENT

    (A) ALFRESCO
    (B) ENFANT TERRIBLE
    (C) VENDETTA
    (D) IN LOCO PARENTIS

    CHALLENGE

13. ISTANBUL : CONSTANTINOPLE :: HO CHI
    MINH CITY : _____

    (A) BELIZE
    (B) CHAD
    (C) SAIGON
    (D) STALINGRAD

14. EDISON : PHONOGRAPH :: _____ :
    LIGHTNING ROD

    (A) FRANKLIN
    (B) WHITNEY
    (C) DIESEL
    (D) MARCONI

15. 2/5 : 40% :: _____ : 62.5%

    (A) 1/3
    (B) 5/8
    (C) 4/5
    (D) 1/6

16. LOUVRE : PARIS :: METROPOLITAN :
    _____

    (A) ISTANBUL
    (B) BERLIN
    (C) NEW YORK
    (D) MADRID

17. KINGDOM : _____ :: SPECIES : SAPIENS

    (A) CHORDATA
    (B) ORDER
    (C) GENUS
    (D) ANIMALIA

18. SPORES : AMPHIBIANS :: MODERN
    MAMMALS : _____

    (A) FERNS
    (B) DINOSAURS
    (C) HUMANKIND
    (D) MARINE ALGAE

19. BOON : _____ :: BENEFACTION :
    PRIVATION

    (A) BLESSING
    (B) DRAWBACK   CHALLENGE
    (C) LARGESS
    (D) DONATION

20. SECEDE : GEORGIA :: UNITE : _____

    (A) ALABAMA
    (B) PENNSYLVANIA
    (C) ARIZONA
    (D) ARKANSAS

21. STADIUM : BLEACHERS :: CHURCH :
    _____

    (A) PEWS
    (B) BENCHES
    (C) SEAT
    (D) CHAIRS

22. ENRAPTURE : _____ :: DISGUST: REPEL

    (A) ENCASE
    (B) CLIMB
    (C) BEWITCH
    (D) DESCEND

23. SPRING : SUMMER :: 75 : _____

    (A) 12
    (B) 125
    (C) 50
    (D) 100

24. LAW : PEOPLE :: GOGGLES : _____

    (A) EYES
    (B) READING
    (C) PROTECTION
    (D) CONFINING

25. PERNICIOUS : HARMLESS :: PESTIFEROUS:
    _____

    (A) FATAL   CHALLENGE
    (B) NOXIOUS
    (C) KIND
    (D) INIQUITOUS

Analogies Sample Test Two Answer Key

1. **A**	6. **A**	11. **B**	16. **C**	21. **A**
2. **C**	7. **B**	12. **D**	17. **D**	22. **C**
3. **B**	8. **A**	13. **C**	18. **C**	23. **D**
4. **C**	9. **C**	14. **A**	19. **B**	24. **A**
5. **D**	10. **C**	15. **B**	20. **B**	25. **C**

ANALOGIES SAMPLE TEST TWO ANSWERS EXPLAINED

1. **(A)** The ovary is the egg-producing organ in the female of a species. The testis is the sperm-producing organ in the male of a species.

2. **(C)** The word *can* indicates an individual or group has the ability to do something. The word *may* indicates an individual or group is seeking permission to do something.

3. **(B)** A stallion is a male horse capable of producing offspring. A rooster is a male chicken capable of producing offspring.

4. **(C)** A butte is a round-topped hill. A canyon is a narrow deep valley.

5. **(D)** In literature, transitional words are used to indicate or allude to the purpose of the presented details. "For example" is an expression that illustrates a general idea or impression. "As well as" is an expression that indicates that additional items are present.

6. **(A)** An allegory is a literary, dramatic, or pictorial piece in which abstract concepts, characters, events, or objects are presented in symbolic, concrete terms. *Pilgrim's Progress* is an example of an allegory. A comedy is a humorous literary, dramatic, or pictorial piece that has a happy ending. *All's Well That Ends Well* is an example of a comedy.

7. **(B)** The fraction 24/36 reduced to its lowest term is 2/3. The fraction 12/64 reduced to its lowest term is 3/16. This is accomplished by dividing both numbers by the largest number that divides evenly into both. Four is the largest number that evenly divides into 12/64.

8. **(A)** Principle and principal are homonyms or words that are pronounced the same but have different spellings and meaning. Meat and meet are also homonyms.

9. **(C)** Pharmacology is the study of drugs and their interactions. Cardiology is the study of the heart.

10. **(C)** A hoe is a hand-held tool used by a farmer. A rod or fishing rod is a hand-held tool used by a fisherman.

11. **(B)** Heterogeneous and mixed are synonyms, as are homogeneous and uniform.

12. **(D)** Many foreign words and phrases have been incorporated in everyday English usage. *Persona non grata* is Latin and means an unwelcome person. *In loco parentis* is Latin and means in the place of a parent.

13. **(C)** The names of many cities have changed over time. Constantinople is the previous name of the modern city of Istanbul, Turkey. Saigon is the previous name of the modern city of Ho Chi Minh City, Vietnam.

14. **(A)** Thomas Edison invented the phonograph. Benjamin Franklin invented the lightning rod.

15. **(B)** Rational numbers may be presented as fractions or decimals. Two fifths and 40% are the same amount or quantity, as are 5/8 and 62.5%. To change a fraction to a percentage, divide the denominator, the bottom number, into the numerator, the upper number.

16. **(C)** The Louvre is in Paris. The Metropolitan is in New York. Both are world famous art museums.

17. **(D)** Living organisms are classified according to taxonomy or taxonomic groups. Kingdom is the largest taxonomic unit. Animalia is an example found within this unit. The smallest taxonomic unit is the species of which *sapiens* is an example.

18. **(C)** According to geologic time, spores, as life forms, appeared prior to amphibians. Modern mammals, as life forms, appeared prior to humankind.

19. **(B)** Boon and drawback are antonyms, as are benefaction and privation. Boon and benefaction are synonyms, as are drawback and privation.

20. **(B)** During the Civil War, Georgia was one state to secede, or split away, from the Union. The state of Pennsylvania remained united with the Union.

21. **(A)** Individuals sit in bleachers at a stadium. Bleachers are typically a part of a stadium. Individuals sit in pews in a church. Pews are typically a part of a church.

22. **(C)** Enrapture and bewitch are synonyms, as are disgust and repel.

23. **(D)** The season spring comes before summer, or summer follows spring. The number 75 comes before 100, the number 100 follows 75. Choice B is incorrect because 125 follows 100, not 75.

24. **(A)** The purpose of the law is to protect people. The purpose of goggles is to protect the eyes.

25. **(C)** Pernicious and harmless are antonyms, as are pestiferous and kind. Pernicious and pestiferous are synonyms, as are harmless and kind.

Reading Comprehension 4

Reading, whether conscious or unconscious, is an important part of our lives from the time we learn to read in elementary school until we die. In our everyday lives, we read almost continuously and probably never give much thought to what we have read because it has little importance for us. Nursing requires reading for understanding, learning, correctly applying, and evaluating your actions in the care of patients.

Comprehension is the most basic skill. Reading comprehension is the capability to read printed material, process it, and grasp its meaning. An individual's ability to understand text is affected by his or her individualities and skills, one of which is the ability to make interpretations and conclusions. Understanding and applying information is imperative in nursing. A nurse constantly reads—nurses' notes from other shifts, health care provider orders, laboratory results, special instructions for administering medications, and numerous other documents.

Recognizing the meanings of the words you read is central to understanding and applying what you have read to everyday life. Medicine and nursing have their own unique vocabulary you will have to learn in order to understand content in your textbooks, in lecture, and in the clinical setting. Success in your nursing program depends heavily upon understanding the terminology and correctly applying it.

Critical reading, as reading comprehension is sometimes called, is not as easy as it sounds. Material you are familiar with is the easiest to understand since you have previous information or knowledge about the topic. Material beyond your scope of reference is more difficult both to read and to understand. It may have its own vocabulary and writing style. It's possible that you may have problems grasping the meaning and purpose of this material. Using a dictionary is always good, but if the majority of your time is spent looking up words, will you be able to remember what you have already read? Therefore, use every opportunity to familiarize yourself with words in this book that may be new to you.

QUESTIONS TO ASK YOURSELF ABOUT READING COMPREHENSION

This chapter can enhance your test-taking skills through practice with reading passages from areas such as literature, social studies, and science. Each sample reading passage in this chapter is different. Regardless of what type of material you're reading, there are skills that are common to all reading materials. Before attempting the Reading Comprehension Sample Test that follows, ask yourself these important questions:

❑ **When should I look at the questions relating to the reading selection?**

It may seem strange to ask this question first, but there is no consensus as to when to read the passage or questions. One premise is to read the questions before perusing the selected passage. The other is to address the questions after you have examined the passage. Try both of these methods; use what you have been taught or what you are most comfortable with. Employ the method that serves you best.

❏ What is the main idea of the reading selection?

The main idea of a selected passage may be obvious, difficult to locate, or it may not be found, but is implied. It's a good idea to quickly read or scan the passage to get an idea of what it presents. The main idea may be presented anywhere in the passage—there is no rule for placement of the main idea. Try to locate a sentence or two that "sums up" the reading passage. In some instances, the main idea of the passage is repeated again in the conclusion. If you cannot locate a main idea, it may be implied by the entire selection.

❏ What supports the main idea?

Once the main idea is determined, look for words, phrases, or statements that support the main idea. Ask yourself who, what, where, when, why, and how regarding the passage. Finding these supporting details should reinforce that you have captured the main idea.

❏ Do I really understand the words in the passage?

As you examine the passage, are you stumbling over words that have no meaning to you? You are faced with new words every day—when communicating with friends and family, in readings, in lecture, and even when watching television and news broadcasts. You hear words like "stem cell" and its potential to enhance human life, but do you really know what a "stem cell" is? Did you know life is impossible without stem cells?

The need for recognizing words and knowing their meanings cannot be stressed enough. Keep a notebook of new words and their meanings. Study these words on a daily basis and use the words in sentences. Add unknown words from this review book to your list. The science chapter will have numerous words that may be new to you.

❏ What can I infer from the passage?

Try to draw inferences or conclusions from the passage. Does the passage suggest more than it is saying? Consider the last stanza of Robert Frost's poem, *Stopping by the Woods on a Snowy Evening.*

> The woods are lovely, dark and deep,
> But I have promises to keep,
> And miles to go before I sleep,
> And miles to go before I sleep.

What does this stanza literally state? The stanza states that an individual in the woods has promises to keep and miles to go before he sleeps. What does the stanza suggest or imply? The individual is on a journey of some kind that involves promises to someone, and the journey is not yet over—he has many miles to travel before he reaches his destination. This is a simple interpretation of the stanza. There are many others.

Table 4.1. Common Connecting Words in a Passage

Type	Words/Phrases
Compare (Are there similarities between ideas? How are they alike?)	➤ Associate ➤ Comparison ➤ In a manner ➤ Likewise ➤ Relate ➤ Similarly
Contrast (Are there dissimilar ideas? How are they different?)	➤ But ➤ Conversely ➤ However ➤ In contrast to ➤ On the other hand ➤ Notwithstanding ➤ Still
Direction and Place (Are movement and change of place demonstrated?)	➤ Above ➤ Adjacent ➤ Compass directions ➤ Inside of ➤ Opposite ➤ Over ➤ Under
Ordinal Sequence (Is there an order in which ideas are presented?)	➤ 1st, 2nd, 3rd ➤ Finally ➤ Initially ➤ Last ➤ Next ➤ Succession
Time Sequence (Are there changes in time? Does time show progression or regression?)	➤ After ➤ Before ➤ Finally ➤ Tomorrow ➤ While ➤ Yesterday

❑ Are there words or phrases in the passage that tie relationships or ideas together?

There is no standard for how authors present information, but they may use words and/or phrases to more effectively communicate their message. Table 4.1 provides a list of words that may indicate relationships or ideas in a passage.

❑ Why was the passage written? What is its purpose?

After reading and gathering all you can about the passage, ask yourself what the author is trying to do. Is the purpose to provide factual information about life in another part of the world? Is it to sway you to the author's way of thinking? Is the author simply telling a story for the enjoyment of his readers? Could the author's purpose in writing this passage be to teach a moral or ethical lesson?

Authors write for numerous reasons, and it's important to remember not to believe everything you read in print. How do they refer to sources that are supposed to be facts? Does the author refer to "numerous research studies" or "research done in 2014 at Johns Hopkins University on stem cells and tissue regrowth by noted microbiologist, Franklin Eugene Watts, Ph.D."? Which statement is more reliable and adds to the veracity of the passage?

❑ How do I answer the questions?

When preparing to answer the questions at the end of a passage, do not make assumptions about the potential answers and do not argue with the question or potential answers. Your purpose is to answer the question based on your understanding of the material. You may be asked to infer what a word or selected passage means. Again, do not assume. Base your response on logical, critical, unbiased thought.

As you use this review book in preparation for your nursing entrance exam, keep in mind that this entire review book is one form of reading comprehension. It's a review of topics you will be formally tested on. Use a dictionary and your prerequisite course textbooks as you prepare using this review book. Remember, don't just read what you look up. Write it down!

READING COMPREHENSION SAMPLE TEST

Keeping these important questions in mind, proceed to the Reading Comprehension Sample Test. Note that almost any type of writing can be used for reading comprehension. The first reading selection is an adaptation of *The Three Pigs*, a popular children's fairly tale with which you are probably familiar. Selections written in everyday language are the easiest to understand because they employ words used in your daily reading and speech. Their verbiage is also nontechnical. *The Other Three Pigs* is an example of a long selection. The second selection is *The Gettysburg Address* by Abraham Lincoln. This is an example of a historical document that will test your ability to comprehend more difficult language as well as to make inferences about historical events based on the details in the passage. The final selection is a piece called *Heart Failure*. This nonfiction passage presents scientific facts. All of the information that you will need to answer the questions can be found within the passage. The vocabulary may be more difficult, so pay attention to clues within the passage that will help you understand their meaning.

The Reading Comprehension Sample Test that follows is only for practice and is therefore untimed. Take extra time to read through all of the selections carefully and apply the strategies you've learned thus far. This is the time to jot down any words or phrases that you are unfamiliar with. Be aware that the reading comprehension selection in the model tests at the end of this book will be timed.

ANSWER SHEET
Reading Comprehension Sample Test

Section 1: The Other Three Pigs

1. Ⓐ Ⓑ Ⓒ Ⓓ
2. Ⓐ Ⓑ Ⓒ Ⓓ
3. Ⓐ Ⓑ Ⓒ Ⓓ
4. Ⓐ Ⓑ Ⓒ Ⓓ

5. Ⓐ Ⓑ Ⓒ Ⓓ
6. Ⓐ Ⓑ Ⓒ Ⓓ
7. Ⓐ Ⓑ Ⓒ Ⓓ
8. Ⓐ Ⓑ Ⓒ Ⓓ

9. Ⓐ Ⓑ Ⓒ Ⓓ
10. Ⓐ Ⓑ Ⓒ Ⓓ

Section 2: The Gettysburg Address

1. Ⓐ Ⓑ Ⓒ Ⓓ
2. Ⓐ Ⓑ Ⓒ Ⓓ

3. Ⓐ Ⓑ Ⓒ Ⓓ
4. Ⓐ Ⓑ Ⓒ Ⓓ

5. Ⓐ Ⓑ Ⓒ Ⓓ

Section 3: Heart Failure

1. Ⓐ Ⓑ Ⓒ Ⓓ
2. Ⓐ Ⓑ Ⓒ Ⓓ

3. Ⓐ Ⓑ Ⓒ Ⓓ
4. Ⓐ Ⓑ Ⓒ Ⓓ

SECTION 1: THE OTHER THREE PIGS

> For Questions 1–10, read the following passage and select the letter (A, B, C, or D) that best answers the question. Record your answers in Section 1 of the Reading Comprehension Sample Test Answer Sheet on page 87.

Long ago in a land far away, there lived a family of pigs. There was Papa Pig, Mama Pig, and their triplet sons Horace, Kervin, and
Line Calvert. The Pig family was prosperous. Papa
(5) Pig farmed on land left to him by his father, and he hoped his sons would follow in his footsteps.

The Pig boys lived at home after finishing school. Papa and Mama Pig had given each
(10) son a parcel of land as a graduation gift, and the sons were working and saving money to build homes on their land. All three had decided to become farmers.

It's important to note that even though the
(15) Pig boys were identical triplets, their similarities ended there. Horace, the first born of the three, was improvident. His coffer was meager. He enjoyed dressing in the finest available, and flashing his coin about the
(20) village and the pub where he frequently bought drinks for his friends and those who feigned friendship. It wasn't that Horace didn't want to save; he just couldn't help himself when it came to himself—he came
(25) first.

Kervin, the second born of the three, was overly altruistic. He often donated half of his earnings to those less fortunate. He dressed moderately and rarely went to the pub. When
(30) he did, he bought his own drinks or Horace was buying. His coffer was in much better shape. Like Horace, Kervin wanted to save, he just couldn't put himself above those in privation.

(35) Calvert, the youngest, was for the most part, a pinchpenny. On a rare occasion, he

could be charitable, but that was on a really rare occasion. Like Kervin, he dressed modestly, and he never went to the pub
(40) unless Horace was buying. Calvert's coffer was full. He often wondered why he was not more like his brothers, but he never dwelled on it because he knew he needed money to do the things he had envisaged for years.

(45) One evening at supper, Calvert announced that he had reached his savings goal and would soon begin building a house on his land. He had talked with builders in the village about the sturdiest and securest house
(50) to build and decided to build a brick house. With the design he selected, it would be easy to build an addition when he married and had children. He was enthusiastic because he had enough money not only to build his
(55) home, but also a barn.

Weeks later, Horace and Kervin announced that they, too, had reached their savings goals and would soon have their own houses built. They admitted to their parents
(60) they had not done the research Calvert had, but felt they could look into things as they progressed. Both admitted they did not have the money to build anything more than a house.

(65) Horace and Kervin had not been totally honest with Mama and Papa Pig. While they did have money to build, neither could afford a brick house. Horace could only afford a stick house, and Kervin a wood house.

(70) By early fall, the Pig boys were in their homes. Calvert kept his day job, and worked evenings clearing the trees, rocks, and

stumps to have acreage to plant in the spring. Horace worked when he felt like it, but his

(75) behaviors didn't change. Like Calvert, he worked clearing the land for planting, but it was hard, backbreaking work and he accomplished very little. Kervin worked part time and when his boss needed him, but he

(80) still gave to the needy leaving little for himself. After deciding he didn't need to plant a large acreage his first year, he cleared a small patch of land.

The Pig boys had supper with their parents

(85) every Sunday evening. Papa Pig was quiet this evening, and it was obvious he had something on his mind. He finally told them that a big wolf had been seen in the north of the county, and it was rumored the wolf had

(90) torn his way into houses to get to the inhabitants. Mama Pig stated she would worry about the boys and wanted them to stay with them in their big house since there was a wolf in the area. Each son refused her

(95) offer, stating his home could withstand almost anything.

On the way to their homes later that evening, the brothers talked about what their father had told them. The county had been

(100) safe for years. There were children that had never seen a wolf, let alone seen the malevolent destruction a wolf could make. As they parted to go their separate ways, each pledged to make sure their home was safe.

(105) Within weeks, the wolf had ravaged much of the county, and many had lost almost all they had. Among the victims were Horace and Kervin who had lost their homes and everything they owned. Calvert, Mama, and

(110) Papa Pig lost little—the wolf could not get into their brick homes.

Horace and Kervin were able to move in with their parents. They had little interest in anything and were content to sit around and

(115) do nothing. Papa Pig finally told them they must find work and save their money to

restart their lives. This did not please them and they went to Calvert to live with him. They became angry and left when Calvert

(120) told them they had to find work and save their earnings, or live in the barn and work for him. He said he would give them a meager amount to spend each week, but the bulk of their earnings he would hold until

(125) enough was saved for them to rebuild their own houses and start again.

Even though Horace and Kervin were both angry when they left Calvert's, their moods and thinking soon diverged, and they parted

(130) ways. Horace stayed angry and vowed to sell his land and leave the county—he didn't need anyone. Kervin, on the other hand, saw the wisdom of his parents and Calvert and lost his anger. He decided that he couldn't be a

(135) farmer. He found little joy in it and vowed to give his land to Calvert and find his calling. Both were true to their vows.

Horace sold his land and stole away in the middle of the night. The Pig family rarely

(140) heard about him. What they heard saddened them. Horace had squandered the money from selling his land. He had become a slave to drink, spent most his time intoxicated or in the village jail, and only worked when he

(145) had to.

Kervin found happiness and the family often saw him. He gave his land to Calvert, and joined a community of religious individuals who cared for the penurious.

(150) Calvert became the prosperous farmer he'd hoped to be. He eventually married Elizabeth and started a family. Papa and Mama Pig became more prosperous than they had been and enjoyed spoiling their

(155) grand piglets.

P. S. The wolf wasn't killed. He was captured by hunters and taken to a remote mountain area and released. He was never seen again.

1. What is the moral of *The Other Three Pigs?*

   (A) Children need strong role models to become responsible adults.
   (B) Individuals who apply themselves and set aside their earnings are more likely to be affluent than those who do not.
   (C) Parents should help their children financially regardless of their behaviors.
   (D) There is no guarantee that siblings raised in the same fashion will have the same values and standards as adults.

2. What does the word "improvident" in line 17 suggest?

   (A) careful
   (B) miserly
   (C) profligate
   (D) thrifty

3. What is the most applicable definition for "coffer" in lines, 17, 31, and 40?

   (A) a basket
   (B) a hole in the ground for storing valuables
   (C) a treasury
   (D) an ornamental panel in a wall suitable for hiding valuables

4. Based on lines 16–25, Horace could best be described as

   (A) conspicuously dashing and colorful.
   (B) planning prudently for the future.
   (C) an apathetic pig.
   (D) the prodigal son.

5. Why did Horace and Kervin not have enough money to build a brick house like Calvert did?

   (A) They did not realize the value of money.
   (B) They had problems differentiating between reality and fantasy in their lives.
   (C) They were foolish spenders.
   (D) They were not taught, as children, to be savers.

6. What probable reason could Mama Pig have for wanting Horace, Kervin, and Calvert to stay with them (lines 91–94)?

   (A) She does not think Papa Pig could protect her if the wolf attacked their home.
   (B) She does not think her sons' homes had proper security systems if the wolf attacked.
   (C) She wants her children home with her and Papa Pig if the wolf attacked.
   (D) She has control issues.

7. Calvert tells his brothers, in lines 122–126, that he will hold their wages until they have enough money to start over again. Why does he plan to do this?

   (A) He will be able to validate their earnings with their employers.
   (B) He is concerned about their future well-being.
   (C) He is interested in knowing how much they earn.
   (D) He will keep a small portion of their wages for room and board.

8. Horace and Kervin each had a change in mood and thinking after leaving Calvert's house, and they parted ways (lines 127–137). Based on the passage, what does each of their behaviors suggest?

   (A) Horace is narcissistic whereas Kervin is overly philanthropic.
   (B) Horace decides that their chances for success would be better if they parted ways, and Kervin agrees.
   (C) Horace and Kervin cannot agree on the best course of action to take.
   (D) Horace and Kervin do not trust each other.

9. What does the phrase "slave to drink" mean as it relates to Horace in lines 142–145?

    (A) He is ashamed he left his family and drinks to forget that fact.

    (B) He is still as flamboyant as he has always been and enjoys daily drinking.

    (C) He spends all his earnings on drink.

    (D) In all probability, he is an alcoholic.

10. What is the "community of religious individuals," described in lines 147–149?

    (A) an association of village elders intent on improving the lives of the poor in their village

    (B) an enterprise for males involved in caring for the impoverished

    (C) a fraternity for males interested in caring for the indigent

    (D) a group of nuns and monks dedicated to caring for the disadvantaged

SECTION 2: THE GETTYSBURG ADDRESS

For Questions 1–5, read the following passage and select the letter (A, B, C, or D) that best answers the question. Record your answers in Section 2 of the Reading Comprehension Sample Test Answer Sheet on page 87.

The Gettysburg Address by Abraham Lincoln (1863)

Four score and seven years ago our fathers brought forth, on this continent, a new nation, conceived in Liberty, and dedicated
Line to the proposition that all men are created
(5) equal.

Now we are engaged in a great civil war, testing whether that nation, or any nation so conceived, and so dedicated, can long endure. We are met here on a great battlefield
(10) of that war. We have come to dedicate a portion of that field, as a final resting place for those who here gave their lives that that nation might live. It is altogether fitting and proper that we should do this.

(15) But in a larger sense, we cannot dedicate— we cannot consecrate—we cannot hallow— this ground. The brave men, living and dead, who struggled here, have consecrated it far above our poor power to add or detract. The
(20) world will little note, nor long remember, what we say here, but it can never forget what they did here.

It is for us, the living, rather, to be dedicated here to the unfinished work which
(25) they who fought here have, thus far, so nobly advanced. It is rather for us to be here dedicated to the great task remaining before us—that from these honored dead we take increased devotion to that cause for which
(30) measure of devotion—that we here highly resolve that these dead shall not have died in vain—that this nation under God shall have a new birth of freedom—that government of the people, by the people, for the people,
(35) shall not perish from the earth.

1. What historical event is suggested in lines 1–5?
   (A) the beginning of the Revolutionary War in 1775
   (B) the Boston Tea Party in 1773
   (C) the Continental Congress adopts the stars and stripes as the national flag in 1777
   (D) the signing of the Declaration of Independence in 1776

2. The word "proposition" (line 4) is a <u>synonym</u> for
   (A) identify.
   (B) opportunity.
   (C) premise.
   (D) reality.

3. What does the word "fitting" in line 13 mean?
   (A) to be appropriate for a situation
   (B) to be of the right size for something
   (C) to be suitable for a person or object
   (D) to be the correct shape

4. What was the purpose of the gathering in Gettysburg?
   (A) dedicating a cemetery
   (B) emancipating the slaves
   (C) observing the aftermath of a battle
   (D) reconciling differences between political groups

5. Line 29 speaks of having "increased devotion to that cause." What cause is Lincoln referring to?
   (A) to accomplish the great task remaining
   (B) to be dedicated to the task at hand
   (C) to consecrate the ground where so many died
   (D) to preserve the nation

SECTION 3: HEART FAILURE

> For Questions 1–4, read the following passage and select the letter (A, B, C, or D) that best answers the question. Record your answers in Section 3 of the Reading Comprehension Sample Test Answer Sheet on page 87.

Heart failure is a chronic, progressive disorder commonly seen in older adults. Simply put, heart failure is pump failure.
Line Heart failure does not strike out of the blue
(5) like a heart attack, but progresses quietly until symptoms appear. Individuals usually don't seek medical attention until symptoms begin to interfere with their activities of daily living. Without treatment, the heart
(10) continues to fail.

A diagnosis of heart failure does not mean the heart has quit working. It means the heart does not work as effectively as it once did. The diagnosis is also not a death sentence—
(15) with health care provider prescribed management, an individual can live a fairly normal life within limitations. Management includes medications, lifestyle changes, and exercise to control and reduce symptoms.
(20) Heart failure has numerous etiologies. They include coronary artery disease, valvular heart disease, high blood pressure, heart attack, disorders that damage the heart muscle, and other conditions such as
(25) diabetes, thyroid, and kidney disease. Drug and alcohol abuse can also lead to heart failure. In heart failure, the heart gradually loses its ability to pump effectively. This results in the heart not being able to pump
(30) enough blood to meet the body's metabolic needs.

Signs and symptoms of heart failure include: (1) congested lungs, shortness of breath with activity or when lying down
(35) caused by fluid backing up into the

pulmonary veins; (2) swelling in the feet, ankles, lower legs, abdomen and/or sudden weight gain caused by fluid buildup in body tissues; (3) rapid heart rate and increased
(40) respiratory rate caused by the heart trying to play "catch up" to meet the body's metabolic requirements; (4) nausea and anorexia caused by the gastrointestinal system receiving less blood; (5) tiredness or fatigue
(45) that affects the ability to complete everyday tasks (shopping, cleaning house, cooking, dressing, bathing) in a timely fashion; (6) "troublesome" cough or wheezing with or without bringing up white or blood-tinged
(50) sputum brought about by fluid backup into the lungs; and (7) changes in amount of urination, a decrease in the day and increase at night after going to bed.

There are a number of laboratory and
(55) diagnostic studies that can be performed to confirm a diagnosis of heart failure. Among these are (1) an electrocardiogram (EKG) to look at the electrical activity and beating of the heart; (2) a chest x-ray to determine the
(60) size of the heart to show fluid buildup around the heart, if present, and fluid buildup and congestion in the lungs; (3) a pulse oximeter reading to determine oxygen saturation of the blood; (4) blood tests to determine kidney
(65) and thyroid function, the presence or absence of anemia, and brain natriuretic peptide testing (BNP) that increases when heart failure exists or symptoms worsen and decreases when the condition is stable.

1. What does the phrase "out of the blue," in line 4, suggest?

   (A) all of a sudden
   (B) from above
   (C) rapidly building to a crescendo
   (D) with fanfare

2. What can you infer from the article?

   (A) An increase in fluid intake will help the circulatory system meet metabolic demands.
   (B) Heart failure will result in death if left untreated.
   (C) Older adults will develop heart failure.
   (D) Treatment by a competent health care provider will cure heart failure.

3. Synonyms for "control and reduce," as used in line 19, are

   (A) command and condense.
   (B) conduct and render.
   (C) determine and relinquish.
   (D) invigorate and lengthen.

4. You are a junior nursing student at a university that is several hundred miles from your home. You live with your grandmother in the city where the university is located to save money. Your 76-year-old grandmother has always been healthy and is proud of the fact that the sickest she ever remembers being is when she experienced morning sickness when pregnant with your mother over 50 years ago.

   Over the last one to two months, you have noticed changes in your grandmother. Her lower legs and feet look fairly normal in the morning, but are swollen in the evening. She complains of tiredness and fatigue more than she used to, and you're aware that she gets up several times at night to urinate. Based upon the changes you have seen, as well as what you learned in the "Heart Failure" reading passage, what is your best course of action?

   (A) Assume more responsibility with household chores. Less work will reduce her fatigue and give her more time for herself.
   (B) Call your mother and talk with her about the changes you've seen. Ask her to suggest a plan of action.
   (C) Say nothing. Your grandmother will let you know if she is having problems.
   (D) Talk with your grandmother about the changes you've noticed and encourage her to see her health care provider.

Section 1: The Other Three Pigs

1. **B**   3. **C**   5. **C**   7. **B**   9. **D**
2. **C**   4. **D**   6. **C**   8. **A**   10. **D**

Section 2: The Gettysburg Address

1. **D**   2. **C**   3. **A**   4. **A**   5. **D**

Section 3: Heart Failure

1. **A**   2. **B**   3. **A**   4. **D**

ANSWERS EXPLAINED

Section 1: The Other Three Pigs

1. **(B)** Choice B is the only reasonable option. The theme throughout the story is that Calvert is the serious pig who saves his money and ultimately becomes prosperous. The story provides no information on what type of role models Papa and Mama Pig are, as choice A suggests. Choice C is wrong because the passage does not encourage the parents to continue to finance their children when they do not manage their money well. Choice D may seem like a good choice, but it is also incorrect because the passage never directly says that the way the pigs were raised has anything to do with their individual personalities, values, and standards. If you missed this question, you probably made assumptions without verifying the details from the passage.

2. **(C)** Improvident means imprudent, careless, reckless, or irresponsible. Profligate means wasteful, reckless, squandering, or spendthrift. Improvident and profligate are synonyms.

3. **(C)** A coffer, in the sense of this story, is a treasury or strongbox. While choices B and D might both seem like the correct answer, the story does not provide information regarding the architecture of Papa and Mama Pig's home or where the coffers are, making choice C the most correct answer. If you chose choice B or D, you made an assumption.

4. **(D)** Prodigal is an adjective meaning wasteful, extravagant, or uncontrolled. Prodigal describes Horace and his lifestyle. Conspicuously dashing and colorful, choice A, seems like an okay description of Horace, but the question asks for the traits that *best* describe Horace. He is noticeably well-dressed, but the reason that he is so stylish is because of his prodigal or extravagant spending. Choice B is wrong because Horace is the least prepared of all the brothers. Choice C is incorrect because Horace is not indifferent or apathetic about his life. Rather, he spends too much time focused on the "finer" things in life, which gets him into trouble.

5. **(C)** Horace and Kervin were foolish spenders in that they did not have clear direction of their tasks—to earn money to build their homes. Horace was foolish because he was more interested in himself whereas Kervin was foolish enough to completely sacrifice himself for the good of others. Both obviously realized the value of money given that Horace knew it could buy him every extravagant item he wanted and Kervin knew that he could use large sums of money to help the less fortunate. Therefore, choice A is wrong. Choice B has no basis since the passage never discusses reality versus fantasy. The story also doesn't provide information about what they were taught as children, so choice D cannot be correct.

6. **(C)** Mama Pig states she will worry about her sons if they are not at the large family home. The story provides no information on Papa Pig's ability to protect Mama Pig, choice A, the security systems in the sons' homes if the wolf attacked, choice B, or Mama Pig's supposed control issues, choice D.

7. **(B)** Calvert is concerned about his brothers being able to save, rebuild, and get on with their lives. No supporting details suggest that Calvert needs to validate his brothers' earnings, choice A, knows how much they are earning, choice C, or that he will withhold a portion of wages for room and board, choice D.

8. **(A)** Horace is a good example of a vain and self-absorbed individual. Kervin, on the other hand, is the opposite of Horace. Kervin gives away all that he has even to the detriment of himself and his own well-being. When the brothers part ways, Horace continues to be his narcissistic self by spending money on himself only. Kervin, on the other hand, continues to act selflessly by giving away his land to his brother and devoting his life to philanthropic causes, like helping the less fortunate. There is nothing in the story that states or suggests the brothers would do better if parted, choice B, that they are unable to agree on a course of action to take, choice C, or that they do not trust each other, choice D.

9. **(D)** Horace has probably become an alcoholic. As such, his life centers around the ingestion of alcohol and intoxication—he has become a slave to drink and suffers because of it. There is nothing to suggest that he drinks to forget or is still flamboyant, so choices A and B can be eliminated. He probably does spend most or all of his money on drink, as choice C suggests, but it does not match the phrase "slave to drink" as asked about in the question.

10. **(D)** This question calls for a definition of "community of religious individuals." The key word here is "religious." While choices A, B, and C do represent a group or community of individuals, they do not include religious figures specifically. Choice D is the only option that mentions religious figures, nuns and monks, making it the only plausible answer.

Section 2: The Gettysburg Address

1. **(D)** Lincoln is referring to the signing of the Declaration of Independence in 1776 when he speaks of bringing forth a new nation on the continent. Four score and seven years ago is 87 years—the number of years from 1776 when the declaration was signed until 1863 when the Gettysburg Address was given.

2. **(C)** In this line, the word "proposition" could be replaced with "premise." Lincoln is referring to the suggestion, assertion, or idea that all men are created equal as declared by the forefathers of America.

3. **(A)** In order to determine what "fitting" means, it must be analyzed in the context in which it is used. The word "fitting" is paired with "proper" in this sentence. Something that is proper is generally considered appropriate, as choice A suggests. The remaining choices, B, C, and D, are correct *alternate* meanings for "fitting," but they do not fit the context of this sentence.

4. **(A)** The third paragraph (lines 15–22) describes the purpose of the gathering—to dedicate a cemetery for those who died at the Battle of Gettysburg. None of the remaining reasons are directly mentioned in this selection.

5. **(D)** The preservation of the nation is the theme of line 29. Soldiers died trying to do this. Lincoln envisions the nation having a new birth of freedom and a government that shall not perish from Earth.

Section 3: Heart Failure

1. **(A)** Something that happens "out of the blue" happens without warning and all of a sudden, choice A. As the passage states, heart failure is not "out of the blue." It occurs gradually over time.

2. **(B)** According to the passage, heart failure is a chronic, progressive disorder that will result in death if left untreated. The passage does not support choices A, C, or D.

3. **(A)** As used in line 19, "control and reduce" could be interchanged with "command and condense." This sentence is saying that all of these methods can be used to take charge of and lessen the degree of heart failure symptoms. The other choices do not present a pair of words that are synonymous with "control and reduce."

4. **(D)** As a junior nursing student, you are seeing signs and symptoms in your grandmother that are suggestive of a worsening problem. Talking with your grandmother is the most proactive action you can take. Based on the nature of heart failure, it would not help your grandmother to assume more responsibility of the house, as choice A suggests. There is nothing to suggest that your mother knows about the changes you are seeing in your grandmother or would know the best plan of action, so choice B does not work. To say nothing is foolhardy so eliminate choice C as well. Even though your grandmother complains of tiredness and fatigue more than she used to and she seems to know when she is sick, your nursing education should still tell you that she needs medical intervention.

Numerical Ability 5

The ability to use numbers competently is essential in virtually every aspect of our everyday lives. Numerical ability is nothing more than using mathematics effectively in its many different forms.

We are surrounded by numbers. Consider the following examples that use numbers and require some mathematical ability:

1. You set your alarm clock to get up at a certain time each morning. The time you choose to get up depends on the number of tasks you must accomplish before leaving to get to school or work on time.

2. You purchase a number of items at a store. The clerk tells you the cost of your purchase, and you must know how much money to give to the clerk, as well as how to determine the amount of change you should receive.

3. You want to purchase your first car. You will probably have to see if car payments will fit into your budget. Moreover, a car costs more than the price posted on the window sticker. You must pay for taxes, title, and license as well as the interest on the car loan. You must also see if car insurance will fit into your budget.

4. You decide to paint several rooms in your apartment. You must determine how many square feet there are to be painted before you can buy the correct amount of paint.

5. You have volunteered to bake 100 dozen chocolate chip cookies for a charity bazaar. Your chocolate chip cookie recipe yields three dozen cookies approximately three inches in diameter. You will need to determine the total amount of ingredients to purchase in order to bake this large amount of cookies.

In nursing, just as in everyday life, good numerical skills are as important as having good communication skills. Nurses use many levels of mathematics from simple arithmetic to more advanced algebra in all aspects of patient care. Consider that nurses are responsible for their own actions, and a nurse with poor numerical ability may harm or kill a patient. For example, a patient may receive medication based on body weight and the nurse is responsible for not only knowing what the patient weighs but also figuring the amount of medication the patient is to receive based on the physician's order. The patient could get too much or too little medication if the nurse's numerical skills are not up to par.

To complicate matters even more, a number of measuring systems are currently in use. In the United States, the English system is commonly used. Much of the rest of the world uses the metric system. The health care system in the United States also uses the metric system.

Converting from the English system of measurement to the metric or from the metric system to the English when you do not know the equivalents can easily be done using the ratio and proportions formula presented later in this chapter. Ratio and proportions can also be used when going from one unit of measure to another within each system. Common metric measurements you may need to know are presented in Table 5.1.

Table 5.1. Common Metric Measurements

Gram (Mass)[a]	Equivalents in Other Units
1000 mcg	1 mg
1000 mg	1 g
1000 g	1 kg[d]
1000 kg	1 metric ton

Liter (Volume)[b]	Equivalents in Other Units
1000 ml	1 L
1000 L	1 kl

Meter (Length)[c]	Equivalents in Other Units
1000 mm	100 cm
100 cm	10 dm
10 dm	1 m
1 m	10 dam
10 dam	100 hm
100 hm	1000 km

[a]mcg = microgram, mg = milligram, g = gram, kg = kilogram.
[b]ml = milliliter, L = liter, kl = kiloliter.
[c]mm = millimeter, cm = centimeter, dm = decimeter, m = meter, dam = dekameter, hm = hectometer, km = kilometer.
[d]1 kg = 2.2 lbs.

Just as it is difficult to conceive of life without using numbers in one form or another, it is difficult to think of many situations where measurements of one type or another are not used. Measurements are presented in numerical format, and you should be familiar with a number of measurements, many of which are shown in Table 5.2 on page 103.

Nurses use measurements in numerous aspects of patient care. In many instances nurses use the metric system of measurement. For example, a record may be kept of the amount of fluids a patient takes in orally and the amount of urine a patient puts out. Nurses calculating a patient's intake and output would need to be able to convert from the liquid measurement system to the metric system. Table 5.3 on page 104 lists the most common nursing measurements.

It is beyond the scope of this book to present all aspects of mathematics, so we assume that you have basic mathematical reasoning abilities and can competently add, subtract, multiply, and divide numbers *without* a calculator.

A number of different mathematical symbols may be used with any type of mathematical problem. You should be familiar with these symbols, which are given in Table 5.4 on page 104.

CALCULATOR USE

The uses of handheld calculators are commonplace in schools, homes, and businesses. Although calculators have made life easier when it comes to computations, they have also been detrimental. Some individuals have a weakness with paper-and-pencil calculations; others may not be able to do computations without calculators.

The use of handheld calculators in nursing has eased the workload of nurses caring for patients. There are numerous formulas that nurses must be familiar with in order to correctly administer medications to patients.

Table 5.2. Units of Measurement

Unit	U.S. Equivalent	Metric Equivalent
Length		
foot	12 inches	0.305 meters
yard	3 feet (36 inches)	0.914 meters
rod	5.5 yards	5.029 meters
statute mile	1,760 yards (5,280 feet)	1.609 kilometers
nautical mile	1,151 statute miles	1.852 kilometers
Area		
square foot	144 square inches	929.030 square centimeters
square yard	9 square feet	0.836 square meters
acre	4,840 square yards	4,072 square meters
section	1 square mile (640 acres)	2,590 square kilometers
Capacity		
ounce	8 drams	29.573 milliliters
cup	8 ounces	0.237 liter
pint	16 ounces	0.473 liter
quart	2 pints	0.946 liter
gallon	4 quarts	3.785 liters
peck	8 quarts	8.810 liters
bushel	4 pecks	35.239 liters
Weight		
ounce	16 drams	28.350 grams
pound	16 ounces	0.45 kg (1 kg = 2.21 lbs.)
ton	2,000 pounds	0.907 metric tons

Unit	U.S. and Metric Equivalents
Time	
minute	60 seconds
hour	60 minutes
day	24 hours
year	365 days or 12 months
decade	10 years
century	100 years
millennium	1000 years

Table 5.3. Common Nursing Measurements[a]

Household Equivalent	English Equivalent	Metric Equivalent
1 gtt (drop)	1 m (minum)	0.06 ml (milliliter)
	15 or 16 m	1 ml
60 gtt = 1 tsp = 5 ml	1 fluid dram	5 ml
3 tsp = 1 tbsp	4 fluid drams	15 or 16 ml
2 tbsp	1 fluid ounce	30 ml
1 glass = 1 measuring cup	8 fluid ounces = 1/2 pint	240 ml
	1/300 gr	0.2 mg
	1/200 gr	0.3 mg
	1/150 gr	0.4 mg
	1/100 gr	0.6 mg
	1/60 gr	1 mg = 1000 mcg
	1/10 gr	6 mg
	1/8 gr	8 mg
	1/6 gr	10 mg
	1/4 gr	15 mg
	1 gr	60 mg

[a]gtt = drop, m = minum, ml = milliliter, tsp = teaspoon, tbsp = tablespoon, gr = grain, mg = milligram, mcg = microgram.

Table 5.4. Mathematical Symbols

Symbol	Meaning	Example
$+$	Add	$10 + 15 = 25$
$-$	Subtract	$60 - 40 = 20$
$\times$ or $\cdot$ or $(\,)$	Multiply	$6 \times 5 = 30$ or $(6)(5) = 30$
		$7 \cdot 5 = 35$
		$(12)(4) = 48$
$\div$ or $\dfrac{a}{b}$	Divide	$15 \div 3 = 5$ or $\dfrac{15}{3} = 5$
		$\dfrac{50}{5} = 10$
$=$	Is equal to	$12 = 12$
$\neq$	Is not equal to	$8 \neq 15$
$\geq$	Is equal to or greater than	$a \geq b$
$\leq$	Is equal to or less than	$c \leq d$
$>$	Is greater than	$7 > 2$
$<$	Is less than	$9 < 13$
$\perp$	Is perpendicular to	$b \perp d$
$\parallel$	Is parallel to	$a \parallel c$
$\sqrt{}$	Square root	$\sqrt{64} = 8$
$\sqrt[3]{}$	Cube root	$\sqrt[3]{216} = 6$
$(\,)$	Parentheses	$8(6 + 4) = 80$
$[\,]$	Brackets	$7 + [8(6 + 4) - 2] = 85$
$\{\,\}$	Braces	$119 + 7 - \{2 + [8(6 + 4) - 8] + 3\} = 49$
$\angle$	Angle	$\angle ABC + 80° = 165°$

Your entrance examination may or may not allow the use of *personal* calculators. Simple calculators, with addition, subtraction, multiplication, and division only, may be built into the testing program if your test is on a computer. You may be provided with a simple calculator if your test is paper-and-pencil.

Information regarding calculator use should be included with the materials you receive about your test. If not, call the testing center or the nursing program to find out.

BASIC ARITHMETIC REVIEW

Whole Numbers

Whole numbers are composed of digits. Each digit has a place value that helps us "translate" the amount of the number. The American number system is based on ten, and the place or position of each digit indicates what the digit is worth. Figure 5.1 demonstrates our number system using whole and partial numbers. Commas are used as place holders and are placed every three digits beginning with the first whole number to the left of the decimal. Numbers to the left of the decimal are whole numbers, and those to the right are parts of whole numbers in tenths.

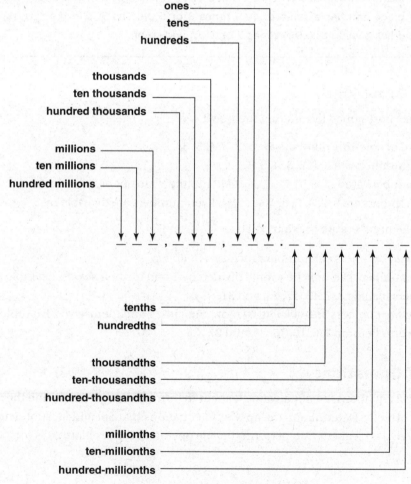

Figure 5.1. Tens Number System

Using the information in Figure 5.1, consider the following examples:

EXAMPLE 1

734,815,690

The 0 is in the ones place and has a value of 1 times 0 or 0. The 9 is in the tens place and has a value of 10 times 9 or 90. The 6 is in the hundreds place and has a value of 100 times 6 or 600. The 5 is in the thousands place and has a value of 1,000 times 5 or 5,000. The 1 is in the ten-thousands place and has a value of 10,000 times 1 or 10,000. The 8 is in the hundred-thousands place and has a value of 100,000 times 8 or 800,000. The 4 is in the millions place and has a value of 1,000,000 times 4 or 4,000,000, and so on.

EXAMPLE 2

0.6874

The 6 is in the tenths place and has a value of 0.1 times 6 or 0.6. The 8 is in the hundredths place and has a value of 0.01 times 8 or 0.08. The 7 is in the thousandths place and has a value of 0.001 times 7 or .007, and so on.

Number Groupings

Numbers may be grouped by different methods:

- *Natural* or *counting* numbers are 1, 2, 3, 4, 5, 6, . . . , ∞.
- *Whole* numbers are 0, 1, 2, 3, 4, 5, 6, . . . , ∞.
- *Odd* numbers are 1, 3, 5, 7, 9, . . . , ∞. Odd numbers are not divisible by 2.
- *Even* numbers are 0, 2, 4, 6, 8, 10, . . . , ∞. Even numbers are divisible by 2.
- *Rational* numbers are fractions such as $\frac{4}{7}$, $\frac{7}{21}$, and $\frac{10}{6}$.
- *Irrational* numbers are numbers such as $\sqrt{18}$ and π.
- *Prime* numbers can only be evenly divided by 1 and by themselves. Examples of prime numbers include 3, 7, 13, 17, 23, and 31.
- *Composite* numbers are divisible by more than just 1 and themselves. Examples of composite numbers are 2, 6, 10, 15, 21, and 27.

TIP

Mathematical operations must be performed in the prescribed order to obtain a correct answer.

Order of Operations

Mathematical equations are not always clear cut in terms of how to determine the answer to a problem correctly. Determining the answer to equations that are added, subtracted, multiplied, or divided is clear cut. You perform the one operation the problem calls for.

Consider the following equation in which an incorrect answer is determined working from left to right, ignoring the order of operations:

$$8 + 15 \times 3^2 - 6(4 + 4) =$$

$$23 \times 3^2 - 6(4 + 4) =$$

$$23 \times 9 - 6(4 + 4) =$$

$$207 - 6(8) =$$

$$207 - 6 \times 8 =$$

$$201 \times 8 = 1,608$$

For problems that contain more than one operation, there is an order for performing operations encountered with multipart equations. The order of operations is as follows:

(STEP 1) Perform operations within *parentheses*.

(STEP 2) Perform operations with *powers* and *square roots*.

(STEP 3) Perform operations requiring *multiplication* or *division*, whichever comes first working from left to right.

(STEP 4) Perform operations requiring *addition* or *subtraction*, whichever comes first working from left to right.

When using the order of operations, if one of the steps or operations is not indicated, skip to the next. Now consider the same equation as above, only this time the answer is determined following the order of operations:

Equation: $8 + 15 \times 3^2 - 6(4 + 4) =$
(STEP 1) $8 + 15 \times 3^2 - 6(8)$ $=$
(STEP 2) $8 + 15 \times 9 - 6(8)$ $=$
(STEP 3) $8 + 135 - 48$ $=$ (No division required)
(STEP 4) $143 - 48$ $=$
Answer: $143 - 48$ $= 95$

You can see there is a difference in answer when the correct order of operations is followed.

Rounding Numbers

When performing mathematical operations, numbers or answers do not always come out as whole numbers and it may be necessary to round to a whole number. For example, at the end of a course a student has an average of 79.6 percent, but the school's grading system indicates that only whole numbers in the form of percentages may be issued as course grades. What grade does the teacher issue? The average is higher than the next lowest whole number 79, but lower than the next highest whole number of 80. Rounding 79.6 percent allows the teacher to issue a grade of 80 percent.

Rules regarding rounding work with numbers to the left as well as to the right of the decimal place. When rounding numbers, use the following steps:

STEP 1 Determine the place value of the number to be rounded. Circle or underline this number.

STEP 2 Look at the number immediately to the right of your circled or underlined number.

    A. If that number is 5 or greater, round the circled or underlined number up one place value.

    B. If that number is 4 or smaller, leave the circled or underlined number as it is.

EXAMPLES

Round to the nearest one.

$$45.87 = 45\underline{.}87 = 46$$

$$13.49 = 13\underline{.}49 = 13$$

Round to the nearest ten.

$$78.149 = \underline{7}8.149 = 80$$

$$2,963.3888 = 2,9\underline{6}3.3888 = 2,960$$

Round to the nearest hundredth.

$$587.887 = 587.8\underline{8}7 = 587.89$$

$$13,629.74 = 13,629.7\underline{4}0 = 13,629.74$$

Round to the nearest thousandth.

$$5.89765 = 5.89\underline{7}65 = 5.898$$

$$23.37449 = 23.37\underline{4}49 = 23.374$$

Positive and Negative Numbers

The value of a number may be positive or negative. Any number preceded by a plus or minus sign may also be referred to as a signed number. On a number line, all numbers to the right of zero are positive and greater than zero. All numbers to the left of zero are negative and less than zero.

Positive numbers may be written in two different formats. The first with a plus sign preceding the number, such as +4 or +3.76, and the second simply as the number, such as 14 or 10.13. Negative numbers are always written with a minus sign preceding the number, such as – 38 or – 43.4. When working with both positive and negative numbers in the same equation, positive numbers always display the plus (+) sign before the number. See Figure 5.2.

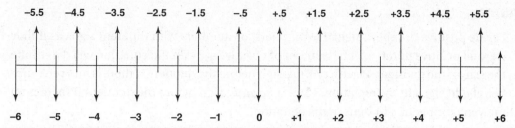

Figure 5.2. Positive/Negative Number Line

There are rules for working with positive and negative numbers that deal with mathematical operations of addition, subtraction, multiplication, and division.

ADDITION

1. When adding numbers with the same sign, perform the operation. Do not change the sign of the sum.

$$+3 + 7 = +10 \quad -17 + (-5) = -22$$

2. When adding numbers with different signs, subtract the smaller number from the larger number. Place the sign of the larger number before the sum.

$$-34 + 18 = -16 \quad 88 + (-100) = -12$$

SUBTRACTION

1. When subtracting positive numbers, negative numbers, or numbers with different signs, change the sign of the subtrahend (the number being subtracted), then add the numbers together. Place the sign of the minuend (top or first number) before the difference.

$$+84 - (+15) = +84 + (-15) = +69$$

$$-43 - (-11) = -43 + (+11) = -32$$

$$+10 - (-6) = +10 + (+6) = +16$$

$$-23 - (+15) = -23 + (-15) = -38$$

MULTIPLICATION

1. Multiply positive numbers, negative numbers, or numbers with different signs as if they were all positive numbers. The number of negative signs in the equation will determine the sign of the product. Place a *positive* sign before the product if there is an even number of similar signs in the equation. Place a *negative* sign before the product if there is an odd number of odd signs in the equation.

$$(-7)(+4)(+3)(-2) = +168$$

$$(+5)(-2)(-3)(+2)(-2) = -120$$

DIVISION

1. Divide positive numbers, negative numbers, or numbers with different signs as if they were all positive numbers. The number of negative signs in the equation will determine the sign of the quotient. Place a *positive* sign before the quotient if there is an even number of odd signs in the equation. Place a *negative* sign before the quotient if there is an uneven number of odd signs in the equation.

$$-14 \div (-2) = +7$$

$$[(-4)(-3)(+2)] \div (+2)(-3) = -4$$

Fractions

Fractions are parts of a whole and are composed of two segments. The numerator, the number before or above the dividing line, tells how many parts are available, and the denominator, the number after or below the dividing line, tells how many pieces are in the whole.

TYPES OF FRACTIONS

Proper fractions are fractions in which the numerator is smaller than the denominator. A proper fraction is less than one whole.

EXAMPLE 1

$$\frac{6}{42} \quad \frac{15}{100} \quad \frac{18}{53}$$

Improper fractions are fractions in which the numerator is equal to or larger than the denominator. An improper fraction is equal to one whole or more than one whole.

EXAMPLE 2

$$\frac{8}{5} \quad \frac{42}{7}$$

Mixed numbers are composed of a natural number and a fraction. Mixed numbers are greater than one whole.

EXAMPLE 3

$$2\frac{4}{5} \quad 16\frac{32}{72}$$

REDUCING FRACTIONS

Reducing a fraction to its lowest terms means dividing the numerator and denominator by a number that divides evenly into both.

$$\frac{5}{10} = \frac{5 \div 5}{10 \div 5} = \frac{1}{2} \qquad \frac{32}{48} = \frac{32 \div 16}{48 \div 16} = \frac{2}{3}$$

RAISING FRACTIONS

Raising a fraction to higher terms is the opposite of reducing a fraction to its lowest terms. Both the numerator and denominator are multiplied by the same number.

$$\frac{3}{4} = \frac{3 \cdot 5}{4 \cdot 5} = \frac{15}{20} \qquad \frac{15}{34} = \frac{15 \cdot 2}{34 \cdot 2} = \frac{30}{68}$$

FACTORS

Whole numbers are composed of factors. Factors are numbers that, when multiplied together, equal the whole number. Some numbers have numerous factors whereas others have only one or two.

The factors of 36 are 1, 2, 3, 4, 6, 9, 12, 18, and 36.

$$36 = 1 \times 36$$
$$= 2 \times 18$$
$$= 3 \times 12$$
$$= 4 \times 9$$
$$= 6 \times 6$$

The factors of 81 are 1, 3, 9, 27, and 81.

$$81 = 1 \times 81$$
$$= 3 \times 27$$
$$= 9 \times 9$$

COMMON FACTORS

Common factors are those factors that are common to two or more whole numbers.

EXAMPLE 7

1 and 2 are the common factors for 6, 10, and 12. They are the only factors common to all three numbers.

$$6 = \underline{1} \times 6 \quad 10 = \underline{1} \times 10 \quad 12 = \underline{1} \times 12$$

$$= \underline{2} \times 3 \quad = \underline{2} \times 5 \quad = \underline{2} \times 6$$

CONVERTING IMPROPER FRACTIONS INTO WHOLE OR MIXED NUMBERS

Improper fractions are converted into whole or mixed numbers by dividing the denominator into the numerator.

EXAMPLE 8

$$\frac{18}{15} = 1\frac{3}{15} = 1\frac{1}{5} \quad \frac{100}{50} = 2$$

CONVERTING MIXED NUMBERS INTO IMPROPER FRACTIONS

Mixed numbers are converted into improper fractions by multiplying the denominator of the fraction times the whole number and adding the numerator. This total becomes the new numerator and is placed over the original denominator.

EXAMPLE 9

$$6\frac{2}{5} = \frac{32}{5} \quad 17\frac{4}{7} = \frac{123}{7}$$

ADDING FRACTIONS

To add fractions, you must be sure that the denominators of all fractions in the equation are the same. To do this, the lowest common denominator (LCD) of each fraction must be determined. The LCD is the smallest number that divides evenly into all denominators. After you determine the LCD, add the numerators but do not add the denominators. They remain the same.

EXAMPLE 10

$$\frac{5}{8} + \frac{3}{4} = \frac{5}{8} + \frac{6}{8} = \frac{11}{8} = 1\frac{3}{8}$$

$$\frac{1}{3} + \frac{3}{7} + \frac{4}{63} = \frac{21}{63} + \frac{27}{63} + \frac{4}{63} = \frac{52}{63}$$

$$3\frac{4}{5} + \frac{1}{10} = 3\frac{8}{10} + \frac{1}{10} = 3\frac{9}{10}$$

SUBTRACTING FRACTIONS

Subtracting fractions is similar to adding fractions. You must determine the LCD before you can subtract.

EXAMPLE 11

$$\frac{7}{8} - \frac{1}{3} = \frac{21}{24} - \frac{8}{24} = \frac{13}{24}$$

$$\frac{3}{5} - \frac{1}{10} = \frac{6}{10} - \frac{1}{10} = \frac{5}{10} = \frac{1}{2}$$

$$7\frac{2}{3} - 2\frac{1}{5} = 7\frac{10}{15} - 2\frac{3}{15} = 5\frac{7}{15}$$

MULTIPLYING FRACTIONS OR MIXED NUMBERS

To multiply fractions or mixed numbers, you need to multiply the numerators together and then multiply the denominators together.

EXAMPLE 12

$$\frac{4}{5} \cdot \frac{3}{7} = \frac{12}{35}$$

$$\frac{8}{15} \cdot \frac{1}{4} = \frac{8}{60} = \frac{2}{15}$$

$$8\frac{2}{3} \times \frac{2}{7} = \frac{26}{3} \times \frac{2}{7} = \frac{52}{21} = 2\frac{10}{21}$$

DIVIDING FRACTIONS

Dividing fractions is similar to multiplying fractions, but it requires an additional step. To divide fractions, you need to invert the fraction you are dividing by and then multiply the two fractions together.

EXAMPLE 13

$$\frac{4}{15} \div \frac{3}{10} = \frac{4}{15} \times \frac{10}{3} = \frac{40}{45} = \frac{8}{9}$$

$$17 \div \frac{3}{4} = \frac{17}{1} \times \frac{4}{3} = \frac{68}{3} = 22\frac{2}{3}$$

Decimals

Decimals and fractions have a very special relationship because decimals are a type of fraction. If you discount the previous section on fractions, the majority of our discussion on numerical ability has dealt with numbers to the left of the decimal in our tens numbering system. We have been talking about whole numbers.

Decimals also refer to numbers to the right of the decimal in our tens numbering system. Look back at Figure 5.1 if you need to review; then consider Table 5.5. Notice that the denominators of the fractions are in tens, which is 1×10; then 100, which is 10×10; then 1,000, which is 100×10; and so on.

Table 5.5. Decimals and Fractions

Places to the Right of the Decimal	Name	Example	Fraction
One	Tenths	0.3	$\dfrac{3}{10}$
Two	Hundredths	0.87	$\dfrac{87}{100}$
Three	Thousandths	0.231	$\dfrac{231}{1,000}$
Four	Ten-thousandths	0.4543	$\dfrac{4,543}{10,000}$
Five	Hundred-thousandths	0.18766	$\dfrac{18,766}{100,000}$
Six	Millionths	0.241296	$\dfrac{241,296}{1,000,000}$

CHANGING FRACTIONS TO DECIMALS

Fractions may be changed into decimals by dividing the denominator into the numerator.

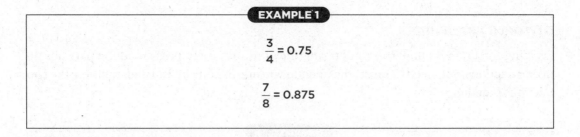

EXAMPLE 1

$$\frac{3}{4} = 0.75$$

$$\frac{7}{8} = 0.875$$

CHANGING DECIMALS TO FRACTIONS

When changing a decimal to a fraction, note the number of places to the right of the decimal to determine the name of the decimal. This determines the denominator of your fraction. Then change the number to a whole number, and use it as the numerator in your fraction.

$$0.85 = \frac{85}{100}$$

$$0.675 = \frac{675}{1,000}$$

ADDING OR SUBTRACTING DECIMALS

Adding or subtracting decimals is no different from adding or subtracting other numbers except that the decimal points must be aligned. As with using the orders of operation, you must follow the rules. You will get an incorrect answer if the decimals are not aligned.

EXAMPLE 3

```
  4,755.000
     18.870
     32.987
     16.400
 +  187.040
  5,010.297


     87.704
 -   16.440
     71.264
```

MULTIPLYING DECIMALS

Multiplying decimals is no different than multiplying other numbers, except that you must take the decimal places into account. Multiply the numbers in the regular fashion. Your answer is a whole number. Count the number of decimal places in the multiplicand and multiplier (the top and bottom numbers). Then count over from the right of the product the number of places that totals the decimal places in the multiplicand and multiplier.

EXAMPLE 4

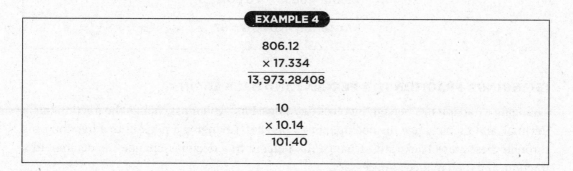

```
    806.12
 ×  17.334
 13,973.28408


       10
 ×  10.14
   101.40
```

DIVIDING DECIMALS

Dividing decimals is no different than dividing any other numbers, except that, once again, you must take the decimals into account before you start to divide. The divisor (the number being divided into another number) must be a whole number. The number of decimal places in the divisor must be moved to the right until you have a whole number. The number of spaces the decimal is moved to the right is the same number of spaces the decimal will be moved to the right in the dividend (the number being divided into). Moving the decimals in the divisor and the dividend will always make them larger numbers.

EXAMPLE 5

$$3.2\overline{)36.0} = 32\overline{)360.00} \quad (11.25)$$

$$103.06\overline{)488.693} = 10,306\overline{)48,869.3000} \quad (4.7418)$$

Percentage

Percents are another form of fractions. Percents are unique in that the denominator is always 100 in the fraction form. The percent sign (%) is used instead of 100 and stands for per hundred. In most cases, 100% is the totality of something. It is possible to have more than 100% of something. If a business increased its profits from $1 million in one year to $5 million the next year, the increase in profits is 500%.

CHANGING A DECIMAL TO A PERCENT AND BACK AGAIN

Move the decimal place two spaces to the right to change a decimal to a percent. The decimal moves two spaces to the left to change a percent to a decimal.

EXAMPLE 1

0.47 = 47% = 0.47

0.6012 = 60.12% = 0.6012

87 or 87.00 = 8700% = 87

CHANGING A FRACTION TO A PERCENT AND BACK AGAIN

Changing a fraction to a percent involves two steps. First, you must change the fraction into a decimal, and then change the decimal into a percent. Changing a percent to a fraction runs through these steps backwards. Change the percent to a decimal, change the decimal to a fraction, and then reduce as necessary.

$$\frac{3}{4} = 0.75 = 75\% = 0.75 = \frac{3}{4}$$

$$\frac{13}{51} = 0.2549 = 25.49\% = 0.2549 = \frac{13}{51}$$

Learning the equivalents can save time and energy. Table 5.6 contains equivalents you should be familiar with.

Table 5.6. Fraction-Decimal-Percentage Equivalents

Fraction	Decimal	Percentage
$\frac{1}{4}$	0.25	25%
$\frac{1}{2}$	0.50	50%
$\frac{3}{4}$	0.75	75%
$\frac{1}{3}$	$0.33\frac{1}{3}$ or $0.33\overline{3}$	$33.\overline{3}\%$
$\frac{2}{3}$	$0.66\frac{2}{3}$ or $0.66\overline{6}$	$66.\overline{6}\%$
$\frac{1}{5}$	0.20	20%
$\frac{3}{5}$	0.60	60%
$\frac{4}{5}$	0.80	80%
$\frac{1}{6}$	$0.16\frac{2}{3}$ or $0.16\overline{6}$	$16.\overline{6}\%$
$\frac{5}{6}$	$0.83\frac{1}{3}$ or $0.83\overline{3}$	$83.\overline{3}\%$
$\frac{1}{8}$	0.125	12.5%
$\frac{3}{8}$	0.375	37.5%
$\frac{5}{8}$	0.625	62.5%
$\frac{7}{8}$	0.875	87.5%

TIP

Memorize these equivalents. They will save time when calculating problems.

Exponents and Powers

An exponent indicates that a number must be multiplied by itself a number of times. It can be either a positive or negative number. The number to be multiplied by itself is called the base, and the exponent is a superscript number to the right of the base. In Example 1, the bases are 5, 7, 4, and 8. The numbers 2, 6, –4, and –3 are exponents.

$$5^2 = 5 \times 5 = 25$$

$$7^6 = 7 \times 7 \times 7 \times 7 \times 7 \times 7 = 117{,}649$$

$$4^{-4} = \frac{1}{4^4} = \frac{1}{4 \times 4 \times 4 \times 4} = \frac{1}{256}$$

$$8^{-3} = \frac{1}{8^3} = \frac{1}{8 \times 8 \times 8} = \frac{1}{512}$$

The following rules apply to exponents:

1. When adding or subtracting exponents with the same or different bases, each base with an exponent must be simplified before the addition or subtraction can take place.

EXAMPLE 2

$$6^3 + 2^4 = 216 + 16 = 232$$

$$8^2 + 4^6 = 64 + 4{,}096 = 4{,}160$$

$$5^3 - 3^2 = 125 - 9 = 116$$

$$7^5 - 7^3 = 16{,}807 - 343 = 16{,}464$$

2. When multiplying or dividing exponents with different bases, each base must be simplified before the multiplication or division can take place.

EXAMPLE 3

$$8^4 \times 2^7 = 4{,}096 \times 128 = 524{,}288$$

$$4^3 \div 2^3 = 64 \div 8 = 8$$

$$6^3 \div 5^3 = 216 \div 125 = 1.728$$

3. Multiply the exponents when raising a power to another power.

EXAMPLE 4

$$(9^5)^2 = 9^{5 \times 2} = 9^{10}$$

$$(2^4)^3 = 2^{4 \times 3} = 2^{12}$$

4. Add the exponents when multiplying powers with the same nonzero bases.

EXAMPLE 5

$$3^4 \times 3^2 = 3^{4+2} = 3^6$$

$$7^3 \times 7^2 \times 7^7 = 7^{3+2+7} = 7^{12}$$
---

5. Subtract the exponents when dividing powers with the same nonzero bases.

EXAMPLE 6

$$4^9 \div 4^6 = \frac{4^9}{4^6} = 4^{9-6} = 4^3$$

$$8^5 \div 8^2 = \frac{8^5}{8^2} = 8^{5-2} = 8^3$$

You should be familiar with the square and cube numbers listed in Table 5.7.

Table 5.7. Square and Cube Numbers

Whole Number	Number Squared	Number Cubed
0	0	0
1	1	1
2	4	8
3	9	27
4	16	64
5	25	125
6	36	216
7	49	343
8	64	512
9	81	729
10	100	1,000
11	121	1,331
12	144	1,728

Square Roots and Cube Roots

There is a relationship between powers and roots. The square of a number is the product of a number multiplied by itself, or twice. The cube of a number is the product of a number multiplied by itself three times.

In $\sqrt{81}$, the $\sqrt{}$ is the radical and 81 is the radicand. When finding the square root of a radicand, you are interested in finding a number that when multiplied by itself equals the radicand. When finding the cube root of a radicand, you are interested in finding a number that when multiplied by itself three times, or cubed, equals the radicand.

EXAMPLE 1

$$\sqrt{81} = 9 = \sqrt{9 \times 9}$$

$$\sqrt{34} = 5.831 = \sqrt{5.831 \times 5.831}$$

$$\sqrt[3]{27} = 3 = \sqrt{3 \times 3 \times 3}$$

$$\sqrt[3]{216} = 6 = \sqrt{6 \times 6 \times 6}$$

Simple Statistics

Simple statistics deals with means, medians, and modes. The mean, also called the average, is determined by adding a series of items or numbers and dividing by the number of items.

EXAMPLE 1

Determine the mean of the numbers 5, 10, 22, and 7.

$$5 + 10 + 22 + 7 = 44 \div 4 = 11.$$

The average of the set of numbers is 11.

The median is the middle number in a set of numbers arranged in ascending or descending order. With an odd set of numbers the median is always the middle number. If there is an even set of numbers, the median is the average of the two middle numbers.

EXAMPLE 2

Determine the median of the following set of numbers: 5, 10, 6, 15, 12, 8, 1, and 22.

$$1, 5, 6, 8, 10, 12, 15, 22$$

$$8 + 10 = 18 \div 2 = 9$$

The median of the set of numbers is 9.

The mode is the number that occurs most often in a series of numbers.

EXAMPLE 3

Determine the mode of the following set of numbers: 3, 7, 9, 16, 16, 18, 22, 54.

The mode of the set of numbers is 16.

ANSWER SHEET
Basic Arithmetic Sample Test

1. Ⓐ Ⓑ Ⓒ Ⓓ

2. Ⓐ Ⓑ Ⓒ Ⓓ

3. Ⓐ Ⓑ Ⓒ Ⓓ

4. Ⓐ Ⓑ Ⓒ Ⓓ

5. Ⓐ Ⓑ Ⓒ Ⓓ

6. Ⓐ Ⓑ Ⓒ Ⓓ

7. Ⓐ Ⓑ Ⓒ Ⓓ

8. Ⓐ Ⓑ Ⓒ Ⓓ

9. Ⓐ Ⓑ Ⓒ Ⓓ

10. Ⓐ Ⓑ Ⓒ Ⓓ

11. Ⓐ Ⓑ Ⓒ Ⓓ

12. Ⓐ Ⓑ Ⓒ Ⓓ

13. Ⓐ Ⓑ Ⓒ Ⓓ

14. Ⓐ Ⓑ Ⓒ Ⓓ

15. Ⓐ Ⓑ Ⓒ Ⓓ

16. Ⓐ Ⓑ Ⓒ Ⓓ

17. Ⓐ Ⓑ Ⓒ Ⓓ

18. Ⓐ Ⓑ Ⓒ Ⓓ

19. Ⓐ Ⓑ Ⓒ Ⓓ

20. Ⓐ Ⓑ Ⓒ Ⓓ

21. Ⓐ Ⓑ Ⓒ Ⓓ

22. Ⓐ Ⓑ Ⓒ Ⓓ

23. Ⓐ Ⓑ Ⓒ Ⓓ

24. Ⓐ Ⓑ Ⓒ Ⓓ

25. Ⓐ Ⓑ Ⓒ Ⓓ

Directions: For each question, select the letter (A, B, C, or D) that corresponds to your answer. Record your answers on the answer sheet on page 121.

1. $6 + 14 - 3(4 + 2) + 2(5^2 - 15) =$

   (A) 35
   (B) 22
   (C) 18
   (D) 58

2. Identify the unique characteristic of the following odd numbers: 3, 7, 13, 21, 59, and 87.

   (A) They are divisible by 3 or 7.
   (B) They are rational numbers.
   (C) They are not divisible by 2.
   (D) They are not prime numbers.

3. Identify the average of the following numbers: 15, 18, 4, 22, 38, 56.

   (A) 6
   (B) 25.5
   (C) 159
   (D) 918

4. Select the rational number: CHALLENGE

   $\sqrt{64}$ $\dfrac{7}{32}$ 8 π

   (A) π
   (B) $\sqrt{64}$
   (C) 8
   (D) $\dfrac{7}{32}$

5. Identify the number in the tenths place: 347.1896

   (A) 7
   (B) 9
   (C) 4
   (D) 1

6. $13 - 2^3 + 4(3 - 1) =$

   (A) 13
   (B) 17
   (C) 16
   (D) 2

7. $-45 + (-7) =$

   (A) 38
   (B) -38
   (C) 52
   (D) -52

8. $-35 \div 5 + 8^2(5 - 3) =$ CHALLENGE

   (A) 135
   (B) 121
   (C) 249
   (D) 505

9. Factors common to 15 and 30 are

   (A) 1, 3, 5, 15.
   (B) 1, 3, 5, 10.
   (C) 2, 3, 5, 15.
   (D) 3, 5, 6, 10.

10. $\dfrac{7}{10} + \dfrac{3}{20} =$

    (A) $\dfrac{13}{20}$
    (B) $\dfrac{17}{20}$
    (C) $\dfrac{10}{30}$ or $\dfrac{1}{3}$
    (D) 1

11. $\dfrac{15}{100} =$

    (A) 150%
    (B) 15%
    (C) 1.5%
    (D) .15%

12. $(17.412)(3.78) =$

   (A) 63.42170
   (B) 51.0
   (C) 65.81
   (D) 65.81736

13. $0.7424 =$

   (A) 74.24%
   (B) 7424%
   (C) 7.424%
   (D) 80.0%

14. $4^3 + 2^5 =$

   (A) 6^8
   (B) 96
   (C) 36
   (D) 6^{-2}

15. $\sqrt{144} =$

   (A) 11
   (B) 14.4
   (C) 12
   (D) 14

16. $\sqrt[3]{64} - 4(15-4) + 7^2 - (-14+14) =$ CHALLENGE

   (A) 13
   (B) 41
   (C) 5.7
   (D) 9

17. $\dfrac{5}{7} \div 3\dfrac{4}{5} =$

   (A) 2.714
   (B) 0.18797
   (C) 38.6114
   (D) 1.896

18. $15^3 =$

   (A) 45
   (B) 5
   (C) 3,375
   (D) 18

19. 58% of 17 yards =

   (A) 29 inches
   (B) 110 inches
   (C) 118.32 inches
   (D) 355 inches

20. $857.42 \div 7.056 =$

   (A) 121.52
   (B) 0.121516
   (C) 0.0082
   (D) 122.42

21. $6^{-4} =$

   (A) $\dfrac{1}{1,296}$
   (B) $-1,296$
   (C) -4
   (D) -24

22. $\dfrac{3}{4}(7+13) \div [4(3\times 2)+15] =$ CHALLENGE

   (A) 15.625
   (B) 585
   (C) 0.3846
   (D) 11.875

23. 2 square miles =

   (A) 4,840 acres
   (B) 1,280 acres
   (C) 2,590 acres
   (D) 929.3 acres

24. 4 pecks =

   (A) 8 quarts
   (B) 3 quarts
   (C) 32 quarts
   (D) 20 quarts

25. Determine the median of the following numbers: 10, 15, 39, 8, 17, 27, and 21.

   (A) 8
   (B) 32
   (C) 7
   (D) 17

Basic Arithmetic Sample Test Answer Key

1. **B**	6. **A**	11. **B**	16. **D**	21. **A**
2. **C**	7. **D**	12. **D**	17. **B**	22. **C**
3. **B**	8. **B**	13. **A**	18. **C**	23. **B**
4. **D**	9. **A**	14. **B**	19. **D**	24. **C**
5. **D**	10. **B**	15. **C**	20. **A**	25. **D**

BASIC ARITHMETIC SAMPLE TEST ANSWERS EXPLAINED

1. **(B)** $6 + 14 - 3(4 + 2) + 2(5^2 - 15)$
   $= 6 + 14 - 3(6) + 2(10)$
   $= 6 + 14 - 18 + 20$
   $= 40 - 18 = 22$

2. **(C)** They are not divisible by 2. Only even numbers are divisible by 2.

3. **(B)** $(15 + 18 + 4 + 22 + 38 + 56) = 153 \div 6 = 25.5$

4. **(D)** Fractions are rational numbers.

5. **(D)** 347.$\underline{1}$896

6. **(A)** $13 - 2^3 + 4(3 - 1)$
   $= 13 - 2^0 + 4(2)$
   $= 13 - 8 + 4(2)$
   $= 13 - 8 + 8$
   $= 21 - 8 = 13$

7. **(D)** $-45 + (-7) = -45 - 7 = -52$

8. **(B)** $-35 \div 5 + 8^2(5 - 3)$
   $= -35 \div 5 + 8^2(2)$
   $= -35 \div 5 + 64(2)$
   $= -35 \div 5 + 128$
   $= -7 + 128 = 121$

9. **(A)** $15 = \underline{1} \times \underline{15}$ $30 = \underline{1} \times 30$
          $= \underline{3} \times \underline{5}$ $= 2 \times \underline{15}$
                          $= \underline{3} \times 10$
                          $= \underline{5} \times 6$

10. **(B)** $\dfrac{7}{10} + \dfrac{3}{20} = \dfrac{14}{20} + \dfrac{3}{20} = \dfrac{17}{20}$

11. **(B)** $\dfrac{15}{100} = 0.15 = 15\%$

12. **(D)** After multiplying the two numbers, count over five decimal places to the left to determine the correct answer.

13. **(A)** $0.7424 = 74.24\%$

14. **(B)** $4^3 + 2^5 = 64 + 32 = 96$

15. **(C)** $\sqrt{144} = \sqrt{12 \times 12} = 12$

16. **(D)** $\sqrt[3]{64} - 4(15-4) + 7^2 - (-14+14)$

   $= \sqrt[3]{64} - 4(11) + 7^2 - (0)$

   $= 4 - 4(11) + 49$

   $= 4 - 44 + 49 = 9$

17. **(B)** $\dfrac{5}{7} \div 3\dfrac{4}{5} = \dfrac{5}{7} \times \dfrac{5}{19} = \dfrac{25}{133} = 0.18797$

18. **(C)** $15^3 = 15 \times 15 \times 15 = 3{,}375$

19. **(D)**　　　1 yard = 36 inches

   17×36 inches = 612 inches

   58% of 612 inches = 0.58×612

   = 354.96 inches = 355 inches

20. **(A)** $7.056\overline{)857.42} =$

   $\dfrac{121.5164399}{7056\overline{)857420.0000000}} = 121.52$

21. **(A)** $6^{-4} = \dfrac{1}{6^4} = \dfrac{1}{6 \times 6 \times 6 \times 6} = \dfrac{1}{1{,}296}$

22. **(C)** $\dfrac{3}{4}(7+13) \div [4(3 \times 2) + 15]$

   $= 0.75(20) \div [4(6) + 15]$

   $= 15 \div [24 + 15]$

   $= 15 \div 39$

   $= 0.3846153 = 0.3846$

23. **(B)** 1 square mile = 640 acres

   2×640 acres = 1,280 acres

24. **(C)** 1 peck = 8 quarts

   4×8 quarts = 32 quarts

25. **(D)** 8, 10, 15, <u>17</u>, 21, 27, 39

ALGEBRA REVIEW

Algebra is similar to arithmetic except that letters are used in the place of some numbers. Much of algebra has to do with solving an equation or an algebraic expression. When solving such an expression, you must find the value of one or more components of the expression. These components, called variables, are generally identified as x or y, but other letters may be used. Variables are equal to a number. The following are algebraic expressions:

$$3a - 5 = 10$$

$$5(x^3 + 4) - x^2 + 3 = 4x$$

$$\frac{3}{4}y + 15 - y = 45$$

$$2(5x + 5) \div 2x^2 - 7 = 0$$

Evaluating Algebraic Expressions

When evaluating algebraic expressions, replace the letters in the expression with their known numerical value; then solve the expression.

EXAMPLE 1

Evaluate $2x + 3y - x^2$, if $x = 5$ and $y = 10$.

$2(5) + 3(10) - 5^2 = 10 + 30 - 25 = 40 - 25 = 15$

In this example the x with $2x$ cannot be combined with the x^2 because they have different exponents. Only variables with like exponents can be combined.

EXAMPLE 2

Evaluate $4 + 8(a + 6) \div b^2$, if $a = 10$ and $b = 2$.

$4 + 8(10 + 6) \div 2^2 = 4 + 8(16) \div 4 = 4 + 128 \div 4 = 4 + 32 = 36$

Solving Equations with Inverse Operations

Algebra has mathematical sentences just as grammatical sentences do. The difference is that mathematical sentences use numbers and letters, whereas grammatical sentences use words and numbers. Mathematical sentences are called equations, and an equation tells us that the two sides of the equation are equal.

The equal sign (=) is important in algebra because it indicates that each side of the equation must be equal as the equation is solved. Consequently, what you do to one side of the equal sign in the equation you must also do to the other side of the equal sign in the equation. Prior to solving an algebraic equation, the unknown variable must be isolated on one side of the equation. The remaining information or constant should be placed on the other side of the equation.

EXAMPLE 1

$3x - 5 = 10$

$3x = 15$

$x = 5$

$4 + 5a - 4 = 30$

$5a = 30$

$a = 6$

EXAMPLE 2

Problem	Answer Check
$3x - 6 = 15$	$3x - 6 = 15$
$3x = 21$	$3(7) - 6 = 15$
$x = 7$	$21 - 6 = 15$
	$15 = 15$
$x + 17 = 30$	$x + 17 = 30$
$x = 13$	$13 + 17 = 30$
	$30 = 30$

There are a number of rules for solving algebraic equations. As with other orders of operation, the rules must be followed in order to obtain the correct answer.

TIP

The order of operations must be followed to obtain a correct answer.

1. Remove all grouping symbols, such as parentheses and brackets. Perform the addition, subtraction, multiplication, or division inside of the groupings prior to removing the grouping symbols.

EXAMPLE 3

Problem	Answer Check
$5(x - 3) - 3 = 30$	$5(x - 3) - 3 = 30$
$5x - 15 - 3 = 30$	$5(9.6 - 3) - 3 = 30$
$5x - 18 = 30$	$5(6.6) - 3 = 30$
$5x = 48$	$33 - 3 = 30$
$x = 9.6$	$30 = 30$

2. Change fractions into whole numbers using the least common denominator of the fractions before solving the equation. Then combine like terms on each side of the equation.

EXAMPLE 4

Problem

$$\frac{1}{2}(x+1) + \frac{3}{5}(x+2) = 0$$

$$\left(\frac{10}{1}\right)\frac{1}{2}(x+1) + \left(\frac{10}{1}\right)\frac{3}{5}(x+2) = 0\left(\frac{10}{1}\right)$$

$$5(x+1) + 6(x+2) = 0$$

$$5x + 5 + 6x + 12 = 0$$

$$11x + 17 = 0$$

$$11x = -17$$

$$x = -1.545$$

Answer Check

$$\frac{1}{2}(x+1) + \frac{3}{5}(x+2) = 0$$

$$5(-1.545 + 1) + 6(-1.545 + 2) = 0$$

$$5(-0.545) + 6(0.455) = 0$$

$$-2.73 + 2.73 = 0$$

$$0 = 0$$

---

3. Starting at the left side of the expression, perform all operations involving multiplication and division. Then moving from the left side of the expression, perform all operations involving addition and subtraction.

EXAMPLE 5

<u>Problem</u>

$$4(6x + 10) - 3[(3x + 7) - (2x - 3)] = 160$$

$$24x + 40 - 3(x + 10) = 160$$

$$24x + 40 - 3x - 30 = 160$$

$$21x + 10 = 160$$

$$21x = 150$$

$$x = 7.14$$

<u>Answer Check</u>

$$4(6x + 10) - 3[(3x + 7) - (2x - 3)] = 160$$

$$4(52.84) - 3[(28.42) - (11.28)] = 160$$

$$4(52.84) - 3(17.14) = 160$$

$$211.36 - 51.42 = 160$$

$$160 = 160$$

<u>Problem</u>

$$5b + 2[(b + 17) + (2b - 5)] = 50$$

$$5b + 2(3b + 12) = 50$$

$$5b + 6b + 24 = 50$$

$$11b = 26$$

$$b = 2.36$$

<u>Answer Check</u>

$$5b + 2[(b + 17) + (2b - 5)] = 50$$

$$5(2.36) + 2[(19.36) + (-0.28)] = 50$$

$$11.8 + 2(19.08) = 50$$

$$11.8 + 38.16 = 50$$

$$50 = 50$$

---

4. Cross multiply if the equation states that one fraction is equal to another fraction. Then solve the problem. Cross multiplying means multiplying the numerator of the first side of the equation with the denominator of the second side of the equation, and multiplying the denominator of the first side of the equation with the numerator of the second side of the equation.

EXAMPLE 6

Problem	Answer Check
$\dfrac{5}{8} = \dfrac{x}{40}$	$\dfrac{5}{8} = \dfrac{x}{40}$
$8x = 200$	$\dfrac{5}{8} = \dfrac{25}{40}$
$x = 25$	$\dfrac{5}{8} = \dfrac{5}{8}$
$\dfrac{1}{2} = \dfrac{a}{50}$	$\dfrac{1}{2} = \dfrac{a}{50}$
$2a = 50$	$\dfrac{1}{2} = \dfrac{25}{50}$
$a = 25$	$\dfrac{1}{2} = \dfrac{1}{2}$

Ratios and Proportions

Ratios are numbers that have something in common. They have some type of relationship. Ratios compare two numbers, and may be written in one of two formats:

$$x : y \text{ or } \frac{x}{y}$$

Both are read "x is to y" with the variable following the "to" as the denominator in the fraction.

EXAMPLE 1

$$6 : 8 \quad \frac{6}{8}$$

$$50 : 1 \quad \frac{50}{1}$$

Proportions are two ratios that are equal to each other. In proportion problems, there is usually one variable that is not known and must be determined. Proportions are written in a format similar to the ratio format.

EXAMPLE 2

$$a : b = c : d \quad \text{or} \quad \frac{a}{b} = \frac{c}{d}$$

The problem is read *a* is to *b* as *c* is to *d*.

$$4 : 8 = 3 : 18 \quad \text{or} \quad \frac{4}{8} = \frac{3}{18}$$

The problem is read four is to eight as three is to eighteen.

When solving proportion problems, the format you use will determine how you go about solving the problem. Either format is acceptable and both will give the correct answer.

EXAMPLE 3

Solve for *x* in this proportion: 5 is to 10 as *x* is to 20.

With the linear format, you multiply the means or numbers nearest the equal sign, and multiply the extremes or the numbers on the outside of the problem.

$$5 : 10 = x : 20$$

$$(10)(x) = (5)(20)$$

$$10x = 100$$

$$x = 10$$

Utilizing the fractions format, you cross multiply and then solve the problem.

$$\frac{5}{10} = \frac{x}{20}$$

$$(10)(x) = (5)(20)$$

$$10x = 100$$

$$x = 10$$

Both algebra and geometry use various formulas when solving word problems or equations. Table 5.8 presents the formula, what each component of the formula means, and a graphic representation. You should be familiar with these formulas.

Table 5.8. Formulas

Name	Formula	Graphic
Area (*A*) of a circle	$A = \pi r^2$, where $\pi = 3.14$ and r = radius	
Area (*A*) of a parallelogram	$A = bh$, where b = base and h = height	
Area (*A*) of a rectangle	$A = lw$, where l = length and w = width	
Area (*A*) of a square	$A = s^2$, where s = side	
Area (*A*) of a trapezoid	$A = \dfrac{1}{2}h\,(b+a)$, where h = height, a = lower base, and b = upper base	
Area (*A*) of a triangle	$A = \dfrac{1}{2}bh$, where b = base and h = height	
Circumference (*C*) of a circle	$C = \pi d$, where $\pi = 3.14$ and d = diameter	
Distance (*D*)	$D = rt$, where r = rate and t = time	
Mean (Average)	$\text{Average} = \dfrac{\text{Sum of the } n \text{ values}}{N}$ where Sum of the n values = all of the numbers in the set added together and N = the total of numbers in the set	
Percent Change (PC)	$PC = \dfrac{\text{Amount of change}}{\text{Original cost}}$	

Table 5.8. Formulas (*Continued*)

Name	Formula	Graphic
Perimeter (*P*) of a parallelogram	$P = 2l + 2w$, where l = length and w = width	
Perimeter (*P*) of a rectangle	$P = 2l + 2w$, where l = length and w = width	
Perimeter (*P*) of a square	$P = 4s$, where s = side	
Perimeter (*P*) of a triangle	$P = a + b + c$, where a, b, and c are the sides	
Perimeter (*P*) of a trapezoid	$P = b_1 + b_2 + s_1 + s_2$, where b_1 = lower base, b_2 = upper base, s_1 = one side, and s_2 = the opposite side	
Probability (*P*)	$P = \dfrac{\text{Number of successful outcomes}}{\text{Number of possible outcomes}}$	
Pythagorean Theorem	$c^2 = a^2 + b^2$, where c = hypotenuse and a and b are legs of a right triangle	
Ratio and proportion	$A = B :: C = D$ or $\dfrac{A}{B} = \dfrac{C}{D} = (AD)(BC)$, where one side of the equation, either A and B or C and D is known and only one component of the remaining equation is known	
Selling price (SP)	$SP = c + o + p$, where c = cost, o = overhead, and p = profit	

Table 5.8. Formulas (*Continued*)

Name	Formula	Graphic
Simple interest (*I*)	$I = P \times R \times T$, where P = principal, R = rate, and T = time	
Surface Area (*SA*) of a cube	$SA = s \times s \times 6$, where s = length of a side	
Surface Area (*SA*) of a cylinder	$SA = 2(\pi r^2) + h(2\pi r)$	
Surface Area (*SA*) of a rectangular solid	$A = 2lw + 2wh + 2lh$, where lw = area of bottom and top, wh = area of sides, and lh = area of back and front	
Volume (*V*) of cube	$V = s \times s \times s$, where s = length of a side	
Volume (*V*) of cylinder	$V = \pi r^2 \times h$, where π = 3.14, r = radius, and h = height	
Volume (*V*) of rectangular solid	$V = l \times w \times h$, where l = length, w = width, and h = height	

ANSWER SHEET
Algebra Sample Test

1. Ⓐ Ⓑ Ⓒ Ⓓ
2. Ⓐ Ⓑ Ⓒ Ⓓ
3. Ⓐ Ⓑ Ⓒ Ⓓ
4. Ⓐ Ⓑ Ⓒ Ⓓ
5. Ⓐ Ⓑ Ⓒ Ⓓ
6. Ⓐ Ⓑ Ⓒ Ⓓ
7. Ⓐ Ⓑ Ⓒ Ⓓ
8. Ⓐ Ⓑ Ⓒ Ⓓ
9. Ⓐ Ⓑ Ⓒ Ⓓ

10. Ⓐ Ⓑ Ⓒ Ⓓ
11. Ⓐ Ⓑ Ⓒ Ⓓ
12. Ⓐ Ⓑ Ⓒ Ⓓ
13. Ⓐ Ⓑ Ⓒ Ⓓ
14. Ⓐ Ⓑ Ⓒ Ⓓ
15. Ⓐ Ⓑ Ⓒ Ⓓ
16. Ⓐ Ⓑ Ⓒ Ⓓ
17. Ⓐ Ⓑ Ⓒ Ⓓ
18. Ⓐ Ⓑ Ⓒ Ⓓ

19. Ⓐ Ⓑ Ⓒ Ⓓ
20. Ⓐ Ⓑ Ⓒ Ⓓ
21. Ⓐ Ⓑ Ⓒ Ⓓ
22. Ⓐ Ⓑ Ⓒ Ⓓ
23. Ⓐ Ⓑ Ⓒ Ⓓ
24. Ⓐ Ⓑ Ⓒ Ⓓ
25. Ⓐ Ⓑ Ⓒ Ⓓ

Directions: For each question, select the letter (A, B, C, or D) that corresponds with your answer. Record your answers on the answer sheet on page 137.

1. If $5x - 6 = 24$, then $x + 5 =$

   (A) 11
   (B) 7
   (C) 15
   (D) 12

2. If $x + 7x - 16 = 0$, then $x =$

   (A) 2.29
   (B) 3
   (C) 2
   (D) 4

3. If $7(b + 7) - 5b - 13 = 0$, then $3b =$

   (A) 13
   (B) −15
   (C) −54
   (D) 31

   CHALLENGE

4. If $\frac{1}{6}x + \frac{1}{5}x + \frac{3}{10}x = 90$, then $x =$

   (A) 60
   (B) 85
   (C) 105
   (D) 135

5. Solve for a in the proportion: a is to 10 as 6 is to 20.

   (A) 12
   (B) 20
   (C) 3
   (D) 6

6. If $3(5 \cdot 2) = 6(x + 3)$, then $x =$

   (A) 1.66
   (B) 2
   (C) 8
   (D) 4

7. Evaluate $x^3 - x^2 + 15$ if $x = 2$.

   (A) 19
   (B) 15
   (C) 0
   (D) 10

   CHALLENGE

8. If $15 - x = 13$, then $x =$

   (A) 28
   (B) 2
   (C) −2
   (D) 14

9. If $5x + 6 = 3x$, then $x =$

   (A) 0.75
   (B) 3.6
   (C) −3
   (D) 0.10

10. If $\frac{4}{5}x = 50$, then $x =$

   (A) 40
   (B) 400
   (C) 10
   (D) 62.5

11. Solve $\frac{x + y}{5} + 5x - 3y$ if $x = 8$ and $y = 10$.

   (A) 29
   (B) 26
   (C) 73.3
   (D) 13.6

12. Solve for x in the proportion: 15 is to 80 as x is to 10.

   (A) 53.33
   (B) 1.875
   (C) 120
   (D) 64

13. If $8x - 7 = 3x + 10$, then $x =$
    (A) 3.4
    (B) 0.6
    (C) 27.2
    (D) 6

14. If $x + 15 = 95$, then $x =$
    (A) 110
    (B) −15
    (C) 80
    (D) 40

15. If $\frac{3}{4}b + 15 = 50$, then $b =$
    (A) 2.92
    (B) 46.7
    (C) 65
    (D) 35

16. If $\frac{b}{5} = 7$, then $b =$
    (A) 35
    (B) 5
    (C) 40
    (D) 12

17. If $(4x + 7) \div 5 = 58$, then $x =$
    (A) 12.75
    (B) 1.15
    (C) 74.25
    (D) 70.75

18. Evaluate $5ab^2 + 3(a^2 + b^3)$ when $a = 4$ and $b = 7$.
    (A) 1,175   CHALLENGE
    (B) 1,400
    (C) 2,057
    (D) 1,682

19. If $4x + 3(7x + 15) = 195$, then $x =$
    (A) 5
    (B) 6
    (C) 7.5
    (D) 8.4

20. If $5a - 10 = 3a + 4$, then $a =$
    (A) −0.75
    (B) 7
    (C) 3
    (D) 4.5

21. If $\frac{2}{3}x + \frac{4}{5}(x - 5)$, then $x =$
    (A) 57.3
    (B) 51.82
    (C) 6.36
    (D) 2.97

22. If $8x - 17 = 425$, then $x =$
    (A) 62.74
    (B) 51
    (C) 47.89
    (D) 55.25

23. If $8 + 4(x - 15) = 42$, then $x =$
    (A) −2.5
    (B) 23.5
    (C) 25.5
    (D) 12.5

24. If $(7b + 3) \div 3 = 80$, then $2b =$ CHALLENGE
    (A) 67.72
    (B) 22.86
    (C) 38.86
    (D) 45.71

25. If $\frac{3}{7} = \frac{b}{15}$, then $b =$
    (A) 1.4
    (B) 6.43
    (C) 35
    (D) 7

Algebra Sample Test Answer Key

1. **A**		6. **B**		11. **D**		16. **A**		21. **A**
2. **C**		7. **A**		12. **B**		17. **D**		22. **D**
3. **C**		8. **B**		13. **A**		18. **C**		23. **B**
4. **D**		9. **C**		14. **C**		19. **B**		24. **A**
5. **C**		10. **D**		15. **B**		20. **B**		25. **B**

ALGEBRA SAMPLE TEST ANSWERS EXPLAINED

1. **(A)** $5x - 6 = 24$
$$5x = 30$$
$$x = 6$$
$$6 + 5 = 11$$

2. **(C)** $x + 7x - 16 = 0$
$$8x - 16 = 0$$
$$8x = 16$$
$$x = 2$$

3. **(C)** $7(b + 7) - 5b - 13 = 0$
$$7b + 49 - 5b - 13 = 0$$
$$2b + 36 = 0$$
$$2b = -36$$
$$b = -18$$
$$3(-18) = -54$$

4. **(D)** $\dfrac{1}{6}x + \dfrac{1}{5}x + \dfrac{3}{10}x = 90$
$$\dfrac{5}{30}x + \dfrac{6}{30}x + \dfrac{9}{30}x = 90$$
$$\dfrac{20}{30}x = 90$$
$$x = 135$$

5. **(C)** $a : 10 = 6 : 20$
$$(a)(20) = (10)(6)$$
$$20a = 60$$
$$a = 3$$

6. **(B)** $3(5 \cdot 2) = 6(x + 3)$
$$3(10) = 6x + 18$$
$$30 = 6x + 18$$
$$12 = 6x$$
$$2 = x$$

7. **(A)** $x^3 - x^2 + 15 = (2 \cdot 2 \cdot 2) - (2 \cdot 2) + 15$
$$= 8 - 4 + 15 = 19$$

8. **(B)** $15 - x = 13$

$x = 2$

9. **(C)** $5x + 6 = 3x$

$2x + 6 = 0$

$2x = -6$

$x = -3$

10. **(D)** $\frac{4}{5}x = 50$

$x = 62.5$

11. **(D)** $\frac{x+y}{5} + 5x - 3y =$

$\frac{8+10}{5} + 5(8) - 3(10) =$

$\frac{18}{5} + 40 - 30 =$

$3.6 + 40 - 30 = 13.6$

12. **(B)** $15 : 80 = x : 10$

$(80)(x) = (15)(10)$

$80x = 150$

$x = 1.875$

13. **(A)** $8x - 7 = 3x + 10$

$5x - 7 = 10$

$5x = 17$

$x = 3.4$

14. **(C)** $x + 15 = 95$

$x = 80$

15. **(B)** $\frac{3}{4}b + 15 = 50$

$\frac{3}{4}b = 35$

$b = 46.7$

16. **(A)** $\frac{b}{5} = 7$

$b = 35$

17. **(D)** $\frac{4x+7}{5} = 58$

$4x + 7 = 290$

$4x = 283$

$x = 70.75$

18. **(C)** $5ab^2 + 3(a^2 + b^3) =$

$5(4)(7^2) + 3(4^2 + 7^3) =$

$5(4)(49) + 3(16 + 343) =$

$980 + 1,077 = 2,057$

19. **(B)** $4x + 3(7x + 15) = 195$
$$4x + 21x + 45 = 195$$
$$25x + 45 = 195$$
$$25x = 150$$
$$x = 6$$

20. **(B)** $5a - 10 = 3a + 4$
$$5a = 3a + 14$$
$$2a = 14$$
$$a = 7$$

21. **(A)** $\dfrac{2}{3}x + \dfrac{4}{5}(x - 5) = 80$
$$10x + 12(x - 5) = 1,200$$
$$10x + 12x - 60 = 1,200$$
$$22x = 1,260$$
$$x = 57.3$$

22. **(D)** $8x - 17 = 425$
$$8x = 442$$
$$x = 55.25$$

23. **(B)** $8 + 4(x - 15) = 42$
$$8 + 4x - 60 = 42$$
$$4x - 52 = 42$$
$$4x = 94$$
$$x = 23.5$$

24. **(A)** $\dfrac{7b + 3}{3} = 80$
$$7b + 3 = 240$$
$$7b = 237$$
$$b = 33.86$$
$$2b = 67.72$$

25. **(B)** $\dfrac{3}{7} = \dfrac{b}{15}$
$$7b = 45$$
$$b = 6.43$$

GEOMETRY REVIEW

Geometry is the study of shapes and figures in either two or three dimensions. Plane geometry studies shapes and figures in two dimensions, whereas solid geometry studies shapes and figures in three dimensions.

Lines and Points

In geometry the word *line* always indicates a straight line. A line extends indefinitely in one or two directions. Straight lines are actually composed of an indefinite number of points. The following illustration is a line with three points. An arrow or arrows at one or both ends of the line indicate the direction of the line.

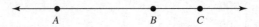

The line is *AC* and is written $\overleftrightarrow{AC}$. Lines may also be identified by using an italicized lowercase letter as in the following illustration. When identified in lowercase, one or two directional arrows are used.

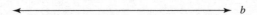

Since lines are made up of infinite points, it is possible to identify a portion or part of a line. This identified part of a line is called a *line segment*. Such segments are identified in one of two formats. A line without arrows may be drawn above the letters identifying the segment, or simply the letters without a line may indicate the line segment. In the following illustration, *AB*, *BC*, and *CD* are line segments of the line *AD*.

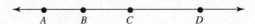

A *ray*, unlike a straight line, has a definite endpoint and proceeds only in one direction. A ray is identified by the letter placed at the end point or any other point on the ray. The symbol placed above the letter identifying the ray indicates the direction of the ray. The ray illustrated here is written $\overrightarrow{GH}$.

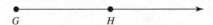

Lines are more than just single entities. There are a number of ways in which lines can be presented. *Intersecting lines* are just what the words indicate—the lines intersect or cross each other. In the next diagram the lines $\overleftrightarrow{AB}$ and $\overleftrightarrow{CD}$ intersect at *Y*.

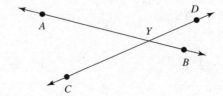

Perpendicular lines also intersect, but as opposed to intersecting lines, perpendicular lines always form 90° angles where they intersect.

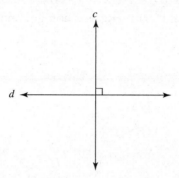

The small box (□) where lines *c* and *d* intersect denotes a 90° angle. The box is used with diagrams. When writing about perpendicular lines, the symbol ⊥ is used.

A third type of lines are parallel lines. *Parallel lines* do not intersect but continue with a constant, unchanging distance between them. Lines *s* and *t* in the following diagram are parallel lines.

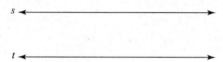

Parallel lines may be intersected or crossed by another or *transverse line*. With transverse lines, both parallel lines must be crossed by a straight line. In the following diagram, the line *z* crosses the parallel lines *s* and *t*.

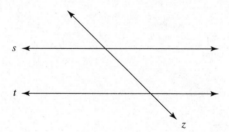

Geometric Figures

Shapes and figures used in geometry determine the type of geometry present. As mentioned earlier, plane geometry is two dimensional and is represented by flat figures. Solid geometry is represented by figures that have three dimensions or shape. We live in a three-dimensional world.

Angles

Angles are two rays that have a common endpoint. An angle has two components, the vertex or point where the two endpoints meet, and the sides of the angle or the rays. Angles are labeled according to their vertex and endpoints, their vertex, or by a numeral or lowercase letter inside the angle. Angles are measured in degrees from 0° to 360°.

SINGLE ANGLE TYPES

There are many types of single angles. You should be able to identify an angle by looking at it. The angle in the next diagram is a *right* angle. Such angles have a measurement of 90°. Angles with more or less than 90° are not right angles. The right angle below could be labeled ∠A, ∠CAB, or ∠BAC.

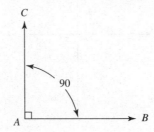

The following angle is an *acute* angle. Such angles have a measure of less than 90°. This acute angle could be labeled ∠E, ∠1, ∠DEF, or ∠FED.

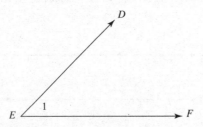

Obtuse angles are angles measuring more than 90° but less than 180°. The following obtuse angle could be labeled ∠T, ∠RTS, ∠2, or ∠STR.

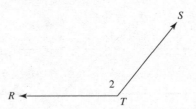

The last type of angle is the *straight* angle. A straight angle has a measure of 180°. If the angle has more or less than 180° it is not a straight angle. The following straight angle is labeled ∠ACE or ∠ECA.

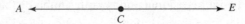

MULTIPLE ANGLE TYPES

Angles may occur with other angles. Just as there are different types of single angles, there are different types of multiple angles. *Adjacent* angles share a common side or ray and have the same vertex or meeting point. In the next diagram, $\overleftrightarrow{AC}$ is the common side of the two angles, and ∠A is the vertex. The diagram indicates that ∠1 and ∠2 are adjacent angles, as are angles ∠BAC and ∠CAD.

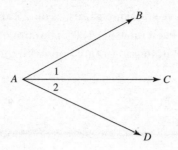

Complementary angles have a total measure of 90°. If two angles are more or less than 90°, they are not complementary angles. In this diagram, ∠1 + ∠2 = 90°; as does ∠ABC since it is a right triangle.

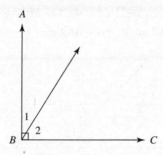

Perpendicular angles are formed when two lines intersect and form right triangles at their common vertex. In the following diagram, ∠1, ∠2, ∠3, and ∠4 each measure 90°. The sum of the four angles is 360°. Each angle is also a right triangle.

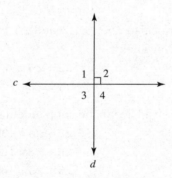

Supplementary angles are two angles whose measure equals 180°. Two angles with a measure of more or less than 180° are not supplementary. In this diagram, ∠1 + ∠2 = 180°. Supplementary angles always form a straight line.

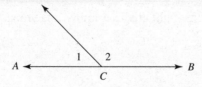

Vertical angles are formed when two lines intersect but do not form 90° angles at their common vertex or meeting point. In vertical angles, opposite angles have equal measures. In the following diagram ∠1 and ∠3 have equal measures, as do ∠2 and ∠4. Also, ∠1 and ∠2, ∠2 and ∠3, ∠3 and ∠4, and ∠4 and ∠1 each measure 180°. The sum of the four measures, that is, ∠1 through ∠4, is 360°. Also note that AB and CD are lines with measures of 180° each.

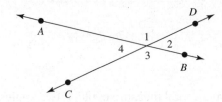

Interior and *exterior* angles are formed when a transversal line intersects with two parallel lines. Interior angles are those angles on the inside of the parallel lines. Exterior angles are those angles outside of the parallel lines. In the next diagram, ∠1, ∠2, ∠7, and ∠8 are exterior angles whereas ∠3, ∠4, ∠5, and ∠6 are interior angles.

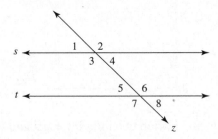

This intersection of one line with two parallel lines forms a number of relationships worth remembering.

1. ∠1, ∠2, ∠3, and ∠4 are identical to ∠5, ∠6, ∠7, and ∠8. In this case, the following angles are identical or corresponding angles:

   ∠1 = ∠5   ∠2 = ∠6
   ∠3 = ∠7   ∠4 = ∠8

2. The following angles are both adjacent and supplementary angles:

   ∠1 + ∠3 = 180°   ∠2 + ∠4 = 180°
   ∠5 + ∠7 = 180°   ∠6 + ∠8 = 180°
   ∠1 + ∠2 = 180°   ∠3 + ∠4 = 180°
   ∠5 + ∠6 = 180°   ∠7 + ∠8 = 180°

3. The following are vertical angles:

   ∠1 and ∠4   ∠2 and ∠3
   ∠5 and ∠8   ∠6 and ∠7

4. If the measure of one of the eight angles is known, the measures of the remaining angles can be determined.

EXAMPLE 1

Using the preceding diagram, assume that ∠5 = 45°. Determine the measures of the remaining angles. There are a number of different approaches to solving the problem. One approach follows:

a. ∠5 and ∠6 are located on line *t*, which has a total measure of 180°. Subtract the measure of ∠5 from 180° to determine the measure of ∠6.

   180° − 45° = 135° = ∠6

b. The angles on line *s* and line *t* are identical, so if ∠5 = 45°, then ∠1 = 45°, and if ∠6 = 135°, then ∠2 = 135°.

c. ∠1 and ∠4, and ∠5 and ∠8 are vertical angles and are, therefore, equal in measurement. If ∠1 and ∠5 are each equal to 45°, then ∠4 and ∠8 are also 45° each.

d. ∠2 and ∠3, and ∠6 and ∠8 are vertical angles and are equal in measurement. If ∠2 and ∠6 are 135° each, then ∠3 and ∠7 are also 135° each.

e. The answer to the problem is if ∠5 = 45°, then

∠1 = 45°	∠2 = 135°
∠3 = 135°	∠4 = 45°
∠6 = 135°	∠7 = 135°
∠8 = 45°	

Circles

Circles, as opposed to lines, come about and join together. They do not extend into space for an indefinite distance. Like the line, the circle is composed of an infinite number of points, but the points in a circle are all equidistant from an imaginary or identified point in the center of the circle. The center of the circle is labeled with an uppercase letter, as are the points around the circle.

A circle has three parts, the circumference (*c*) or distance around the circle, the diameter (*d*) or distance across the circle going through the center point, and the radius (*r*) or half the distance of the diameter going from a point on the circle to its center point.

The area and circumference of a circle can be determined. Refer to Table 5.8 for specific formulas and graphic representations for circular objects.

Polygons

Polygons are closed two-dimensional shapes or figures having three or more sides. Two-dimensional objects are flat objects. Triangles, squares, rectangles, octagons, and hexagons are all examples of polygons.

TRIANGLES

Figures or shapes having three sides are triangles. Triangles have three interior angles that total 180°. A figure or shape measuring more or less than 180° is not a triangle.

There are many types of triangles. Triangles can be classified according to their shape:

- **Isosceles triangles** have two equal sides and, therefore, two equal angles plus an additional angle.
- **Equilateral triangles** have three equal sides, and each of the three angles is equal to 60°.
- **Scalene triangles** have no equal sides or angles.

Triangles can also be classified by their angles:

- **Acute triangles** have each interior angle or measure less than 90°.
- **Obtuse triangles** have one interior angle or measure greater than 90° but less than 180°.
- **Right triangles** have one interior angle or measure of 90°.

SQUARES AND RECTANGLES

Two-dimensional shapes or figures with four sides are squares or rectangles. The total measurement for a square or rectangle is 360°. Both squares and rectangles have four sides with each angle equal to 90°. Squares and rectangles are composed of right angles.

Squares and rectangles differ in the length of their sides. Squares have four sides of equal length, whereas rectangles have two sides of one length and two sides of another length. The equal sides are opposite each other in the rectangle.

The area, or the measure within the figure, and perimeter, or distance around the figure, can be determined for triangles, squares, and rectangles. See Table 5.8 for the formulas for finding the area of various polygons and their graphic representations.

Pythagorean Theorem

The Pythagorean Theorem applies to right triangles only. It states that the sum of the squares of two legs of the triangle is equal to the square of the hypotenuse or third leg. The theorem is employed when working with right triangles when two of the three sides are known, and the third side is unknown. In most instances, the theorem is used for indirect measurement when it is impractical or impossible to measure directly. Refer to Table 5.8 for the formula and graphic representation of the Pythagorean Theorem.

Cubes, Rectangular Solids, and Cylinders

Cubes, rectangular solids, and cylinders are three-dimensional objects. They might be thought of as extensions of the square, rectangle, and circle. For three-dimensional figures, volume is expressed in terms of *cubic* inches, centimeters, or feet. The volume, or amount of space within the object, and surface area, the outer area of the object, of cubes, rectangular solids, and cylinders can be mathematically determined. Refer to Table 5.8 for exact formulas and graphic representations of each three-dimensional object.

ANSWER SHEET
Geometry Sample Test

1. Ⓐ Ⓑ Ⓒ Ⓓ
2. Ⓐ Ⓑ Ⓒ Ⓓ
3. Ⓐ Ⓑ Ⓒ Ⓓ
4. Ⓐ Ⓑ Ⓒ Ⓓ
5. Ⓐ Ⓑ Ⓒ Ⓓ
6. Ⓐ Ⓑ Ⓒ Ⓓ
7. Ⓐ Ⓑ Ⓒ Ⓓ
8. Ⓐ Ⓑ Ⓒ Ⓓ
9. Ⓐ Ⓑ Ⓒ Ⓓ

10. Ⓐ Ⓑ Ⓒ Ⓓ
11. Ⓐ Ⓑ Ⓒ Ⓓ
12. Ⓐ Ⓑ Ⓒ Ⓓ
13. Ⓐ Ⓑ Ⓒ Ⓓ
14. Ⓐ Ⓑ Ⓒ Ⓓ
15. Ⓐ Ⓑ Ⓒ Ⓓ
16. Ⓐ Ⓑ Ⓒ Ⓓ
17. Ⓐ Ⓑ Ⓒ Ⓓ
18. Ⓐ Ⓑ Ⓒ Ⓓ

19. Ⓐ Ⓑ Ⓒ Ⓓ
20. Ⓐ Ⓑ Ⓒ Ⓓ
21. Ⓐ Ⓑ Ⓒ Ⓓ
22. Ⓐ Ⓑ Ⓒ Ⓓ
23. Ⓐ Ⓑ Ⓒ Ⓓ
24. Ⓐ Ⓑ Ⓒ Ⓓ
25. Ⓐ Ⓑ Ⓒ Ⓓ

Directions: For each question, select the letter (A, B, C, or D) that corresponds with your answer. Record your answers on the answer sheet on page 151.

Questions 1–3 refer to the following diagram.

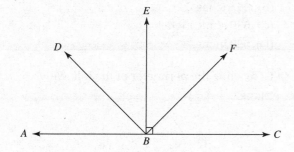

1. The number of degrees in ∠EBA is
   (A) 80°.
   (B) 90°.
   (C) 140°.
   (D) 180°.

2. _____ is an acute angle.
   (A) ∠DBC
   (B) ∠ABC
   (C) ∠ABE
   (D) ∠DBA

3. If ∠EBC is 90°, then ∠FBC is
   (A) 90°.
   (B) 45°.
   (C) 15°.
   (D) 5°.

4. The diameter of a circle is 50 inches. The radius of the circle is
   (A) 100 inches.
   (B) 25 inches.
   (C) 157 inches.
   (D) 45 inches.

5. If two angles of a triangle have a total measure of 95°, the third angle has a measure of
   (A) 180°.
   (B) 265°.
   (C) 90°.
   (D) 85°.

6. An obtuse angle has a measure of
   (A) less than 90° but larger than 45°.
   (B) more than 90° but less than 180°.
   (C) equal to 90° but less than 360°.
   (D) 180°.

7. In the following diagram, ∠ABC is a right triangle. The ∠ABD has a measure of 50° and ∠DBC has a measure of 40°. The two angles are called

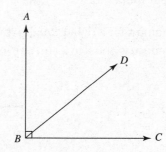

   (A) supplementary angles.
   (B) supporting angles.
   (C) complementary angles.
   (D) pairs of angles.

8. The following diagram is a (an) _____ triangle.

(A) scalene
(B) isosceles
(C) concave
(D) right

9. If, in the following diagram, ∠ABE has a measure of 130°, then ∠y has a measure of

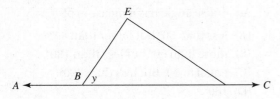

(A) 50°.
(B) y^2.
(C) 230°.
(D) Not enough information is given to make a determination.

10. Determine x for a right triangle where the hypotenuse is equal to 5 and one leg is equal to 4.

(A) 9
(B) 3
(C) 1
(D) 5

CHALLENGE

11. A circle has a radius of 7 inches. Determine the circumference of the circle.

(A) 21.98 inches
(B) 153.86 inches
(C) 138.03 inches
(D) 43.96 inches

12. Determine the volume of the following rectangular solid.

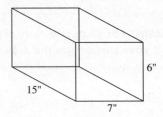

(A) 99 cubic inches
(B) 99 inches
(C) 630 cubic inches
(D) 630 inches

13. Determine the perimeter of the following triangle.

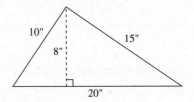

(A) 27″
(B) 53″
(C) 43″
(D) 45″

14. Determine the area of the following trapezoid.

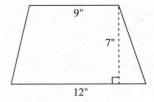

(A) 28 square inches
(B) 73.5 square inches
(C) 756 square inches
(D) 14.3 square inches

15. Determine the area of a circle whose diameter is 8 inches.

    (A) 50.24 square inches
    (B) 50.24 inches
    (C) 200.96 square inches
    (D) 200.96 inches

16. If three angles of a square measure 270°, what is the measure of the fourth angle?

    (A) 90°
    (B) 180°
    (C) 300°
    (D) 30°

17. Determine x in the following right triangle.

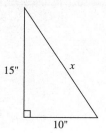

    (A) 25″
    (B) 18″
    (C) 32.5″
    (D) 20″

    CHALLENGE

18. Determine the area of the following parallelogram.

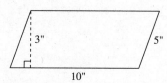

    (A) 18 square inches
    (B) 35 square inches
    (C) 30 square inches
    (D) 25 square inches

19. Determine the volume of a cube whose sides are each 13″.

    (A) 169 cubic inches
    (B) 52 cubic inches
    (C) 109.8 cubic inches
    (D) 2,197 cubic inches

    CHALLENGE

20. A quadrilateral figure has how many sides?

    (A) 3
    (B) 4
    (C) 5
    (D) 6

21. The perimeter of a square is 40 inches. Determine the area of the square.

    (A) 160 square inches
    (B) 10 square inches
    (C) 100 square inches
    (D) 80 square inches

22. Determine the perimeter of the following figure.

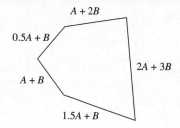

    (A) $A^2 + B^2$
    (B) $0.5(A^2 + B^2)$
    (C) $5(6A + 9B)$
    (D) $6A + 8B$

23. Which object has the greater volume?

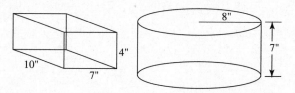

    (A) The volume of the cylinder with 1,406.72 cubic inches is greater.

    CHALLENGE

    (B) The volume of the rectangular solid with 280 cubic inches is greater.
    (C) They will hold equal amounts.
    (D) Rectangular solids and cylinders can't be compared because of the difference in shapes.

24. Which contains the greatest measure of degrees, a circle or a triangle?

    (A) A circle
    (B) A triangle
    (C) Both contain the same measure of degrees since both are two-dimensional figures.
    (D) There is not enough information given to determine an answer.

25. $\triangle ABC$ is a right isosceles triangle. If $\angle A = \angle C$, then $\angle B =$

    CHALLENGE

    (A) 90°
    (B) 35°
    (C) 30°
    (D) 45°

Geometry Sample Test Answer Key

1. **B**	6. **B**	11. **D**	16. **A**	21. **C**
2. **D**	7. **C**	12. **C**	17. **B**	22. **D**
3. **B**	8. **B**	13. **D**	18. **C**	23. **A**
4. **B**	9. **A**	14. **B**	19. **D**	24. **A**
5. **D**	10. **B**	15. **A**	20. **B**	25. **A**

GEOMETRY SAMPLE TEST ANSWERS EXPLAINED

1. **(B)** $\angle EBA$ is a right angle.

2. **(D)** An acute angle is less than 90°.

3. **(B)** One half of a right angle has a measure of 45°.

4. **(B)** The radius of a circle is one half of the diameter.
$$d = 50''$$
$$r = \frac{1}{2}d$$
$$r = \frac{1}{2}(50'')$$
$$r = 25''$$

5. **(D)** The total measure of a triangle is 180°. If two of the angles are equal to 95°, then the remaining angle is 85°.

6. **(B)** Obtuse angles are more than 90° but less than 180°.

7. **(C)** Complementary angles have a total measure of 90°.

8. **(B)** Isosceles triangles have 2 equal sides or angles.

9. **(A)** A straight angle has a measure of 180°. $\overleftrightarrow{AC}$ is a straight angle. If $\angle ABE = 130°$, then $\angle y = 50°$.

10. **(B)** Let side $a = x$, $b = 4$, and $c = 5$.
$$a^2 + b^2 = c^2$$
$$a^2 + 4^2 = 5^2$$
$$a^2 + 16 = 25$$
$$a^2 = 9$$
$$a = \sqrt{9}$$
$$a = 3 = x$$

11. **(D)** $d = 2r = 2 \times 7 = 14''$
$$C = \pi d$$
$$C = (3.14)(14)$$
$$C = 43.96''$$

12. **(C)** $V = lwh$
$$V = (15)(7)(6)$$
$$V = 630 \text{ cubic inches}$$

13. **(D)** $P = s_1 + s_2 + s_3$
$P = 10'' + 15'' + 20''$
$P = 45''$

14. **(B)** $A = \frac{1}{2}(b_1 + b_2)h$

$A = \frac{1}{2}(9'' + 12'')7''$

$A = \frac{1}{2}(21'')7''$

$A = 73.5$ square inches

15. **(A)** $r = \frac{1}{2}d = \frac{1}{2}(8\text{ inches}) = 4\text{ inches}$

$A = \pi r^2$
$A = (3.14)(4\text{ inches})^2$
$A = (3.14)(16\text{ square inches})$
$A = 50.24$ square inches

16. **(A)** A square has four equal sides and four equal angles of 90° each, or a total measure of 360°. If a square has three angles measuring 270°, then the remaining angle has a measure of 90°.

17. **(B)** $a^2 + b^2 = c^2$
$10^2 + 15^2 = c^2$
$100 + 225 = c^2$
$325 = c^2$
$\sqrt{325} = c$
$18\text{ inches} = c$

18. **(C)** $A = bh$
$A = (10\text{ inches})(3\text{ inches})$
$A = 30$ square inches

19. **(D)** $V = s^3$
$V = (13'')^3$
$V = (13'')(13'')(13'')$
$V = 2{,}197$ cubic inches

20. **(B)** Quadrilaterals have four sides.

21. **(C)** $A = s^2$
$A = 10^2$
$A = (10)(10)$
$A = 100$

22. **(D)** $(A + 2B) + (2A + 3B) + (1.5A + B) + (A + B) + (0.5A + B) = 6A + 8B$

23. **(A)** **Volume of rectangular solid**

$V = lwh$

$V = (4\text{ inches})(7\text{ inches})(10\text{ inches})$

$V = 280$ cubic inches

Volume of cylinder

$V = \pi r^2 h$

$V = (3.14)(8\text{ inches})^2(7\text{ inches})$

$V = (3.14)(64\text{ square inches})(7\text{ inches})$

$V = 1,406.72$ cubic inches

24. **(A)** A circle contains 360°, whereas a triangle contains 180°.

25. **(A)** Right isosceles triangles have one angle with a measure of 90°, and the two remaining angles are equal.

$$\angle A = x$$
$$\angle C = x$$
$$x + x + 90° = 180°$$
$$2x + 90° = 180°$$
$$2x = 90°$$
$$x = 45°$$

Therefore, if $\angle A$ and $\angle C$ both equal 45°, then $\angle B$ equals 90°.

VERBAL PROBLEM REVIEW

Verbal problems mirror events or problems encountered in life, and like problems encountered in life, verbal problems can be difficult to solve if you are not sure of what you are doing, get in a hurry, or leave out a step.

Verbal problems can address any life event and can use any type of mathematics. A verbal problem may ask about the interest rate on a loan, how to find the average grade for a course, or how much medication to give a patient. The problem may ask about distance traveled or how far a group of hikers is from their home base after they changed directions and walked a set distance.

With regard to mathematics, a verbal problem may ask for nothing more than simple arithmetic, or it may include several steps and use principles of algebra and geometry. Verbal problems may require specific formulas or units of measurement in order to solve the problem. It's important to go beyond mere memorization of formulas. Know when to use the formula and how to apply it correctly. Learn both English, as well as metric, units of measurement.

When solving verbal problems, take your time, read carefully, and do not become overly anxious if you think you cannot solve the problem. Work the problem one step at a time, and do not try to jump ahead or jump to an answer. Consider the following when working verbal problems:

1. What is the problem asking you to do? If you can write in your test booklet or on your exam, underline or circle what you need to know.

2. What information does the problem give you? The problem must give you a certain amount of information in order for you to solve the problem. Mark this information on your exam if possible. Does the problem give you information in yards and then ask for the answer in inches?

3. Make a simple diagram or sketch of the information the problem gives you and use an X or a question mark to indicate what you need to find out. Label what you know. Some verbal problems may give you more information than what you need, so pay attention to what the problem is asking you to do. Do not waste time trying to make the perfect sketch, but make it good enough so that you understand what you mean.

4. Look for conversions you might need to make before you solve the problem. Do you need to go from ounces to pounds or from the English system to the metric system? Remember that you will not get the correct answer if you are trying to compare feet and inches or milliliters and teaspoons.

5. Consider the expressions or equations you might use to solve the problem. Is there a specific formula that you can use to answer the question the verbal problem poses? If there is a formula, determine which components of the formula are defined. If there is not a specific formula, how will you set up the problem to solve it?

6. Solve the equation or expression. Add, subtract, multiply, and divide carefully. Many errors are caused by a lack of focus or hurrying. Double-check how you worked the problem. If your answers do not agree, look for simple mistakes like $2 + 2 = 5$, $3 \times 3 = 6$, or $30 - 25 = 55$.

7. Look at your answer and then look at what the question asked. Is your answer sensible? Have you answered the question posed in the verbal problem? The majority of verbal problems are based on events occurring in everyday life, so it's doubtful that you would get an answer suggesting a man could run 100 miles per hour.

Age Problems

EXAMPLE 1

Sally and John are brother and sister. Sally is 5 years older than John. Sally was born on their father's 22nd birthday in 1965. In what year was John born?

x = the year that Sally was born or the year 1965

$x + 5$ = the year that John was born since he was born 5 years after Sally was born

$x + 5 = 1965 + 5 = 1970$ = the year of John's birth

The age of Sally and John's father has nothing to do with the problem.

EXAMPLE 2

Martin and Mary are brother and sister. Martin is two times as old as Mary. There is 27 years between their ages. How old are Martin and Mary?

x = Mary's age

$2x$ = Martin's age since he is twice Mary's age

27 = difference in years between Mary and Martin

$2x - x = 27$

$x = 27$

Mary's age = $x = 27$

Martin's age = $2x = 54$

Distance Problems

EXAMPLE 1

Two trains leave from two different cities that are 650 miles apart. They are traveling toward each other. The Prairie Flyer averages 72 miles per hour. The Mountain Breeze averages 55 miles per hour. Both trains left their respective stations at the same time. How many hours will it take for the two trains to meet?

T = the number of hours it will take for the two trains to meet

$R = 72$ = the average speed of the Prairie Flyer

$R = 55$ = the average speed of the Mountain Breeze

650 = the total distance to be covered by both trains

Distance = (Rate)(Time) or $D = RT$

$R \cdot T = D$

$72T + 55T = 650$

$127T = 650$

$T = 5.118$ or 5.12 hours

EXAMPLE 2

Two long-distance runners are 50 miles apart. They start running toward each other at 7:00 A.M. Runner One runs an average 4 miles per hour, and Runner Two runs an average of 1.5 miles per ten minutes. What time will the runners meet?

T = 50 miles or the distance to be covered

4 = the average number of miles run per hour by Runner 1 (R_1)

9 = the average number of miles run per hour by Runner 2 (R_2)

$$1.5 \text{ miles} : 10 \text{ minutes} = x \text{ miles} : 60 \text{ minutes}$$

$$10x = 90$$

$$x = 9 \text{ mph for } R_2$$

$$R \times T = \text{Distance}$$

$$R_1(T) + R_2(T) = \text{Distance}$$

$$4T + 9T = 50$$

$$13T = 50$$

$$T = 3.8 \text{ hours or 3 hr 48 min}$$

The two runners will meet at 10:48 A.M.

Ratio and Proportion Problems

EXAMPLE 1

A cake recipe and its cooked icing call for a total of 11 eggs. You plan to bake 3 cakes with icing for the charity bazaar. How many dozen eggs will you have to buy to bake the 3 cakes and make the icing for each?

$$1 \text{ recipe} : 11 \text{ eggs} = 3 \text{ recipes} : x \text{ eggs}$$

$$33 \text{ eggs} = x$$

$$1 \text{ dozen eggs} : 12 \text{ eggs} = x \text{ dozen eggs} : 33 \text{ eggs}$$

$$12x = 33$$

$$x = 2.75 \text{ or } 3 \text{ dozen eggs}$$

EXAMPLE 2

A doctor gives a patient a prescription that instructs the patient to take 2 tablets every 4 hours. The prescription orders 120 tablets to be issued. How long will the prescription last if the tablets are taken as ordered?

$$2 \text{ tablets every } 4 \text{ hr} = 12 \text{ tablets per } 24 \text{ hr} = 12 \text{ tablets per day}$$

$$12 \text{ tablets} : 1 \text{ day} = 120 \text{ tablets} : x \text{ days}$$

$$12x = 120$$

$$x = 10 \text{ days}$$

Percentage Problems

EXAMPLE 1

Margaret bought a coat on sale. The list price of the coat was $245. She paid $200 for the coat. What was the rate of discount on the coat?

$$\text{Cost of coat} = \$245$$

$$\text{Discount price of coat} = \$200$$

$$\text{Amount of discount} = \$45$$

$$\frac{\text{Amount of discount}}{\text{Cost}} = \frac{45}{245} = 0.1836 = 18.4\%$$

EXAMPLE 2

The Smith family budget allows 15% of monthly income for eating out and entertainment for themselves and their seven children. Mr. Smith contributes $2,400 a month to the budget, and his wife contributes $2,700 a month. How much can the Smith family spend a month on eating out and entertainment?

Mr. Smith = $2,400

Mrs. Smith = $2,700

Total monthly amount to budget = $5,100

Entertainment percentage = 15% = 0.15

(Total amount to budget)(Percentage) = ($5,100)(0.15) = $765.00

Sales Problems

EXAMPLE 1

Basketballs cost a store manager $15 each. He plans to sell the basketballs at a profit of 40% over the cost. His overhead on each basketball is $3. What is the selling price of the basketballs?

Basketball cost = $15

Overhead = $3

Profit = 40% = 0.40

Selling price = Cost + Overhead + Profit

Selling price = $15 + $3 + ($15)(0.40)

Selling price = $15 + $3 + $6

Selling price = $24.00

EXAMPLE 2

The Roundrock Pet Company had sales in the amount of $6,500 for one week. The cost of the merchandise sold was $3,800. The store's overhead was 15% of sales. How much profit was made during the week?

Amount of sales = $6,500

Cost of merchandise = $3,800

Overhead = 15% = 0.15

If Selling price = Cost + Overhead + Profit, then

Profit = Selling price − Cost − Overhead

Profit = $6,500 − $3,800 − (0.15)($6,500)

Profit = $6,500 − $3,800 − $975

Profit = $1,725

Mixture Problems

EXAMPLE 1

The adult dinner theater sold 198 tickets. Adult tickets sold for $15.25 and student tickets for $10.25. If the income for the dinner theater was $2,629.50, how many of each type ticket were sold?

Set up a table to solve this problem.

	Number of Tickets	Cost of Tickets	Total Income
Adult Tickets	x	$15.25	$15.25x$
Student Tickets	$198 - x$	$10.25	$10.25(198 - x)$

Ticket income = Adult ticket income + Student ticket income

$$2,629.50 = 15.25x + 10.25(198 - x)$$

$$2,629.50 = 15.25x + 2,029.50 - 10.25x$$

$$2,629.50 = 5x + 2,029.50$$

$$600 = 5x$$

$$120 = x \text{ (Adult tickets sold)}$$

$$78 = 198 - 120 \text{ (Student tickets sold)}$$

EXAMPLE 2

A jar contains four colors of candy. One fourth of the candy is red in color, one fifth of the candy is green, one fifth of the candy is yellow, and the remaining 30 pieces of candy are orange. How many pieces of candy are in the jar?

$\dfrac{1}{4}$ = red candies $\qquad\qquad$ $\dfrac{1}{5}$ = green candies

$\dfrac{1}{5}$ = yellow candies $\qquad\qquad$ 30 = orange candies

x = total pieces of candy

Total pieces of candy = #red + #green + #yellow + #orange

$$x = \left(\frac{1}{4}x\right) + \left(\frac{1}{5}x\right) + \left(\frac{1}{5}x\right) + 30$$
$$20x = 5x + 4x + 4x + 600$$
$$20x = 13x + 600$$
$$7x = 600$$
$$x = 85.7 = 86 \text{ pieces of candy}$$

Tax Problems

EXAMPLE 1

Jonathan works for Zippies Burgers. His weekly salary is $380. His employer deducts 4% of his salary for Social Security, 5.25% for state withholding tax, and 7% for federal withholding tax. Jonathan uses direct deposit and an additional $50 is deducted and put into a savings account before the money is put into his checking account. How much money goes into Jonathan's checking account each week?

Total weekly salary (WS) = $380

Social Security deduction (SS) = 4% = $380(0.04) = $15.20

State deduction (SD) = 5.25% = 0.0525 = $380(0.0525) = $19.95

Federal deduction (FD) = 7% = $380(0.07) = $26.60

Savings account deduction (SAD) = $50

Checking account deposit = WS − (SS + SD + FD + SAD)

Checking account deposit = $380 − ($15.20 + $19.95 + $26.60 + $50)

Checking account deposit = $380 − $111.75

Checking account deposit = $268.25

EXAMPLE 2

Wanda buys a lamp for $67. The sales tax is 8.7754%. What is the total cost of her purchase?

Total cost = Cost of lamp + tax

Total cost = $67 + ($67)(0.087754)

Total cost = $67 + $5.8795

Total cost = $72.88

Geometry Problems

EXAMPLE 1

In $\triangle ABC$, the measure of $\angle A$ is five times the measure of $\angle B$. The measure of $\angle C$ is three times the measure of $\angle B$. What is the measure of each of the angles of the triangle?

$\angle B = x$

$\angle A = 5x$

$\angle C = 3x$

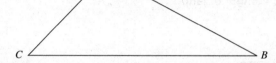

$\angle B + \angle A + \angle C = 180°$

$x + 5x + 3x = 180°$

$9x = 180°$

$x = 20° = \angle B$

$5x = 100° = \angle A$

$3x = 60° = \angle C$

EXAMPLE 2

A carpenter is painting a house and needs access to the second-story windows. The bottom of the windows are 15 feet from the ground. The nearest a ladder can be safely placed to the house is 7 feet. The house is at a right angle to the ground. How long a ladder does the carpenter need to access the second-story windows?

Draw a diagram to help solve the problem.

a = house = 15 feet

b = ground = 7 feet

c = ladder = unknown feet

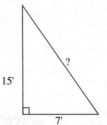

$a^2 + b^2 = c^2$

$15^2 + 7^2 = c^2$

$225 + 49 = c^2$

$274 = c^2$

$\sqrt{274} = 16.6 = c$

16.6 feet = c = length of ladder

Insurance Problems

EXAMPLE 1

Martha is considering purchasing a life insurance policy. The annual premium rate on $10,000 worth of life insurance is $25 per $1,000. What is the annual cost of Martha's premium?

Policy worth = $10,000

Premium rate = $25/$1,000

$25 : $1,000 :: x : $10,000

$1,000x = 250,000$

$x = \$250$

EXAMPLE 2

A boat is insured against fire for 85% of its value. The boat has a value of $85,000 and the premium rate is $15 per $1,000. What is the annual premium for the boat?

Policy = 85% of value of boat = $72,250

Value of boat = $85,000

Premium rate = $15/$1,000

$15 : $1,000 :: x : $72,250$

$1,000x = 1,083,750$

$x = \$1,083.75$

Investment Problems

EXAMPLE 1

Timothy owns 750 shares of Lifelong Computer stock. The stock pays an annual dividend of $22.79 per share. How much will Timothy receive in dividends this year?

number of shares = 750

dividends/share = $22.79

$(750)(\$22.79) = \$17,092.50$

EXAMPLE 2

Joyce bought 110 shares of BioTech Limited at $21 a share. She sold the shares a year later at $27 a share. What is her profit after paying a commission of $40?

Original price = (110 shares)($21) = $2,310

Selling price = (110 shares)($27) = $2,970

Commission = $40

Selling price – Original price – Commission = Profit

$2,970 – $2,310 – $40 = Profit

$620 = Profit

Interest Problems

EXAMPLE 1

What is the simple interest on $15,000 invested at 10% annual rate over 3 years?

Principal = $15,000

Rate = 10% annually

Time = 3 years

Interest = Principal × Rate × Time

Interest = ($15,000)(0.10)(3)

Interest = $4,500

EXAMPLE 2

What is the simple interest on $1,800 at a 5.5% semiannual rate over 6 years?

Principal = $1800

Rate = 5.5% semiannually = 11% annually

Time = 6 years

Interest = Principal × Rate × Time

Interest = $1,800 × 0.11 × 6

Interest = $1,188

Average Problems

EXAMPLE 1

Mike has the following points on pop quizzes: 10, 15, 21, 7, 27, 32, 50, 50, and 50. Each quiz is worth 50 points. If 70% is a passing grade, does Mike have a passing average on quizzes?

$$\left(\frac{10 + 15 + 21 + 7 + 27 + 32 + 50 + 50 + 50}{9} \right) = 29.11 \text{ points}$$

70% of 50 = 35 points

Mike does not have a passing average on pop quizzes.

EXAMPLE 2

Tickets for the All School Play sell for $1.50, $2.50, $5.00, and $10.00. What is the average price of a ticket?

$$\frac{\$1.50 + \$2.50 + \$5.00 + \$10.00}{4} = \$4.75$$

Dosage Problems

EXAMPLE 1

A patient is receiving cough medicine (liquid), 500 milligrams (mg) by mouth every 6 hours. The medication label reads: 250 milligrams/5 milliliters (mL). How many mL will the nurse administer for one dose?

Formula:

$$\frac{Desired \times Volume}{Available} = mL \text{ per dose}$$

$$\frac{500 \text{ mg} \times 5 \text{ mL}}{250 \text{ mg}} = 10 \text{ mL}$$

EXAMPLE 2

A dentist has his nurse administer a one time antibiotic dose to a patient with a tooth infection. The dose is 7.5 milligrams (mg) intramuscularly (IM). The medication concentration mix is 10 milligrams/milliliters (mL). How many milliliters will the nurse give to the patient for the one time dose?

Formula:

$$\frac{Desired \times Volume}{Available} = mL \text{ per dose}$$

$$\frac{7.5 \text{ mg} \times 1 \text{ mL}}{10 \text{ mg}} = 0.75 \text{ mL}$$

EXAMPLE 3

A nurse practitioner orders ABD 20 milligrams (mg) intravenous (IV) every 8 hours for an 18-month-old child weighing 22 pounds (lb). The *Pediatric Drug Handbook* states: Maximum daily dosage of ABD for a child is 6.0 – 7.5 mg/kg/24 hours divided into 1 dose every 8 hours.

STEP 1 Convert the child's weight from pounds to kilograms (kg)

$$1 \text{ kg} = 2.2 \text{ lb} :: x \text{ kg} = 22 \text{ lb}$$

$$2.2x = 22$$

$$x = 10 \text{ kg}$$

STEP 2 Calculate the safe dosage range for 24 hours.

Low range = 6 mg/kg/24 hr

10 kg × 6 mg/24 hr = 60 mg/24 hr ÷ 3 doses/24 hr = 20 mg/dose

High range = 7.5 mg/kg/24 hr

10 kg × 7.5 mg/24 hr = 75 mg/24 hr ÷ 3 doses/24 hr = 25 mg/dose

The dosage is within a safe range for the child at 60 mg ABD/24 hr or 20 mg ABD/8 hr.

EXAMPLE 4

A physician orders D5%NS 1,000 milliliters (mL) to infuse over 8 hours. The nurse plans to run the infusion by intravenous (IV) pump. An infusion pump delivers the solution in mL per hour. What rate will the nurse set the IV pump to infuse at?

Formula:

$$\frac{\text{Total volume}}{\text{Hours}} = \frac{1,000 \text{ mL}}{8} = 125 \text{ mL/hour}$$

GRAPHS AND CHARTS

Using graphs and charts is one method used to easily present information on virtually any topic. Both communicate information visually. Information presented in graphs and charts comes from data or information gathered over time or for a specific event. Sometimes, complicated information that is difficult to understand needs a drawing. Graphs or charts can enhance understanding by getting a point across quickly and visually.

Graphs and charts are "read" by understanding what data is represented, such as time, finances, research results, and numerous other things. They will provide information on exactly what is being looked at. A representation showing the different properties presented on a graph is displayed on the next page.

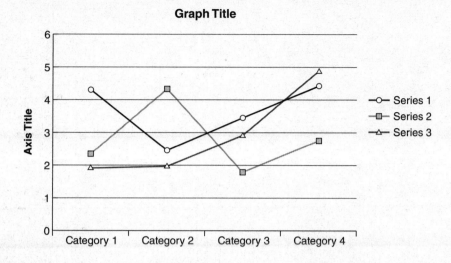

Graph Title

Look at the graph. It has information that must be understood in order to interpret the data correctly. First, there is the title, which tells us exactly what we are looking at. Second, there are two axes. In this graph, the horizontal axis consists of four categories, and the vertical axis ranges in numeral values from zero to six. Third, we have the legend. In this case, it's three "Series." Note that Series 1 has a circular or round symbol, Series 2 is represented by a square symbol, and Series 3 is represented by a triangular symbol. Last, there are the actual data points. Each of the four categories has three data points.

When looking more carefully, there are a number of things we can determine: the sum of each category using the data points, the lows and highs in a category or series, which series demonstrated the steadiest growth, and which category was the most unstable.

Now see what you can do with the two graphs on the following Graphs and Charts Sample Test. Examine the graphs and answer the questions referring to them. Pay attention to how each graph is set up, what the data points present, and what the questions ask.

ANSWER SHEET
Graphs and Charts Sample Test

1. Ⓐ Ⓑ Ⓒ Ⓓ   3. Ⓐ Ⓑ Ⓒ Ⓓ   5. Ⓐ Ⓑ Ⓒ Ⓓ

2. Ⓐ Ⓑ Ⓒ Ⓓ   4. Ⓐ Ⓑ Ⓒ Ⓓ   6. Ⓐ Ⓑ Ⓒ Ⓓ

For Questions 1–3, analyze the graph, and select the letter (A, B, C, or D) that best answers the question. Record your answers on the Graphs and Charts Sample Test Answer Sheet on page 175.

Aaron and Marsha have five male children, all 13 years old. Their children are quintuplets. Aaron and Marsha decide to record their sons' Grade Point Averages (GPAs) over the course of four weeks to see if the boys' grades are improving.

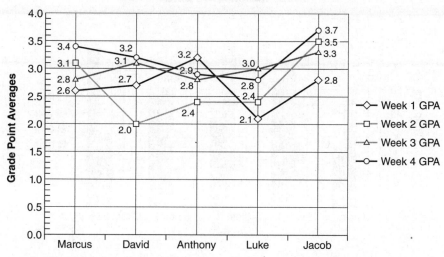

April Grade Point Averages

1. How many data points are on the chart?

   (A) 9
   (B) 14
   (C) 20
   (D) 29

2. Which of the children had the highest GPA in the third week?

   (A) Anthony
   (B) David
   (C) Jacob
   (D) Luke

3. Which of the children had the highest GPA for the entire month of April?

   (A) Anthony
   (B) David
   (C) Jacob
   (D) Luke

Rocky Point Candy Company is preparing to introduce a new product to the mainland United States. Marketing believes buyers of candy are influenced by the color of the candy wrapper, and suggests that a colored wrapper be used. Research supports Marketing's viewpoints, but suggests a study to determine if one color wrapper is more likely to sell the product than another color wrapper. Five states are selected and the new product is made available in each packaging color (red, yellow, green, and blue). The chart below provides information about the study.

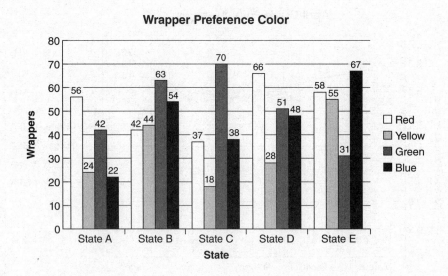

4. What category had the lowest wrapper color preference?

(A) State A
(B) State B
(C) State C
(D) State D

5. In what category did the blue wrapper receive the greatest preference?

(A) State B
(B) State C
(C) State D
(D) State E

6. If you were an employee of Rocky Point Candy Company, what color wrapper would you select for State A?

(A) Red
(B) Yellow
(C) Green
(D) Blue

Graphs and Charts Sample Test Answer Key

1. **C**
2. **C**
3. **C**
4. **C**
5. **D**
6. **A**

GRAPHS AND CHARTS SAMPLE TEST ANSWERS EXPLAINED

1. **(C)** Data points are information regarding what is being addressed—in this case, the grade point averages for the month of April. There are five children whose names appear on the horizontal axis of the chart. The children (five in total) each have one data point for each week (four in total). Five children multiplied by four data points each is equal to 20 data points.

2. **(C)** The third week on the chart is represented by the symbol of a triangle. Tracking the triangle symbol across the chart reveals that Marcus had a 2.8 grade point average, David had a 3.1 GPA, Anthony had a 2.8 GPA, Luke had a 3.0 GPA, and Jacob had the highest GPA of 3.3 during the third week. You must pay attention to what you are being asked as well as how the information on the chart is presented.

3. **(C)** There are a number of ways to determine a correct response. The first, and most time-consuming, is to manually figure out each boy's grade point average for the month, and Jacob clearly has the highest with a 3.3. Another method that requires critical thinking is to "eyeball" each boy's grade point averages and make a determination. With this method, Marcus has grade point averages of 3.4, 3.1, 2.8, and 2.6. David has grade point averages of 3.1, 3.2, 2.7, and 2.0. Anthony has grade point averages of 3.2, 2.9, 2.8, and 2.4. Luke has grade point averages of 3.0, 2.8, 2.4, and 2.1. Looking at the numbers, Marcus, David, Anthony, and Luke will have their grade point average in the 2.0 to 3.0 point range. Jacob's averages for the month are 3.7, 3.5, 3.3, and 2.8. His grade point average for the month will be the highest. He has three weeks where his averages were above 3.0 and one week with a 2.8. He has had grade point averages higher than most of his brothers for three of the four weeks. He must have the highest grade point average for the month.

4. **(C)** Determining the correct response requires looking at each of the five categories and selecting the one with the lowest preference. The question doesn't ask for the color of the wrapper, just the lowest preference of wrappers.

5. **(D)** Again looking at all five categories, where does the blue wrapper have the greatest preference? The greatest number of blue wrappers is found in State E.

6. **(A)** Based on the study findings, the preferred color is red in State A. Therefore, it makes the most sense to give the people what they want, in this case a red color wrapper.

Now, take the Numerical Ability test that follows to review everything that you learned in this chapter.

ANSWER SHEET
Numerical Ability Sample Test

1. Ⓐ Ⓑ Ⓒ Ⓓ
2. Ⓐ Ⓑ Ⓒ Ⓓ
3. Ⓐ Ⓑ Ⓒ Ⓓ
4. Ⓐ Ⓑ Ⓒ Ⓓ
5. Ⓐ Ⓑ Ⓒ Ⓓ
6. Ⓐ Ⓑ Ⓒ Ⓓ
7. Ⓐ Ⓑ Ⓒ Ⓓ
8. Ⓐ Ⓑ Ⓒ Ⓓ
9. Ⓐ Ⓑ Ⓒ Ⓓ

10. Ⓐ Ⓑ Ⓒ Ⓓ
11. Ⓐ Ⓑ Ⓒ Ⓓ
12. Ⓐ Ⓑ Ⓒ Ⓓ
13. Ⓐ Ⓑ Ⓒ Ⓓ
14. Ⓐ Ⓑ Ⓒ Ⓓ
15. Ⓐ Ⓑ Ⓒ Ⓓ
16. Ⓐ Ⓑ Ⓒ Ⓓ
17. Ⓐ Ⓑ Ⓒ Ⓓ
18. Ⓐ Ⓑ Ⓒ Ⓓ

19. Ⓐ Ⓑ Ⓒ Ⓓ
20. Ⓐ Ⓑ Ⓒ Ⓓ
21. Ⓐ Ⓑ Ⓒ Ⓓ
22. Ⓐ Ⓑ Ⓒ Ⓓ
23. Ⓐ Ⓑ Ⓒ Ⓓ
24. Ⓐ Ⓑ Ⓒ Ⓓ
25. Ⓐ Ⓑ Ⓒ Ⓓ

> **Directions:** For each question, select the letter (A, B, C, or D) that best corresponds to your answer. Record your answers on the answer sheet on page 181.

1. A cooking class is baking cookies for the annual county bazaar. Recipes A and C each yield 4 dozen cookies and require two eggs per recipe. Recipe B yields 2 dozen cookies and requires one egg per recipe. One-fifth of the total dozen of cookies will be Recipe A; two-fifths of the total dozen will be Recipe B; and 20 dozen cookies will be Recipe C. What is the total number of eggs needed to make cookies for the bazaar?

   (A) 5 eggs   CHALLENGE
   (B) 12 eggs
   (C) 16 eggs
   (D) 25 eggs

2. Sarah and Rachael are sisters. Rachael is younger than Sarah by 3 years. Sarah is 5 years older than her brother, Tom, who was born in 1996. In what years were Rachael and Sarah born?

   (A) Sarah was born in 2001;   CHALLENGE
   Rachael was born in 1998.
   (B) Sarah was born in 2005; Rachael was born in 2003.
   (C) Sarah was born in 1999; Rachael was born in 1996.
   (D) Sarah was born in 1991; Rachael was born in 1994.

3. Directions on your bottle of cough syrup read: "Take 15 ml every six hours as needed for cough." How many teaspoons (tsp) of cough medicine will you take for your cough?

   (A) 3 tsp
   (B) 9 tsp
   (C) 12 tsp
   (D) 15 tsp

4. A discount store has a video game for $76.95. A retail store has the same game for $99.00 with a 20% markdown at checkout. Which store is offering the best buy?

   (A) The retail store has better price savings by $19.80.
   (B) The discount store has better price savings by $2.25.
   (C) The retail store has a better price of $6.95.
   (D) With the retail store discount, the price is the same at both stores.

5. A map has a scale of 1 inch = 75 miles. Donnerville and Wright's Point are $5\frac{3}{4}$ inches apart. What is the distance, in miles, between the two locations?

   (A) 370.40 miles
   (B) 355.35 miles
   (C) 450.07 miles
   (D) 431.25 miles

6. Glynnis has $45.00 for the purchase of a lamp. She finds a lamp with a price tag of $69.99 marked 25% off today only. Sales tax is 6.788%. Does Glynnis have enough money to make the purchase?

   (A) No, Glynnis needs $3.05 to purchase the lamp.
   (B) Yes, Glynnis will have one cent remaining after the lamp purchase.
   (C) No, Glynnis needs $11.05 to purchase the lamp.
   (D) Yes, Glynnis will have $13.94 remaining after the lamp purchase.

7. Tuition at a community college increased from $55.00 to $62.00 per semester hour. What is the percentage of increase?

   (A) 1.13%
   (B) 7.0%
   (C) 8.87%
   (D) 12.73%

8. A nurse has gauze to dress 3 wounds. He has a length of gauze 5 feet long that needs to be cut into three pieces with two of the three pieces 2 inches longer than the remaining piece. Determine the appropriate lengths of the three pieces.

   (A) 1 length = 10 inches; 2 lengths = 25 inches each

   CHALLENGE

   (B) 1 length = 18.7 inches; 2 lengths = 20.7 inches each
   (C) 1 length = 20.0 inches; 2 lengths = 22.0 inches each
   (D) 1 length = 26 inches; 2 lengths = 28 inches each

9. A large photograph measuring 12 inches in length and 8 inches in width needs to be reduced so the length will be 8 inches. Determine the width of the photograph when reduced.

   (A) $5\frac{1}{3}$ inches
   (B) 4 inches
   (C) $3\frac{1}{3}$ inches
   (D) 2 inches

10. Two runners start running toward each other from different points in the county at the same time. The two points are 34 miles apart. Runner A averages 3 miles per hour and reaches the meeting point in 5 hours. Runner B misses a turn and runs 10 extra miles. What distance did each runner cover?

    (A) Runner A runs 15 miles; Runner B runs 19 miles.
    (B) Runner A runs 15 miles; Runner B runs 29 miles.
    (C) Runner A runs 11.3 miles; Runner B runs 22.7 miles.
    (D) Runner A runs 11.3 miles; Runner B runs 32.7 miles.

11. The ratio of concentrated liquid hair color to the mixing agent is 2:5. If 3 ounces of hair color are in the package, how many ounces of the mixing agent are needed to prepare the hair coloring solution?

    (A) 4 ounces
    (B) 7.5 ounces
    (C) 10 ounces
    (D) 15.6 ounces

12. A student wants to know what grade he needs to get on the final exam to achieve a grade of 80% in a course. His grade on the first exam was 65%, second exam was 85%, and third exam was 77%. The first three exams are each worth 20% of the overall grade with the final exam worth 40%. What grade does the student need to get on the final exam to achieve a grade of 80% in the course?

    (A) 54.6%
    (B) 75.6%
    (C) 80.0%
    (D) 86.5%

13. A farmer needs to buy chicken wire for a coop he is building for his pigeons. The front, floor, and roof of the coop will be wood with the remaining three sides (2 long sides and 1 short side) in chicken wire. The length of the coop is 15 feet, with the width and height each 10 feet. Rolls of chicken wire are 5 feet in height and 100 feet in length. What length of chicken wire does the farmer need to purchase for his pigeon coop?

(A) 20 feet
(B) 40 feet
(C) 80 feet
(D) 100 feet

CHALLENGE

14. An ancient statue is insured for 90% of its value. The statue has a value of $100,000. The annual premium rate is $20.00 per $1,000 of value. What is the annual premium for the statue?

(A) $20,000
(B) $9,000
(C) $4,500
(D) $1,800

15. Martin is planning to paint the surface area of a rectangular solid. Side one is 3 inches by 4 inches, side two is 3 inches by 5 inches, and side three is 4 inches by 4 inches. Determine the total number of square (sq) inches to be painted.

(A) 23 square inches
(B) 43 square inches
(C) 86 square inches
(D) 196 square inches

CHALLENGE

16. The physician ordered Demerol 45 milligrams (mg) intramuscularly (IM) every 6 hours (hr) for pain. The medication label reads 75 mg/ mL. How many milliliters (mL) will the nurse administer to the patient?

(A) 2 mL
(B) 1 mL
(C) 0.7 mL
(D) 0.6 mL

17. The medication label reads Zantac 150 milligrams (mg) per tablet. The patient's order is written for 0.3 grams (gm) by mouth (PO) daily. How many tablets will the nurse administer to the patient?

(A) $\frac{1}{2}$ tablet
(B) 1.5 tablets
(C) 2 tablets
(D) 2.5 tablets

18. A patient is to receive Heparin 15,000 units. The medication is available as 25,000 units/ mL. How many milliliters (mL) of Heparin will the patient receive?

(A) 0.45 mL
(B) 0.5 mL
(C) 0.56 mL
(D) 0.6 mL

CHALLENGE

19. The nurse is starting an intravenous (IV) on a patient who is to receive sodium chloride 1,000 milliliters (mL) of solution to infuse over 12 hours by IV pump. The IV will infuse at how many mL per hour? Round your answer to the nearest whole number.

(A) 83 mL/hr
(B) 82 mL/hr
(C) 80 mL/hr
(D) 79 mL/hr

20. Two trucks leave their home base traveling in opposite directions on straight, flat roads. Because of his load, the driver of the first truck drives 20 mph faster than the driver of the second truck. After six hours of driving, they are 475 miles from each other. How many miles per hour is each driving? (Round your answer for each driver to the nearest whole number.)

(A) The driver of the first truck is driving 43 mph, and the driver of the second truck is driving 36 mph.

(B) The driver of the first truck is driving 50 mph, and the driver of the second truck is driving 30 mph.

(C) The driver of the first truck is driving 70 mph, and the driver of the second truck is driving 50 mph.

(D) The driver of the first truck is driving 81 mph, and the driver of the second truck is driving 61 mph.

21. Sarah is making a quilt. She needs the following: 15 squares of red at $1.50/square, 15 squares of blue at $1.80/square, 30 squares of stripes with $\frac{2}{3}$ costing $2.00/square and the remainder costing $3.00/square. Batting costs $22.50, and 2 yards of backing material is $8.50/yd. The tax rate is 9.875%. What will Sarah pay for her quilting supplies?

(A) $159.00
(B) $165.42
(C) $169.75
(D) $174.70

22. A physician's order reads: "Morphine gr. $\frac{1}{6}$ intramuscular every 4–6 hours as needed for pain." Available in the narcotic box is injectable Morphine in strengths of 8 mg, 10 mg, and 15 mg. Which Morphine strength is the most appropriate to select for administration?

(A) 8 mg.
(B) 10 mg.
(C) 15 mg.
(D) All three strengths are appropriate for administration.

The Ladies Aid Society of the local church is beginning preparation for its annual Charity Bazaar. The Food Subcommittee is presenting a report analyzing the Mexican dinner introduced five years ago. Dinners sell for $5.00 each including a drink. Area grocers donate everything needed for the dinner including cups, paper plates, plastic ware, and napkins. The first three years were dismal. Complaints about the quality of the food increased each year. In 2013, a new cook began preparing the Mexican dinners.

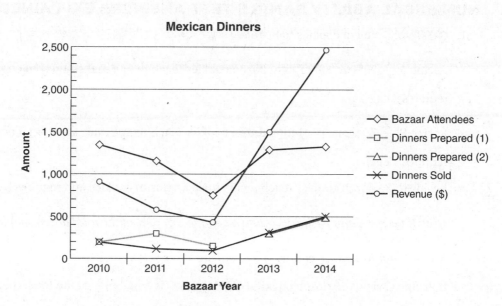

23. Which year had the lowest number of both attendees and revenue?

(A) 2010

(B) 2011

(C) 2012

(D) 2013

24. What could be the cause of the greatest surge in dinners prepared and dinners sold? In what year did this occur?

(A) Better advertising, 2011

(B) Better economy, 2014

(C) Different grocers supplying food, 2012

(D) Hiring a new cook, 2013

25. What was the approximate revenue in 2011?

(A) $500.00

(B) $600.00

(C) $700.00

(D) $800.00

Numerical Ability Sample Test Answer Key

1. **D**	6. **C**	11. **B**	16. **D**	21. **D**
2. **A**	7. **D**	12. **D**	17. **C**	22. **B**
3. **A**	8. **B**	13. **C**	18. **D**	23. **C**
4. **B**	9. **A**	14. **D**	19. **A**	24. **D**
5. **D**	10. **B**	15. **C**	20. **B**	25. **B**

NUMERICAL ABILITY SAMPLE TEST ANSWERS EXPLAINED

1. **(D)** Total dozen of cookies to be made = x

Recipe A: $\frac{1}{5}$ (20% or .20) of total dozen cookies (each recipe makes 4 dozen cookies and requires 2 eggs)

Recipe B: $\frac{2}{5}$ (40% or .40) of total dozen cookies (each recipe makes 2 dozen cookies and requires 1 egg)

Recipe C: 20 dozen cookies (each recipe makes 4 dozen cookies and requires 2 eggs)

Hint: If Recipe A and Recipe B combined equal $\frac{3}{5}$ or 60% of the total dozen cookies, Recipe C has to equal $\frac{2}{5}$ or 40% of the total dozen cookies.

If Recipe C yields 20 dozen cookies, and Recipe C is equal to $\frac{2}{5}$ of the total, then Recipe B must also yield 20 dozen cookies, since Recipe B is also equal to $\frac{2}{5}$ of the total. Recipe A is equal to the remaining $\frac{1}{5}$, or 10 dozen, cookies. Therefore, there are 50 dozen cookies total.

$x = .20x + .40x + 20$

$50 = .20(50) + .40(50) + 20$

$50 = 10 + 20 + 20$

$50 = 50$

Recipe A: 10 dozen cookies $= \frac{10}{4} = 2.5$ recipes $\times$ 2 eggs = 5 eggs

Recipe B: 20 dozen cookies $= \frac{20}{2} = 10$ recipes $\times$ 1 egg = 10 eggs

Recipe C: 20 dozen cookies $= \frac{20}{4} = 5$ recipes $\times$ 2 eggs = 10 eggs

Total eggs needed = 5 eggs + 10 eggs + 10 eggs = 25 eggs

2. **(A)**

Name	Age (yrs)	Year Cal.	Year Born
Sarah	$x + 5$	$1996 + 5$	2001
Rachael	$(x + 5) - 3$	$2001 - 3$	1998
Tom			$x = 1996$

3. **(A)** 1 tsp = 5 ml

x = teaspoons of cough syrup to administer

1 tsp : 5 ml = x tsp : 15 ml

$x = 3$ tsp

4. **(B)** Discount store price = $76.95

Retail store price = $99.00 with 20% discount at checkout

$99.00 \times 20\% = 99 \times .20 = \$19.80$

$99.00 - \$19.80 = \$79.20$

$79.20 - \$76.95 = \$2.25$

5. **(D)** 1 inch = 75 miles

x = distance in miles between locations

$5\frac{3}{4}$ inches = measured distance from Donnerville to Wright's Point

1 inch : 75 miles = 5.75 inches : x miles

$x = 431.25$ miles

6. **(C)** <u>Amount</u> of money Glynnis has to spend = $45.00

Price of lamp = $69.99

Sale price of lamp = $52.49

Sale mark down = 25% or ($17.50)

Sales tax = 6.788% or ($3.56)

Total cost = [Sale price of lamp] + Sales tax

Total cost of lamp = $56.05

Cost of lamp – Amount Glynnis has to spend = $56.05 – $45.00 = $11.05

Glynnis does not have enough money for the purchase.

7. **(D)** Original tuition = $55.00 per semester hour

New tuition = $62.00 per semester hour

New tuition – Original tuition = $62.00 – $55.00 = $7.00 increase in tuition

$\dfrac{\text{Increase in tuition}}{\text{Original tuition}} = \dfrac{7}{55} = 12.727 = 12.73\%$ increase in tuition

8. **(B)** Length of gauze = 5 feet or 60 inches

Length of one shorter piece in inches = x inches

Lengths of two longer pieces in feet or inches = $2(x + 2 \text{ inches})$

$x + 2(x + 2 \text{ inches}) = 60 \text{ inches}$

$x + 2x + 4 = 60$

$3x + 4 = 60$

$3x = 56$

$x = 18.66 = 18.7$ inches

$x + 2 = 20.7$ inches

9. **(A)** <u>Original</u> photo = 12 inches by 8 inches
Reduced photo length = 8 inches
Reduced photo width = x

Original length : Original width = Reduced length : Reduced width
$$12 : 8 = 8 : x$$
$$12x = 64$$
$$x = 5.33 \text{ inches}$$

10. **(B)** Distance between 2 points = 34 miles
Runner A average rate = 3 mph
Runner A time = 5 hr
Runner A distance = D_A
Runner B distance = D_B

Runner A : $D_A = R \cdot T$ Runner B: $D_B = 34 - D_A + 10$
$\qquad\quad D_A = 3 \cdot 5$ $D_B = 29$ miles
$\qquad\quad D_A = 15$ miles

11. **(B)** <u>Hair</u> color = 2 parts
Mixing agent = 5 parts
Hair color in package = 3 ounces
Ounces of mixing agent needed = x

2 parts : 3 ounces = 5 parts : x ounces
$$x = 7.5 \text{ ounces}$$

12. **(D)** Exam 1 = 65%
Exam 2 = 85%
Exam 3 = 77%
Weight of each exam = 20%
Weight of final exam = 40%
Final exam grade = x

(*Exam* 1 · 20%) + (*Exam* 2 · 20%) + (*Exam* 3 · 20%) + (x · 40%) = 80%
$$x = 86.5\%$$

13. **(C)** Draw a diagram to help solve the problem.
<u>Length of each</u> long <u>side</u> = 15 feet
Width of one short side = 10 feet
Height = 10 feet
Roll of chicken wire = 100 feet by 5 feet
$x = (P \cdot 2)$ = Length of chicken wire

Perimeter = 2(length) + width
$\qquad$ P = 2(15) +10
$\qquad$ P = 40 feet

$x = P \cdot 2 = 40 \cdot 2 = 80$ feet

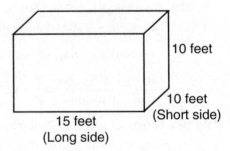

10 feet

10 feet
(Short side)

15 feet
(Long side)

14. **(D)** Value of statue = $100, 000

Insured value = 90%

Annual premium rate = $20.00/$1,000

x = annual premium

$100,000 \cdot 90\% = \$90,000.00$

$\$20.00 : \$1,000.00 = x : \$90,000.00$

$1,000x = 1,800,000$

$x = \$1,800$

15. **(C)** $lw = 3 \text{ in} \times 4 \text{ in}$

$wh = 5 \text{ in} \times 3 \text{ in}$

$lh = 4 \text{ in} \times 4 \text{ in}$

$SA = (lw)(2) + (wh)(2) + (lh)(2)$

$SA = (3)(4)(2) + (5)(3)(2) + (4)(4)(2)$

$SA = 24 + 30 + 32$

$SA = 86$ square inches to be painted

16. **(D)** $\dfrac{\text{Desired} \times \text{Volume}}{\text{Available}} = \text{mL per dose}$

$\dfrac{45 \text{ mg} \times 1 \text{ mL}}{75 \text{ mg}} = 0.6 \text{ mL}$

17. **(C)** Convert 0.3 gm to mg

mg means "milligram;" 0.3 gm = 300 mg

$\dfrac{\text{Desired} \times \text{Volume}}{\text{Available}} = \text{mL per dose}$

$\dfrac{300 \text{ mg} \times 1 \text{ tab}}{150 \text{ mg}} = 2 \text{ tablets}$

18. **(D)** $\dfrac{\text{Desired} \times \text{Volume}}{\text{Available}} = \text{mL per dose}$

$\dfrac{15,000 \text{ units} \times 1 \text{ mL}}{25,000 \text{ units}} = 0.6 \text{ mL}$

19. **(A)** Sodium chloride IV solution 1,000 mL to infuse over 12 hours. The IV will infuse by IV pump. The rate will be set by the nurse.

$\dfrac{1,000 \text{ mL}}{12 \text{ hr}} = 83.3 \text{ mL}$

20. **(B)**

Driver	Rate	Time	Distance
#1	$R + 20$	6	475
#2	R	6	475

Time (Rate) + Time (Rate + 20) = Distance

$6R + 6(R + 20) = 475$

$6R + 6R + 120 = 475$

$12R + 120 = 475$

$12R = 355$

$R = 29.58$ mph ≈ 30 mph

$R + 20 = 49.58 \approx 50$ mph

21. **(D)**

Red = 15($1.50)   Blue = 15 ($1.80)

Stripes = 20($2.00) & 10($3.00)   Batting = $22.50

Backing = 2($8.50)   Tax = 9.875% = 0.09875

$[15(1.50) + 15(1.80) + 20(2.00) + 10(3.00) + 22.50 + 2(8.50)] \times 0.09875 =$

$[22.50 + 27.00 + 40.00 + 30.00 + 22.50 + 17.00] \times 0.09875 =$

$159 \times 0.09875 = 15.70$

$\$159.00 + \$15.70 = \$174.70$

22. **(B)** gr. $\dfrac{1}{6}$ = 10 mg. Eight milligrams is less than the amount ordered, 15 mg is more than the amount ordered and requires wasting medication. The patient would pay for 15 mg of morphine while only receiving 10 mg.

$1 \, gr = 60 \, mg :: \dfrac{1}{6} gr = x \, mg$

$x = \left(\dfrac{60}{6}\right) = 10 \, mg$

23. **(C)** The year with the lowest number of attendees and revenue was 2012. This was also the last year that the original cook worked on the meals. These results were likely why a new cook was brought in in 2013.

24. **(D)** The greatest surge occurred in 2013 when the new cook was hired. The passage and graph do not support choices A, B, or C.

25. **(B)** Based on the graph, the approximate revenue in 2011 was $600.00. Be sure to read what the question is asking for, in this case revenue in 2011.

Science

6

How do you feel about having to take science courses? It can be difficult at times to try to figure out why science courses are needed. As a college student with a definite career choice in mind, science courses should seem more sensible. Can you envision a modern nurse who knows nothing about science?

Let's step back and look at you specifically. How did you do in your high school science courses? How did you do in the prerequisite science courses needed for the nursing entrance exam of your selected nursing program? If you have weaknesses in these courses, there is the potential you may have difficulties with the science section of the entrance exam. It's also a red flag that you may have difficulties when studying disease processes and their pathophysiology in your nursing courses. If you have weaknesses, a thorough review is imperative! This means going back to your course textbook, class notes, and handouts.

This chapter reviews biology, chemistry, and anatomy and physiology. Biology and chemistry set the stage and provide a foundation for anatomy and physiology. The foundation for pathophysiology that you will study in your nursing courses is also set by anatomy and physiology. These courses provide a foundation for pharmacology. Nursing is built upon knowledge from all of these and more.

In preparation for your science review, it is important to remember that biology, chemistry, anatomy, and physiology are stand-alone disciplines. It is beyond the scope of this book to cover every detail of each of these disciplines.

It is also beyond the scope of this book to cover every detail of what was covered in your prerequisite courses. There are, perhaps, hundreds of biology, chemistry, and anatomy and physiology textbooks available, and colleges do not all use the same books. Some colleges have specific science courses for nursing majors. These courses have a different focus than the non-nursing science courses.

So, how do you prepare for the science section of your nursing entrance test? First, have faith you can successfully complete the science review. Second, do not be overwhelmed by the amount of material covered in the review. You've taken the courses, and you should have a fair to strong command of the information. Third, you have the materials you need—this review book, a medical dictionary, your textbooks from courses covered in the review, and your notes and handouts from your prerequisite courses. Lastly, use study suggestions presented earlier in this book or, if you have a proven study method, use it.

This chapter is divided into sections. Biology and chemistry comprise one section. Each body system in anatomy and physiology has its own section. Each section in the chapter has its own exam with answers. This material is lengthy and may take you extra time to read and review. Be sure to look up words you're not sure of. Use your course textbooks, and make sure you understand each concept before continuing your review.

NOTE: You'll notice in the sample test answers explained that follow each sample test that some explanations require more detail than others. Questions where the stem and correct answer provide the information do not have detailed explanations. Instead, we have advised which sections in the book you should review again if you missed that question. An example of this type of question may ask where the spleen is located. More in-depth explanations are provided for questions that may require higher levels of critical thinking or may be areas where individuals typically have more questions. An example of this type of question could ask you to differentiate between types of immunity.

As with earlier chapters, answer sheets, tests, and answer explanations follow the biology/chemistry section and each section of anatomy and physiology. Tests in this chapter are not timed. Even so, you need to realize that if you cannot determine the correct answer in one minute, you may have weaknesses in the content area and need more review.

As you review, remember to have faith in yourself that you will be successful in your endeavors. You've successfully completed your science courses. Now strengthen your knowledge base!

OVERVIEW

- Biology is a science that seeks to understand the activities of living things. It may be referred to as the science of life.
- Basic biological concepts:
  1. Metabolism
  2. Homeostasis
  3. Adaptation
- Sciences, including biology, are dynamic and ever expanding as new discoveries come in from research centers around the world.
  - From the perspective of health care professionals, biology is one small phase of professional preparation.

THE SCIENTIFIC METHOD

- An **organized** group of techniques for investigating phenomena, acquiring new knowledge, or correcting and integrating previous knowledge
  - A way to ask and answer **scientific** questions by making observations and performing experiments
- Follows defined steps or processes, including:
  1. Ask a question.
  2. Complete background research of **scientific** literature.
  3. Develop a hypothesis.
  4. Test your hypothesis by performing **scientific** experimentation.
  5. Analyze your data and draw a conclusion based on **facts**.
  6. Communicate your results in a **scientific** fashion.

BASIC BIOLOGICAL CONCEPTS

- Adaptation
  - The **modification** of an organism, or one or more of its parts, that makes it more fit for existence under the conditions of its environment
- Homeostasis
  - A tendency toward a stable state between different, but interdependent elements or groups of elements of an organism, population, or group
- Metabolism
  - A highly integrated network of chemical reactions by which living cells grow and sustain themselves
- Pathways
  - **Anabolism** uses energy stored in the form of adenosine triphosphate (ATP) to build larger molecules from smaller molecules.
  - **Catabolic** reactions degrade larger molecules in order to produce ATP and raw materials for anabolic reactions.

CHARACTERISTICS OF LIVING MATTER

- Overview
  - There is no prevailing definition of life because it is impossible to define life in a few sentences or paragraphs.
  - For each definition created, there are exceptions to be found.
  - **Life is best defined in terms of the functions performed by all living things.**
  - Functions necessary for life are not necessarily the same for each kind of organism.
  - Consider how the human functions to survive and how the human cells function to survive.
- Life functions
  - **To sustain life, all living organisms must be able to competently carry out biochemical and biophysical activities.**
  - Nutrition
    - ➤ Nutrition, nourishment, or aliment, is the supply of materials or food required by organisms and cells to stay alive.
    - ➤ Processes included with nutrition:
      - – Ingestion: Not always an oral process
      - – Digestion: Chemical changes take place in the body
      - – Assimilation: Changing certain nutrients into the protoplasm of cells
      - – Conveyance or transport: Absorption of materials by living organisms; Active transport
    - ➤ Diffusion: Flow of molecules from areas of **higher** to **lower** concentrations
    - ➤ Circulation: **Movement** of fluid and other materials throughout the organism
  - Respiration
    - ➤ Is a complex process
    - ➤ Consists of breathing and cellular respiration
      - – Involves the taking in of a substance and the letting out of another substance
  - Excretion
    - ➤ Process of removing waste products
  - Synthesis
    - ➤ Biochemical process
    - ➤ The production of a substance by the **coming together** of chemical elements, groups, of simpler compounds or by the degradation of a complex compound where simple molecules are built larger and more complex
  - Regulation
    - ➤ Consists of all processes that control, coordinate, or adjust to numerous activities of the organism
    - ➤ Allows for adaptation to the internal or external environment
    - ➤ Growth
      - – **Coordinated, orderly growth** in cells, resulting in the growth of the organism
  - Reproduction
    - ➤ Reproduction of a new being by parent organisms
    - ➤ Highly complex process
    - ➤ Types of reproduction
      1. **Asexual** requiring a **single** parent
      2. **Sexual** requiring **two** parents
    - ➤ **Without reproduction, the species or organism becomes extinct.**

NOTE

Active transport is the movement of molecules *powered* by energy.

NATURE OF LIVING MATTER

- Protoplasm
  - Living matter composed of protoplasm
    - ➤ **Found only in living matter**
  - Chemical composition varies from organism to organism
    - ➤ Includes proteins, carbohydrates, lipids, water, and nucleic acids
- Growth
  - Living matter is separated from nonliving matter by its distinctive method of growth.
  - Every living thing converts food into more living matter with a consequent increase in size.
- Cellular organization
  - Living matter is usually divided into small units known as cells.
  - Cells vary in size, shape, and function, yet all have important characteristics in common.
- Cell respiration
  - Life cannot be maintained without the release of energy.
  - **Oxygen** is required for food breakdown—the term respiration is used to describe it.
- Favorable response to the environment (Adaptation)
  - Living organisms tend to respond to their environment in ways that are **advantageous** to themselves.
  - The response time and duration varies.
  - Natural selection
  - Inherited adaptations to the environment occur slowly over time.
  - Adaptations are necessary for survival.
- Overproduction of offspring
  - All living organisms produce more offspring than are necessary to replace the parents if all should live.
- Inherited variation within a species
  - All members of one species that are living in one region generally have similar characteristics.
- Struggle for survival
  - Organisms may compete with their surrounding environment, or other organisms, for survival.
- Survival of the fittest
  - Among many species, only the strong survive.
- Reproduction
  - It is necessary because living organisms do not live indefinitely.

CHEMICAL BACKGROUND OF LIVING MATTER

- The nature of matter
  - Anything that has weight and occupies space
  - May be a gas, liquid, or solid
  - Gases
    - ➤ Considered fluids
    - ➤ Have high kinetic energy
    - ➤ Have no definite shape

- ➤ Have no definite volume
- ➤ Volume depends upon the size of the container
- ➤ Examples: hydrogen, methane, nitrogen, oxygen
  - ○ Liquids
    - ➤ They can take the shape of any container they're placed in.
    - ➤ Volume always remains constant.
    - ➤ Examples: metal mercury, nonmetal bromine, glass
  - ○ Solids
    - ➤ Maintain shape
    - ➤ Occupy volume
    - ➤ Have identifying density
    - ➤ Cannot be forced into a smaller space
    - ➤ Do not increase under pressure
    - ➤ Examples: metals (except mercury), nonmetals, carbon, phosphorus, sulfur
  - ○ May change from one state to another as conditions change
  - ○ The state in which matter exists depends upon the moving speed of the molecules it composes.
- ■ Divisions of matter
  - ○ Elements
    - ➤ The simplest form of matter that cannot be changed further by chemical or physical methods
    - ➤ Cannot be broken down into two or more different kinds of atoms
    - ➤ Examples: iron, sulfur, oxygen, iodine, calcium
  - ○ Compounds
    - ➤ Formed by a combination of two or more elements which are chemically united
    - ➤ Examples: water, glucose, alcohol, salt, ethanol, acetic acid, butane, methane, baking soda, citric acid, camphor, octane
  - ○ Mixtures
    - ➤ Combinations of different elements or compounds in which there is little, if any, chemical union of the combined parts
    - ➤ Solutions
      - – **Homogeneous** mixtures
      - – A mixture of two or more substances in a single phase
      - – At least two substances must be mixed in order to have a solution.
      - – The substance that makes up the smallest amount, and the one that dissolves or disperses, is called the **solute**.
      - – The substance that makes up the larger amount is called the **solvent**.
      - – In most common instances, **water** is the solvent. The gases, liquids, or solids dissolved in water are the solutes.
      - – Examples: beer, wine, vinegar, saline solution, sugar solution, hard water, carbonated water, ammonia solution, water in air, smog
    - ➤ Suspensions
      - – Mixtures where the particles are heavy enough to settle out of solution, scatter light, and can be filtered
      - – Examples: snow globe, Italian salad dressing

All matter in the universe may be divided into elements, compounds, and mixtures.

▸ Colloids
  – Mixtures with particle sizes that consist of clumps of molecules with dimensions between 2 and 1,000 nanometers.
  – Appear homogeneous to the naked eye
  – Frequently appear "murky" or "opaque"
  – Particles are large enough to scatter light
  – Generally do separate on standing
  – Not separated by filtration
  – Examples: fog, milk
■ Acids and Bases
  ○ Groups of compounds that react with each other to form a third type of compound salt
    ▸ Acids and bases are opposites.
  ○ Salts are ionic compounds produced by the reaction of an acid with a base.
    ▸ Examples: sodium chloride (table salt), calcium chloride
  ○ Acids
    ▸ Release hydrogen ions in water solutions
    ▸ Sour like lemons or limes
    ▸ Burn to the touch
    ▸ Turn litmus paper red
    ▸ React with metals to release hydrogen gas
    ▸ React with carbonates to release carbon dioxide gas
  ○ Bases
    ▸ Accept hydrogen atoms
    ▸ Bitter like baking soda
    ▸ Slippery like soap
    ▸ Turn litmus paper blue
    ▸ Do not react with metals
    ▸ Do not react with carbonates
  ○ pH
    ▸ A lower amount of hydrogen ions = a higher amount of hydroxyl ions.
    ▸ pH of 0 to 6.9 have a greater amount of hydrogen ions and a lower amount of hydroxyl ions.
    ▸ pH of 7.0 has an equal amount of hydrogen and hydroxyl ions.
    ▸ pH of 7.1 to 14.0 have a lower amount of hydrogen ions and a higher amount of hydroxyl ions.

CELLS—BASIC UNITS OF LIVING MATTER

■ Cell Concepts
  ○ **Living matter is generally organized into units known as cells**.
    ▸ Unicellular organisms are composed of one cell.
    ▸ Multicellular organisms are composed of numerous, specialized cells.
  ○ Unit of structure
    ▸ Cells provide structure and form to an organism.
    ▸ Cells assume varied shapes and sizes as they become specialized to perform specific duties.

- Unit of function
  - ➤ Each cell is a living unit, a biological chemical factory.
  - ➤ Each cell provides for repair of tissues, growth, energy, and reproduction.
- Unit of Growth
  - ➤ All living organisms begin life as a single cell.
  - ➤ Multicellular organisms have a single cell that grows to a certain size and then divides and redivides.
  - ➤ As the number of cells increases, the size of the organism increases.
- Unit of heredity
  - ➤ Dividing cells produce identical cells.
  - ➤ Cells carry hereditary information that is passed on when cells divide. Hereditary information is passed along from generation to generation.
  - ➤ Information is coded in molecules of DNA.
- Parts of a cell (see Figure 6.1)

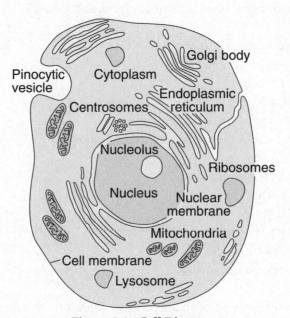

Figure 6.1. Cell Diagram

- Cellular reproduction
  - ➤ The cell cycle consists of four repeating phases.
    - – M (mitosis) phase
    - – G (gap) –1 phase
    - – S (synthesis) phase
    - – G (gap) –2 phase
  - ➤ Mitosis is the process by which cells become duplicated. (see Figure 6.2)

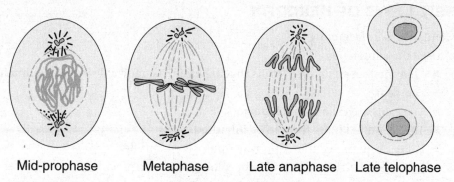

Mid-prophase   Metaphase   Late anaphase   Late telophase

Figure 6.2. Mitosis

➤ Meiosis is a special type of mitosis in which the chromosome number is halved. (see Figure 6.3)

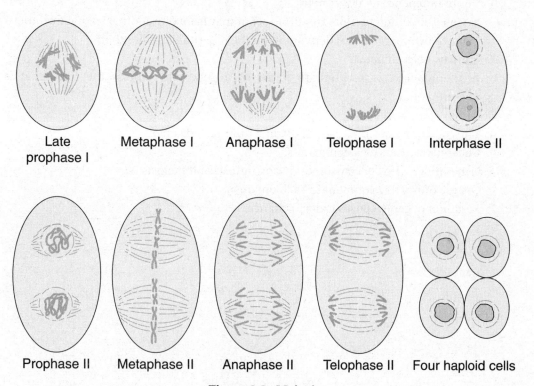

Late prophase I   Metaphase I   Anaphase I   Telophase I   Interphase II

Prophase II   Metaphase II   Anaphase II   Telophase II   Four haploid cells

Figure 6.3. Meiosis

○ Cellular respiration
  ➤ Anaerobic respiration (Glycolysis)
    – Does not require oxygen to carry on respiration
    – Takes place in the cytoplasm of cells
  ➤ Aerobic respiration (Krebs citric acid cycle)
    – Requires free oxygen to maintain life processes
    – Takes place inside the mitochondria of the cell

CLASSIC LAWS OF HEREDITY

- Mendel's Laws of Heredity
  - Used the garden pea
    - Identified seven different traits that are easily recognizable in self-pollinating garden peas
    - The traits are called unit characters.
    - The identified traits seem to be inherited.
    - For each identified trait, opposite traits were identified.
    - Examples: height (short and tall), color (yellow and green)
- Laws of Heredity
  - Law of Segregation
    - Each inherited trait is defined by a gene pair.
    - Parental genes are randomly separated to the sex cells so that sex cells contain only one gene of the pair. Offspring inherit one genetic allele from each parent when sex cells unite in fertilization.
  - Law of Independent Assortment
    - Genes for different traits are sorted separately from one another so that the inheritance of one trait is not dependent on the inheritance of another.
  - The Law of Dominance
    - An organism with alternate forms of a gene will express the form that is dominant.
- Genes
  - Chromosomes are composed of distinct units called genes.
  - Genes are carriers of specific traits.
  - Genes move with chromosomes during mitosis and meiosis.
  - Genes control development in each organism.
  - Mutation of genes causes traits to change.

OVERVIEW

- Chemistry is a physical science that studies the composition, properties, and reactions of substances.
- Everything is either matter or energy.
  - **Energy is the ability to do work.**
  - Matter is defined by physical characteristics of mass and volume.

MASS AND WEIGHT

- Mass is the amount of matter in an object.
  - Kilogram is the basic unit of mass.
  - Mass can be measured.
- Weight is a measure of the pull or acceleration of gravity on an object's mass.
  - The mass of an object does not change.

VOLUME

- The space an object occupies
- Measured in dimensions of length, height, and width

DENSITY

- Amount of matter in a given space
- Can be used to identify genuine solid or liquid substances

ATOMIC THEORY

- Atoms
  - Essentially made of matter
  - Smallest particle into which a chemical element can be divided and still retain its unique properties
  - Consists of a central nucleus composed of protons and neutrons
    - ➤ Protons and neutrons break down into quarks.
    - ➤ Atoms are encircled by one or more electrons.

CHEMICAL REACTIONS

- Occur when atoms **rearrange** for new substances
  - Matter is neither created nor destroyed during the reaction.
  - Only involves valence of electrons
  - Requires energy
- Chemical change results in the formation of a new substance
  - Energy is needed for the reaction to take place.
  - Chemical change may absorb or release energy, usually a heat.
- Signs of chemical reaction
  - Release of light energy
  - Formation of gas

- o Change in pH
- o Change in odor
- o Formation of a precipitate
- o Change in color
- o Change in temperature

PERIODIC TABLE OF ELEMENTS

- An arrangement, usually in table format, of the chemical elements
  - o Organized on the basis of their atomic number (number of protons in the nucleus), electron configurations, and recurring chemical properties
  - o The standard form of the table consists of a grid of elements laid out in 18 columns and 7 rows, with a double row of elements below.
- Groups and Families
  - o Group 1, family of alkali metals
  - o Group 2, family of alkaline earth metals
  - o Groups 3–12, family of transition metals
  - o Groups 13–16, family of mixed groups
  - o Group 17, family of halogens
  - o Group 18, family of noble gasses
  - o Rare earth metals
    - ➤ Lanthanides (elements 57–70)
    - ➤ Actinides (elements 89–102)

ANSWER SHEET
Biology/Chemistry Sample Test

1. Ⓐ Ⓑ Ⓒ Ⓓ
2. Ⓐ Ⓑ Ⓒ Ⓓ
3. Ⓐ Ⓑ Ⓒ Ⓓ
4. Ⓐ Ⓑ Ⓒ Ⓓ
5. Ⓐ Ⓑ Ⓒ Ⓓ
6. Ⓐ Ⓑ Ⓒ Ⓓ
7. Ⓐ Ⓑ Ⓒ Ⓓ

8. Ⓐ Ⓑ Ⓒ Ⓓ
9. Ⓐ Ⓑ Ⓒ Ⓓ
10. Ⓐ Ⓑ Ⓒ Ⓓ
11. Ⓐ Ⓑ Ⓒ Ⓓ
12. Ⓐ Ⓑ Ⓒ Ⓓ
13. Ⓐ Ⓑ Ⓒ Ⓓ
14. Ⓐ Ⓑ Ⓒ Ⓓ

15. Ⓐ Ⓑ Ⓒ Ⓓ
16. Ⓐ Ⓑ Ⓒ Ⓓ
17. Ⓐ Ⓑ Ⓒ Ⓓ
18. Ⓐ Ⓑ Ⓒ Ⓓ
19. Ⓐ Ⓑ Ⓒ Ⓓ
20. Ⓐ Ⓑ Ⓒ Ⓓ

For Questions 1–20, select the letter (A, B, C, or D) that best answers the question. Record your answers on the Biology/Chemistry Sample Test Answer Sheet on page 205.

1. Which of the following mature blood cells does not have a nuclei and dies without undergoing replication?

   (A) erythrocytes
   (B) hemoglobin
   (C) leukocytes
   (D) plasma proteins

2. Chemical reactions require

   (A) atoms.
   (B) energy.
   (C) heat.
   (D) valence neutrons.

3. A neutral substance has a pH of

   (A) 6.5
   (B) 7.0
   (C) 7.5
   (D) 8.0

4. A weather inversion

   (A) is more likely to form when temperatures are in excess of 80 degrees.
   (B) is the catalyst for ground-level ozone formation.
   (C) releases particles that have the ability to cause an explosion.
   (D) traps cooler, denser air below warmer, less dense air.

5. Chromosomes composed of distinct units are called

   (A) complex carbohydrates.
   (B) genes.
   (C) organic catalysts.
   (D) substrates.

6. All of the following are units of cell life EXCEPT

   (A) function.
   (B) growth.
   (C) membrane.
   (D) structure.

7. The "powerhouse" of a human cell is the

   (A) chloroplast.
   (B) cytoplasm.
   (C) mitochondria.
   (D) nucleus.

8. Cells are generally classified as

   (A) cellular or noncellular.
   (B) reproductive or nonreproductive.
   (C) squamous or cuboidal.
   (D) unicellular or multicellular.

9. The basic unit of mass is the

   (A) gram.
   (B) kilogram.
   (C) pound.
   (D) ounce.

10. During the prophase stage of mitosis, chromosomes do which of the following?

    (A) become shorter and thicker
    (B) move away from the equator of the cell
    (C) "overpower" the nuclear membrane
    (D) split apart

11. How many haploid nuclei are formed during the telophase II of meiosis?

    (A) 2
    (B) 4
    (C) 6
    (D) 8

12. What is the fundamental difference between mitosis and meiosis?

(A) Mitosis is the manner in which a primary sex cell splits into two, followed by the division of the parent cell into four daughter cells. Meiosis, or reduction division, occurs in primary sex cells, and the chromosome number is halved.

(B) Mitosis is the manner in which a eukaryotic cell nucleus splits into two, followed by the division of the parent cell into two daughter cells. Meiosis, or reduction division, occurs in primary sex cells, and the chromosome number is halved.

(C) Mitosis is the manner in which a noneukaryotic cell nucleus splits into four, followed by the division of the parent cell into four daughter cells. Meiosis, or reduction division, occurs in primary sex cells, and the chromosome number is doubled.

(D) Mitosis is the manner in which a cell nucleus splits into two, followed by the addition of the parent cells into four daughter cells. Meiosis, or reduction division, occurs in primary sex cells, and the chromosome number is doubled.

13. _____ transport requires heat energy within the cell to increase the frequency with which molecules move.

(A) Active
(B) Connective
(C) Diffuse
(D) Passive

14. NaCl has a _____ ratio of sodium to chloride.

(A) 1 to 1
(B) 1 to 2
(C) 2 to 1
(D) 2 to 2

15. The periodic table can best be defined as

(A) an arrangement, usually in table format, of the chemical elements.
(B) an arrangement, usually in linear format, of the chemical elements.
(C) a list of elements found only in nature.
(D) a list of elements chemically influenced by biology and chemistry.

16. All of the following are considered acids EXCEPT

(A) gastric juice.
(B) oven cleaner.
(C) sour milk.
(D) tomato juice.

17. All of the following are steps of the Scientific Method EXCEPT

(A) Analyze your data and draw a conclusion based on opinions.
(B) Ask a question.
(C) Complete background research of scientific literature.
(D) Develop a hypothesis.

18. An early scientist who worked with garden peas was

(A) Aristotle.
(B) Mendel.
(C) Linnaeus.
(D) Schwann.

19. Solids, gases, and liquids are collectively known as

(A) compounds.
(B) molecules.
(C) matter.
(D) mass.

20. In a structural formula, the line between two atoms, as with H—H, represents

(A) a double bond.
(B) a biatomic bond.
(C) a covalent bond.
(D) a relationship bond.

Biology/Chemistry Sample Test Answer Key

1.	**A**	5.	**B**	9.	**B**	13.	**D**	17. **A**
2.	**B**	6.	**C**	10.	**A**	14.	**A**	18. **B**
3.	**B**	7.	**C**	11.	**B**	15.	**A**	19. **C**
4.	**D**	8.	**D**	12.	**B**	16.	**B**	20. **C**

BIOLOGY/CHEMISTRY SAMPLE TEST ANSWERS EXPLAINED

1. **(A)** Mature erythrocytes (RBCs) do not have a nucleus and the majority of cellular organelles. This makes the best use of the cell's volume and its ability to carry hemoglobin and to transport oxygen.

2. **(B)** In most instances, chemical reactions involve a change in energy between products and reactants.

3. **(B)** A solution that has an exact pH of 7.0 is neutral (neither acidic nor alkaline). A pH of less than 7.0 is acidic. A pH above 7.0 is alkaline.

4. **(D)** Normally, air temperature decreases at a rate of 3.5°F for every 1,000 feet you climb into the atmosphere. When this normal cycle is present, air constantly flows between the warm and cool areas. During an inversion episode, temperatures increase with increasing altitude. The warm inversion layer then acts as a cap and stops atmospheric mixing.

5. **(B)** Genes are working units of heredity. They occupy a specific place (locus) on a chromosome. Humans normally have 46 chromosomes.

6. **(C)** In biology, a membrane is a thin, flexible layer of tissue, covering surfaces or dividing or attaching regions, structures, or organs of a living organism, or a semipermeable layer that confines a cell or an organelle, typically consisting of lipids and proteins. In chemistry, a membrane is a thin layer of natural or synthetic material that is pervious to substances in solution.

7. **(C)** Mitochondria are organelles in the cytoplasm of cells that produce energy for the cells to perform their various functions.

8. **(D)** Cells are the basic unit of living things. Cells are organisms. Unicellular organisms are composed of one single cell. Multicellular organisms are composed of many specialized cell types. The human body is multicellular.

9. **(B)** As a unit of mass, a kilogram is 1,000 grams or 2.2 pounds.

10. **(A)** Review the definitions of mitosis and meiosis, and their respective phases, on pages 200–201.

11. **(B)** Haploid refers to the number of chromosomes found in cells after meiosis reduction division. When four haploid nuclei are formed, each nuclei has one part of each original chromosome prior to the first meiosis.

12. **(B)** *Mitosis* is the process by which cells become duplicated whereas *meiosis* is the process by which the chromosome number is halved.

13. **(D)** Passive transport does not require the cell's chemical energy to move molecules. It does, however, depend on the heat energy within the cell to increase the frequency or rate with which molecules move.

14. **(A)** NaCl, a compound, will always have one sodium atom and one chloride atom—a 1:1 ratio. If either Na or Cl had a different number of atoms, it would no longer be NaCl.

15. **(A)** The periodic table is a tabular arrangement of the chemical elements that is organized by increasing atomic numbers that display the elements so that one may see trends in their properties.

16. **(B)** Oven cleaner is alkali and has a pH of 13. The remaining choices are acids with a pH from 0–6.

17. **(A)** Make sure to read each answer choice carefully. Choice A may seem like a correct step of the Scientific Method if you only read the first half of the choice. Part of the Scientific Method involves analyzing data and drawing conclusions, but those conclusions should be based on *facts*, not *opinions*. Choices B, C, and D are all steps of the Scientific Method.

18. **(B)** Gregor Mendel (1822–1884) was an Austrian monk and biologist whose work on heredity became the basis of today's theory of genetics. Mendel used the common garden pea in his work.

19. **(C)** Matter consists of solids, liquids, and gases. Review the properties of each on pages 197–198.

20. **(C)** Covalent bonds arise from the sharing of electrons between two atoms. Each single covalent bond consists of two shared electrons, as in H—H.

THE CARDIOVASCULAR, BLOOD VESSEL, AND LYMPHATIC SYSTEMS

OVERVIEW

- Responsible for transporting nutrients and oxygen to tissue cells and taking away their metabolic waste products
- Composed of a pump (heart) and a system of various-sized tubes or channels (blood vessels) carrying blood between the heart, cells, and tissues of the body

THE HEART

- Components of the Heart
  - Heart, arteries, arterioles, capillaries, venules, and veins
- Basic Function of the Heart
  - The heart is a **pump** that circulates **oxygenated** blood, via the **arterial system**, and perfuses all body cells, providing oxygen, nutrients, and hormones.
  - **Deoxygenated** blood, via the **venous system**, carries carbon dioxide and unwanted materials to be eliminated.
- Position of the Heart
  - Located in the mediastinum of the thorax, approximately between the second and fifth ribs
  - Rests on the diaphragm, lies posterior to the sternum, and is bordered by lungs that overlie it
  - Lies anterior to the vertebral column
- Structures of the Heart
  - Pericardium
    - ➤ The heart sits in a thin, saclike membrane composed of parietal pericardium and visceral pericardium.
    - ➤ The space between the pericardial layers contains approximately 20–30 ml of fluid that protects the heart and provides lubrication.
- Walls of the Heart
  - Epicardium—outer layer
  - Myocardium—middle layer
  - Endocardium—inner layer
- Chambers of the Heart
  - Consists of four chambers (see Figure 6.4)
    - ➤ Left and right atria
      - Low pressure chambers
    - ➤ Left and right ventricles
      - Right chamber is low pressure
      - Left chamber is high pressure

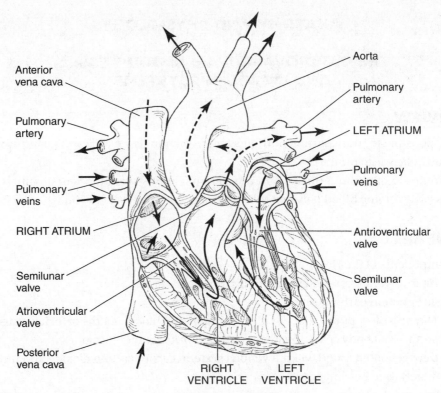

Labels on figure:

Anterior vena cava

Pulmonary artery

Pulmonary veins

RIGHT ATRIUM

Semilunar valve

Atrioventricular valve

Posterior vena cava

Aorta

Pulmonary artery

LEFT ATRIUM

Pulmonary veins

Antrioventricular valve

Semilunar valve

RIGHT VENTRICLE

LEFT VENTRICLE

Figure 6.4. Heart

- Blood Flow Through the Heart
    - The cardiovascular system has two circuits or systems (see Figure 6.4)
        - ➤ Pulmonary circuit
            - Blood travels from the right ventricle to the lungs and into the left ventricle.
        - ➤ Systemic circuit
            - Blood travels from the left ventricle to the body and back to the right atrium.
    - Vena cava ⇒ right atria through tricuspid valve ⇒ right ventricle through pulmonic valve ⇒ pulmonary artery ⇒ lungs ⇒ pulmonary veins ⇒ left atrium through mitral valve ⇒ left ventricle to the aortic valve ⇒ aorta
- Blood Supply to the Heart
    - The left and right coronary arteries perfuse the heart.
        - ➤ The left coronary artery and its branches supply blood to the left heart wall.
        - ➤ The right coronary artery and its branches supply blood to the right heart wall.
    - The coronary artery originates from the aorta.
        - ➤ Receives blood primarily during diastole (ventricular relaxation)
- Conduction System of the Heart
    - Series of pathways via specialized cells that conduct electrical impulses throughout the heart muscle as a precursor to a heart beat
    - SA node ⇒ AV node ⇒ Bundle of His (splits into left and right bundle) ⇒ Purkinje fibers
        - ➤ Seen as waves on an electrocardiogram (EKG)
- Cardiac Cycle
    - **One cardiac cycle = One heart beat**
    - Has two phases

- ➤ Systole
  - – Contraction phase brought about by depolarization and contraction of the ventricles
  - – Blood pumped into pulmonary and systemic circulation
  - – Peak pressure applied against artery walls as the heart contracts
- ➤ Diastole
  - – Relaxation phase brought about by repolarization and refilling of the ventricles
  - – Remaining pressure within the arterial system during cardiac relaxation
- ■ Cardiac Output
  - ○ Volume of blood pumped out of the right and left ventricles in **one minute**
  - ○ CO (cardiac output) = HR (heart rate) × SV (stroke volume)
    - ➤ Stroke volume is the amount of blood pumped out of the left ventricle during one cardiac cycle. The formula for stroke volume is:

$$\text{Stroke Volume (SV)} = \left(\frac{\text{Cardiac Output (CO)}}{\text{Heart Rate (HR)}} \right) \times 1{,}000$$

    - ➤ **Preload** is the volume of blood at the end of diastole.
    - ➤ **Afterload** is the resistance that the left ventricle must exert to circulate blood.
    - ➤ ⇑ Afterload = ⇑ cardiac workload
- ■ Autonomic nervous system
  - ○ Regulates heart rate and blood pressure
    - ➤ Stimulation of sympathetic nervous system
      - – Release of **norepinephrine** and **epinephrine** results in arteriolar vasoconstriction, increased heart rate, and increased arterial blood pressure
    - ➤ Stimulation of parasympathetic nervous system
      - – Release of **acetylcholine**, decreased heart rate, decreased blood pressure, bronchoconstriction, increased intestinal and glandular activity, relaxed sphincter muscles
    - ➤ Baroreceptor Response
      - – Clusters of **neurons** located in the atria, aortic arch, carotid sinus, pulmonary artery, and vena cava
      - – Sends impulses to increase or decrease activity of cardiac muscle (slow or increase heart rate), bringing about changes in blood pressure
      - – Sends impulses to vasomotor center and indirectly controls blood flow by vasodilation or constriction
    - ➤ Chemoreceptor Response
      - – Clusters of **neurons** located in aortic and carotid bodies
      - – React to **abnormal** levels of hydrogen, carbon dioxide, and oxygen in the blood
      - – Reduces O_2 and raises CO_2 concentrations to increase heart rate
      - – Sends impulses to vasomotor center that regulates blood flow

THE BLOOD VESSELS

- ■ Vessels
  - ○ Arteries
    - ➤ Carry oxygenated blood
    - ➤ Composed of three layers
      - – Outer layer is connective tissue (tunica adventitia)

NOTE

Changes in cardiac output affect every body system!

- Middle layer is muscle (tunica media). This layer is able to withstand higher pressures than veins and has the ability to dilate or constrict.
- Inner layer is endothelial cells (tunica intima)
➤ Pump high pressure blood to the body (pulse)
➤ Have the ability to vasoconstrict and vasodilate
○ Arterioles
➤ Smaller than arteries
➤ Walls are similar to arteries
➤ Can adjust blood flow by dilation or constriction
○ Capillaries
➤ Microscopic
➤ Found in almost all cells
○ Venules
➤ Smallest veins
➤ Formed when several small capillaries join together
○ Veins
➤ Carry deoxygenated blood
➤ Similar in structure to arteries except outer layer is thicker and middle layer is thinner
➤ Vein walls not as strong as artery walls
➤ Pressure is much lower than arteries
➤ Valves prevent backflow of blood
➤ Flow of blood is smooth
■ Circulation
○ Composed of two systems or circuits (see Figure 6.5)
➤ Arterial system
- Composed of **high pressure** vessels
- Largest vessel is the aorta
- Delivers **oxygenated** blood from the left ventricle to tissues for nutrition and aids in tissue temperature regulation
➤ Venous system
- Composed of thin walled, **low pressure** vessels
- Vena cava is the largest vein
- Carries **deoxygenated** blood and waste products to the right atrium
- Reservoir for approximately **60%** of blood volume
○ Regulated or adjusted by
➤ Compliance
- Veins are more accommodating than arteries and can serve as storage areas in the circulatory system.
➤ Pressure
- Arterial side has higher pressures than the venous side.
➤ Resistance
- ⇑ Resistance = ⇓ blood flow
- Resistance is determined by the length and diameter of the vessel and blood viscosity.

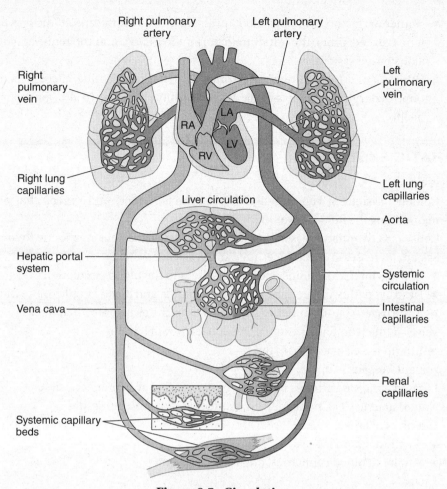

Figure 6.5. Circulation

➤ Velocity
  – Velocity is the distance blood moves with respect to time. **Do not confuse velocity with flow, which is the volume of blood moving per unit of time.**
○ Blood volume coursing through the body's circulatory system is approximately **five liters**
○ Heart ⇒ arteries ⇒ arterioles ⇒ capillaries ⇒ venules ⇒ veins ⇒ heart
■ Pulse and Blood Pressure
  ○ Pulse
    ➤ Created when the left ventricle contracts and pushes blood into the systemic circulation
    ➤ **Heart rate**
      – Number of times the heart beats in one minute
      – Rate constantly varies
  ○ Blood Pressure
    ➤ The measurement of the force of blood against arterial vessel walls
    ➤ Systolic pressure
      – Peak or highest pressure exerted against arterial walls during contraction of the heart
      – ⇑ Cardiac output = ⇑ blood pressure

- ➤ Numerous factors influence blood pressure, including the automatic nervous system, baroreceptors, the antidiuretic hormone (ADH), and the renin-angiotensin-aldosterone system.
- ➤ Other factors include environmental temperature, nicotine, alcohol consumption, dietary salt, older age, genetics, obesity, physical health, and emotional health.

LYMPHATIC SYSTEM

- Overview
  - ○ Complex system of capillary-like vessels, ducts, nodes, and organs that assist in maintaining the fluid environment of the body
  - ○ Consists of lymphatic vessels, lymph, lymph nodes, the spleen, and the thymus
  - ○ System increases and enhances the cardiovascular system
    - ➤ Collects interstitial fluids and returns them to the blood circulation
    - ➤ Destroys pathogens, removes articulate matter, and inactivates toxins in the lymph
    - ➤ Absorbs fat-soluble material and lipids from the gastrointestinal tract
  - ○ Valves in the lymphatic system prevent backflow of lymph.
    - ➤ Lymph is a clear, colorless fluid.
- Lymphatic Vessels
  - ○ Located alongside arteries in the viscera or veins in subcutaneous tissues
  - ○ Nonexistent in CNS, bone marrow, teeth, and nonvascular tissues
  - ○ Lymph capillaries
    - ➤ Smallest lymph vessels
    - ➤ Similar to blood capillaries, but are more porous
  - ○ Lacteals
    - ➤ Specialized lymph capillaries that project finger-like extending into the small intestine
      - – Absorbs creamy white liquid called chyle. The color and consistency of chyle is from the presence of fats in the small intestine.
  - ○ Lymphatic-collecting vessels form where lymph capillaries come together.
  - ○ Lymphatic trunks
    - ➤ Develop from the merger of collecting vessels
    - ➤ Major trunks are bronchomediastinal, jugular, lumbar, and subclavian
  - ○ Lymphatic ducts
    - ➤ Largest lymphatic vessels
    - ➤ Ducts drain lymph into the right and left subclavian veins in the neck.
    - ➤ The right thoracic duct collects lymph from the upper right side of the body.
    - ➤ The left thoracic duct collects lymph from the left side of the body and the right side below the thorax.
  - ○ Lymphoid cells
    - ➤ Connective tissue based
    - ➤ Lymphocytes are WBCs
      - – T-lymphocytes originate in red bone marrow and mature in thymus.
      - – B-lymphocytes originate and mature in red bone marrow.
    - ➤ Macrophages
    - ➤ Reticular cells and their fibers

○ Lymphatic Tissue and Organs
- ➤ **Diffuse**, unencapsulated bundles of lymphatic cells
  - Macrophages
  - Lymphocytes
  - Found in lamina propria of mucous membranes of the gastrointestinal and respiratory tracts
- ➤ **Discrete** unencapsulated bundles of lymphatic nodules or follicles
  - Clear separate boundaries
  - Contain macrophages, lymphocytes
  - Found in lamina propria of mucous membranes of the gastrointestinal, respiratory, reproductive, and urinary tracts
  - May occur as solitary nodules, or cluster as patches (i.e., Peyer's patches) or aggregates (i.e., tonsils). The appendix is lined with aggregates of nodules.
- ➤ Encapsulated organs have lymphatic nodules and diffuse lymphatic cells, and they are surrounded by a capsule of dense connective tissue.
  - Lymph nodes are small oval bodies that occur along lymphatic vessels. They are abundant in the groin, armpits, and mammary gland areas.
  - Spleen
  - Thymus gland

ANSWER SHEET
The Cardiovascular, Blood Vessel, and Lymphatic Systems Sample Test

1. Ⓐ Ⓑ Ⓒ Ⓓ
2. Ⓐ Ⓑ Ⓒ Ⓓ
3. Ⓐ Ⓑ Ⓒ Ⓓ
4. Ⓐ Ⓑ Ⓒ Ⓓ
5. Ⓐ Ⓑ Ⓒ Ⓓ
6. Ⓐ Ⓑ Ⓒ Ⓓ
7. Ⓐ Ⓑ Ⓒ Ⓓ
8. Ⓐ Ⓑ Ⓒ Ⓓ

9. Ⓐ Ⓑ Ⓒ Ⓓ
10. Ⓐ Ⓑ Ⓒ Ⓓ
11. Ⓐ Ⓑ Ⓒ Ⓓ
12. Ⓐ Ⓑ Ⓒ Ⓓ
13. Ⓐ Ⓑ Ⓒ Ⓓ
14. Ⓐ Ⓑ Ⓒ Ⓓ
15. Ⓐ Ⓑ Ⓒ Ⓓ
16. Ⓐ Ⓑ Ⓒ Ⓓ

17. Ⓐ Ⓑ Ⓒ Ⓓ
18. Ⓐ Ⓑ Ⓒ Ⓓ
19. Ⓐ Ⓑ Ⓒ Ⓓ
20. Ⓐ Ⓑ Ⓒ Ⓓ
21. Ⓐ Ⓑ Ⓒ Ⓓ
22. Ⓐ Ⓑ Ⓒ Ⓓ
23. Ⓐ Ⓑ Ⓒ Ⓓ

For Questions 1–23, select the letter (A, B, C, or D) that best answers the question. Record your answers on The Cardiovascular, Blood Vessel, and Lymphatic Systems Sample Test Answer Sheet on page 219.

1. Select the response that demonstrates the circulation of blood through the heart.

    (A) Vena cava ⇒ right atria through tricuspid valve ⇒ right ventricle through pulmonic valve ⇒ pulmonary artery ⇒ lungs ⇒ pulmonary vein ⇒ left atrium through mitral valve ⇒ left ventricle to the aortic valve ⇒ aorta

    (B) Vena cava ⇒ right atria through tricuspid valve ⇒ right ventricle through pulmonic valve ⇒ pulmonary vein ⇒ lungs ⇒ pulmonary artery ⇒ left atrium through mitral valve ⇒ left ventricle to the aortic valve ⇒ aorta

    (C) Vena cava ⇒ right atria through mitral valve ⇒ right ventricle through pulmonic valve ⇒ pulmonary artery ⇒ lungs ⇒ pulmonary vein ⇒ left atrium through tricuspid valve ⇒ left ventricle to the aortic valve ⇒ aorta

    (D) Vena cava ⇒ left atria through tricuspid valve ⇒ left ventricle through pulmonic valve ⇒ pulmonary vein ⇒ lungs ⇒ pulmonary artery ⇒ right atrium through mitral valve ⇒ right ventricle to the aortic valve ⇒ aorta

2. The middle layer of the heart wall is the

    (A) endocardium.
    (B) epicardium.
    (C) pericardium.
    (D) myocardium.

3. Which of the following is a primary function of lymph nodes?

    (A) carry lymph from the peripheral system to the veins of the cardiovascular system
    (B) control lymph development
    (C) maintain T-lymphocytes
    (D) monitor lymph composition

4. Which of the following chambers of the heart has the thickest wall?

    (A) left atrium
    (B) left ventricle
    (C) right atrium
    (D) right ventricle

5. Select the true statement.

    (A) ⇑ Cardiac output = ⇑ blood pressure
    (B) ⇑ Cardiac output = ⇓ blood pressure
    (C) ⇓ Cardiac output = ⇑ blood pressure
    (D) The relationship between cardiac output and blood pressure depends upon individual physiology or pathophysiology.

6. An individual at rest has a cardiac output of 4.745 liters/minute with a heart rate of 65 beats/minute. What is his stroke volume?

    (A) 73 milliliters/minute
    (B) 84 milliliters/minute
    (C) 137 milliliters/minute
    (D) 140 milliliters/minute

7. Coronary arteries branch off of the _____ to supply oxygenated blood to the heart.

    (A) aorta
    (B) inferior vena cava
    (C) pulmonary artery
    (D) right coronary vein

8. In regulating heart function, the sympathetic nervous system releases _____ when stimulated.

    (A) baroreceptors
    (B) chyme
    (C) enzymes
    (D) norepinephrine

9. The distance that blood moves with respect to time is

    (A) diastole.
    (B) flow.
    (C) preload.
    (D) velocity.

10. All blood in the veins of the body flows

    (A) around the spleen.
    (B) away from the heart.
    (C) toward the heart.
    (D) toward the lungs.

11. The only vein that carries oxygenated blood is the

    (A) aortic vein.
    (B) myocardial vein.
    (C) pulmonary vein.
    (D) superior vena cava.

12. Which of the artery layers is able to withstand higher pressures than veins and has the ability to dilate or constrict?

    (A) the inner layer (tunica intima)
    (B) the middle layer (tunica media)
    (C) the outer layer (tunica adventitia)
    (D) None of the above

13. Which system(s) helps protect the body from infection?

    (A) biliary system
    (B) endocrine/metabolic systems
    (C) hematologic system
    (D) lymphatic system

14. The inferior vena cava receives blood from the

    (A) kidneys and lungs.
    (B) thyroid and adrenal glands.
    (C) liver and pancreas.
    (D) upper extremities and head.

15. The largest artery in the body is the

    (A) abdominal aorta.
    (B) common carotid.
    (C) external jugular.
    (D) superior vena cava.

16. Blood pressure is brought about by

    (A) cardiac output and resistance to blood flow.
    (B) elasticity and turgor within the venous system.
    (C) heart rate and pulmonary pressures.
    (D) medulla oblongata and the parasympathetic nervous system.

17. Valves in the circulatory system

    (A) prevent backflow of blood in the venous system.
    (B) prevent increases in preload in the arterial system.
    (C) work to balance pressures in the arterial system.
    (D) work with neurons in the venous system.

18. Heart rate

    (A) decreases with age.
    (B) is activity dependent.
    (C) is static.
    (D) constantly varies.

19. What is created when the left ventricle contracts and forces blood into the systemic circulation?

(A) afterload
(B) cardiac cycle
(C) preload
(D) vasodilation

20. Antidiuretic hormone (ADH), released by the posterior pituitary gland, brings about reabsorption of water by the kidneys that results in

(A) increased blood pressure.
(B) an increase in urinary output.
(C) the release of aldosterone from the adrenal glands.
(D) suppression of rennin.

21. _____ can be defined as a complex system of capillary-like vessels, ducts, nodes, and organs that assist in maintaining the fluid environment of the body.

(A) Active transport processes
(B) Circulatory pathways
(C) Hormonal regulation
(D) The lymphatic system

22. The primary functions of the spleen are all of the following EXCEPT

(A) carries lymph from the peripheral tissues to the veins of the cardiovascular system
(B) monitors circulating blood
(C) acts as the site of cells that engulf pathogens
(D) acts as the site of cells that regulate the immune response

23. What kind of a system is the lymphatic system?

(A) one-way
(B) two-way
(C) depends upon the presence of disease that can influence direction
(D) Valvular incompetence can cause stasis and temporary reversal of direction.

The Cardiovascular, Blood Vessel, and Lymphatic Systems
Sample Test Answer Key

1. **B**	6. **A**	11. **C**	16. **A**	21. **D**
2. **D**	7. **A**	12. **B**	17. **A**	22. **A**
3. **D**	8. **D**	13. **D**	18. **D**	23. **A**
4. **B**	9. **D**	14. **D**	19. **A**	
5. **A**	10. **C**	15. **A**	20. **A**	

THE CARDIOVASCULAR, BLOOD VESSEL, AND LYMPHATIC SYSTEMS SAMPLE TEST ANSWERS EXPLAINED

1. **(B)** Review cardiac circulation through the heart on page 212.

2. **(D)** There are three walls of the heart. The epicardium is the outermost layer. The middle layer is the myocardium, a muscle layer, and the innermost layer is the endocardium.

3. **(D)** The primary functions of lymph nodes are monitoring the composition of lymph, acting as the site of cells that overwhelm pathogens, and controlling the immune responses.

4. **(B)** The left ventricle is the pumping chamber or compartment for systemic circulation. Increased pressure is required to pump blood through the larger, more complicated systemic circulation. The left chamber is larger and its walls are thicker than those of the right ventricle, which only pumps blood into the pulmonary circulation.

5. **(A)** Cardiac output is determined by heart rate and stroke volume. At rest, these are relatively constant. With exercise, however, the heart beats faster and more blood is pumped with each beat. These factors both contribute to a rise in BP, as would any other factor that causes the heart to speed up.

6. **(A)**

$$\text{Stroke (SV)} = \left(\frac{\text{Cardiac Output (CO)}}{\text{Heart Rate (HR)}} \right) \times 1{,}000$$

CO = 4.745 liters/minute

HR = 65 beats/minute

$$SV = \left(\frac{4.745}{65} \right) \times 1{,}000 = 0.073 \times 1{,}000 = 73 \text{ milliliters/minute}$$

7. **(A)** Review the role of coronary arteries and the aorta in relation to blood supply to the heart as discussed on page 212.

8. **(D)** Review the section on the stimulation of the sympathetic nervous system on page 213.

9. **(D)** Velocity is the *distance* an object (solid, liquid, or gas) moves with respect to time. Flow, if you selected it, is the *volume* of a liquid or gas that is moving with respect to time.

10. **(C)** Review arteries and veins in the outline for direction of blood flow on pages 213–214.

11. **(C)** The pulmonary artery carries deoxygenated blood from the right ventricle to the lungs. The pulmonary vein carries oxygenated blood from the lungs to the left ventricle.

12. **(B)** The tunica media, or middle layer, is composed of primarily smooth muscle cells. It is the thickest of the three arterial layers. The muscle contracts and relaxes to control blood pressure and flow in the artery, increasing the elasticity and strength of the wall of the artery.

13. **(D)** The lymphatic system is part of the circulatory system and a vital part of the immune system, comprising a network of lymphatic vessels that carry a clear fluid called lymph toward the heart.

14. **(D)** Understanding the human anatomy is the key to answering this question. Recognizing the word *inferior* is the clue. Choices A, B, and C all flow into the superior vena cava.

15. **(A)** The aorta is the largest vessel (artery) in the body. The size of the aorta is noteworthy—all oxygenated blood bound for the entire body first flows through the aorta. On the venous side, the superior and inferior vena cava are large vessels (veins) that receive all deoxygenated blood from the body that is taken to the heart.

16. **(A)** Changes in blood pressure are brought about by cardiac output and resistance to blood flow. Cardiac output is equal to stroke volume times heart rate. Resistance to blood flow can be altered by vasoconstricted or vasodilated vessels, blood viscosity, and the distance blood has to flow.

17. **(A)** Valves are found in the venous system, and they regulate backflow.

18. **(D)** Choice B seems like it is a true statement, and it is to a point. The heart rate does increase with activity. However, it will also increase without activity. Taking an exam is not considered an activity, but realizing there is not enough time remaining to complete the test causes anxiety that increases one's heart rate. Receiving news, whether it is good or bad, will also increase one's heart rate. The most correct answer is therefore choice D.

19. **(A)** Afterload is the resistance the left ventricle must overcome in order to circulate or pump blood into the systemic circulation. Increased afterload equals increased cardiac workload.

20. **(A)** Vasopressin, or the antidiuretic hormone (ADH), stimulates the tightening of the muscular tissues of the capillaries and arterioles and raises blood pressure. It also increases peristalsis (muscle contractions), exerts some influence over the uterus, and has an effect on the reabsorption of water by the kidneys (concentrating urine). Plasma osmolarity regulates the secretion of ADH from the pituitary.

21. **(D)** The stem of the question is the definition of the lymphatic system.

22. **(A)** The lymph vessels carry lymph from the peripheral tissues to the veins of the cardiovascular system, not the spleen.

23. **(A)** The role or function of the lymphatic system is to return lymph fluid to the circulatory system from the intercellular tissue spaces. It is a one-way system because the flow is in one direction, and there is no direct return flow of these fluids.

THE ENDOCRINE SYSTEM

OVERVIEW

- Endocrinology is the study of communication and management within a living organism using chemical messages produced within the organism.
- Metabolism is a subclass of endocrinology that studies biochemical mechanisms, such as those concerned with obtaining, storing, and mobilizing energy.
- Glands
  - Categorized as endocrine or exocrine glands
  - Endocrine deals with the "**ductless**" secretion of hormones
    - ➤ Hormones regulate fluid and electrolyte balance, reproduction, growth and development, adaptation to stress, and metabolism.
    - ➤ Endocrine glands secrete two types of hormones **directly into the blood stream** to act on specific target cells.
      - – Steroid hormones are lipids synthesized from cholesterol and include cortisol, cortisone, estrogen, progesterone, and testosterone.
      - – Nonsteroid hormones include amines, proteins, and peptides.
  - Exocrine deals with secretions delivered **outside the body** or through "**ducts**"
    - ➤ Exocrine glands secrete enzymes and other substances into ducts.
    - ➤ Glands are classified by the type of secretion they produce:
      - – Mucus producing (respiratory, reproductive, and urinary tracts)
      - – Serous secreting (serous fluid)
      - – Seromucous producing (salivary glands)
      - – Merocrine (sweat glands, salivary glands)

STRUCTURE AND FUNCTION OF THE ENDOCRINE SYSTEM

- Pineal Gland
  - Located in the midbrain on the roof of the third ventricle and attached to the thalamus
  - Produces melatonin
  - Targets reproductive organs, especially the ovaries
  - May influence the sleep-wake cycle
- Pituitary Gland
  - Considered the **master gland**
  - Located in the inferior aspect of the brain within the sella turica behind the optic chiasma
  - Release of hormones regulated by the hypothalamus gland
  - Consists of two lobes—the anterior (adenohypophysis) and the posterior (neurohypophysis)
  - Anterior Lobe
    - ➤ Adrenocorticotropic hormone (ACTH)
      - – Targets the cortex of the adrenal gland, mammary gland, skin, and liver
      - – Stimulates the adrenal cortex to produce primarily cortisol; increases metabolic rate; promotes the deposition of liver glycogen; darkens skin; milk production

- ➤ Follicle-stimulating hormone (FSH)
  - – Targets the ovarian follicle in females and seminiferous tubules of the testes in males
  - – Stimulates the growth of follicles and secretion of estrogen; stimulates the development of the seminiferous tubules and performs spermatogenesis.
- ➤ Growth hormone (HGH) or somatotropic hormone
  - – Targets body tissues, bones, and muscles
  - – Promotes growth
- ➤ Luteinizing hormone (LH)
  - – Targets ovaries and testes
  - – Stimulates the formation of the corpus luteum from follicle; stimulates the production of testosterone by the testes, and the production of progesterone by the ovaries
- ➤ Melanocyte-stimulating hormone (MSH)
  - – Targets skin melanocytes
  - – Controls pigmentation of skin
- ➤ Prolactin (PRL)
  - – Targets female mammary gland
  - – Stimulates the production of milk after birth
- ➤ Thyroid-stimulating hormone (TSH)
  - – Targets the thyroid gland
  - – Stimulates thyroid hormone production
- ○ Posterior lobe
  - ➤ Oxytocin
    - – Produced by hypothalamus and released by posterior pituitary
    - – Targets the uterus and the ducts of the mammary gland
    - – Stimulates the contraction of the uterus when primed by ovarian hormones and mammary glands to stimulate milk production
  - ➤ Antidiuretic hormone (ADH) or vasopressin
    - – Targets smooth muscles (arterioles and tubules of the kidney)
    - – Release rate of ADH is controlled by plasma osmolality
    - – Stimulates the distal renal tubule to increase reabsorption of water; constricts blood vessels (increases blood pressure)
- ■ Adrenal gland
  - ○ Located on the upper surface of the kidneys
  - ○ Contains two types of endocrine tissue:
    - ➤ Adrenal Medulla
      - – Located in the center of the gland
      - – Produces/secretes epinephrine (adrenaline) and norepinephrine
      - – Prepares body for fight or flight response
    - ➤ Adrenal cortex
      - – Located on the outer part of the gland
      - – Produces glucocorticoids and regulates sugar and protein metabolism
      - – Mineralocorticoids control sodium and mineral balance
      - – Influences secondary sex hormones

- Hypothalamus
  - Regulates blood pressure, respiration, and temperature
  - Affects emotional states of anxiety, anger, fear, pain, pleasure, and rage
  - Produces hypothalamic-stimulating hormones
    - Affects inhibition and release of the pituitary hormone
- Gonads
  - Called testes in the male and ovaries in the female
  - Both regulate secondary sexual characteristics and reproduction
  - In the female, estrogen stimulates cells to develop secondary sexual characteristics and behaviors, follicle maturation, and growth of the uterine lining
    - Stops secretion of FHS in the anterior pituitary gland by giving negative feedback
  - In the male, androgens, primarily testosterone, stimulate cells for secondary sexual characteristics and behaviors, maturation of sperm, and protein synthesis.
    - Inhibin provides negative feedback to the anterior pituitary gland to inhibit FSH secretion
  - Both males and females produce FSH and gonadotropin-releasing hormone (GnRH), and inhibin prevents this release in both genders.
    - In women, the hormone produced in the gonads, placenta, and pituitary gland accomplishes this goal.
    - In males, testicular Sertoli cells secrete the needed inhibin. Males also use this in the testes as a means of regulating sperm production. The presence of androgen increases inhibin levels, which in turn seems to promote spermatogenesis.
- Pancreas
  - Located behind the stomach in the posterior abdomen
  - The pancreas functions as both an endocrine and exocrine gland.
    - Endocrine
      - Controls alpha, beta, and delta cells of the Islets of Langerhans
    - Exocrine
      - Secretion of pancreatic digestive enzymes
  - The Islets of Langerhans beta cells
    - Produce insulin
    - Help with cellular glucose uptake, chiefly in the liver
- Parathyroid Gland
  - Seated in posterior surface of the thyroid gland
  - Produces the parathyroid hormone
  - Controls the activity of the osteoclasts and increases calcium concentration in the circulatory system
- Thyroid Gland
  - Anterior and below the larynx
  - Thyroxine and triiodothyronine
  - Targets tissue cells
  - Calcitonin
    - Lowers blood calcium levels by rapidly increasing calcium deposits in the bone

ANSWER SHEET
The Endocrine System Sample Test

1. Ⓐ Ⓑ Ⓒ Ⓓ
2. Ⓐ Ⓑ Ⓒ Ⓓ
3. Ⓐ Ⓑ Ⓒ Ⓓ
4. Ⓐ Ⓑ Ⓒ Ⓓ
5. Ⓐ Ⓑ Ⓒ Ⓓ
6. Ⓐ Ⓑ Ⓒ Ⓓ
7. Ⓐ Ⓑ Ⓒ Ⓓ

8. Ⓐ Ⓑ Ⓒ Ⓓ
9. Ⓐ Ⓑ Ⓒ Ⓓ
10. Ⓐ Ⓑ Ⓒ Ⓓ
11. Ⓐ Ⓑ Ⓒ Ⓓ
12. Ⓐ Ⓑ Ⓒ Ⓓ
13. Ⓐ Ⓑ Ⓒ Ⓓ
14. Ⓐ Ⓑ Ⓒ Ⓓ

15. Ⓐ Ⓑ Ⓒ Ⓓ
16. Ⓐ Ⓑ Ⓒ Ⓓ
17. Ⓐ Ⓑ Ⓒ Ⓓ
18. Ⓐ Ⓑ Ⓒ Ⓓ
19. Ⓐ Ⓑ Ⓒ Ⓓ
20. Ⓐ Ⓑ Ⓒ Ⓓ

For Questions 1–20, select the letter (A, B, C, or D) that best answers the question. Record your answers on The Endocrine Sample Test Answer Sheet on page 229.

1. _____ control(s) the functions of cells.

   (A) Autonomic nervous system
   (B) Thyroid gland
   (C) Hormones
   (D) Metabolism

2. The pineal gland is located

   (A) anterior to the spleen.
   (B) behind the stomach in the posterior abdomen.
   (C) in the midbrain on the roof of the third ventricle, attached to the thalamus.
   (D) on the upper surface of the kidneys.

3. Steroidal hormones are lipids synthesized from

   (A) amines.
   (B) cholesterol.
   (C) cortisol.
   (D) holocrine.

4. The follicle stimulating hormone (FSH) induces which of the following in males?

   (A) excitation of smooth muscles in the genitalia
   (B) inactivation of spermatogenesis
   (C) regulation of bulbourethral gland fluid
   (D) stimulation of seminiferous tubules of the testes

5. Vasopressin is also known as the

   (A) antidiuretic hormone (ADH)
   (B) corticotrophin-releasing hormone (TRH)
   (C) luteinizing hormone (LH)
   (D) mammary hormone (MH)

6. What gland is located on the upper surface of the kidneys?

   (A) adrenal
   (B) gonads
   (C) pancreas
   (D) thyroid

7. The adrenal medulla produces

   (A) epinephrine and norepinephrine.
   (B) glucocorticoids.
   (C) mineralocorticoids.
   (D) sex hormones.

8. Prolactin (PRL) targets/stimulates

   (A) female mammary glands.
   (B) production of testosterone by the testes.
   (C) suppression of milk production prior to birth.
   (D) uterine contractions.

9. The growth hormone (HGH) targets/stimulates

   (A) endocrine hormones.
   (B) mineral balance.
   (C) spermatogenesis.
   (D) tissues, bones, and muscles of the body.

10. Androgens are responsible for regulating/stimulating

    (A) the breakdown of glycogen in the liver.
    (B) ductless systems.
    (C) skin pigment.
    (D) cells for secondary sexual characteristics in the male.

11. The exocrine function of the pancreas
    (A) controls delta cells in the Islets of Langerhans.
    (B) controls osteoclasts.
    (C) produces insulin.
    (D) secretes pancreatic digestive enzymes.

12. The parathyroid hormone regulates
    (A) calcium.
    (B) mineral balance.
    (C) prolactin.
    (D) phospholipase C.

13. Luteinizing hormone (LH) stimulates all of the following EXCEPT
    (A) the formation of corpus luteum from follicle.
    (B) the production of testosterone by the testes.
    (C) the production of secondary sexual characteristics.
    (D) the production of progesterone by the ovaries.

14. Insulin is produced in the
    (A) anterior portion of the pancreas.
    (B) beta cells of the Islets of Langerhans.
    (C) thymus gland.
    (D) posterior lobe of the thyroid gland.

15. Hormone secretion is regulated by the
    (A) antidiuretic hormone (ADH).
    (B) feedback mechanisms.
    (C) parasympathetic nervous system.
    (D) response modifiers.

16. The _____ prepares the body for the "fight or flight" response.
    (A) adrenal medulla
    (B) apocrine gland
    (C) pineal gland
    (D) posterior lobe of the pituitary gland

17. Hormones
    (A) are classified by the type of secretion they produce.
    (B) determine the release of the antidiuretic hormone (ADH) by plasma osmolality to decrease water absorption.
    (C) regulate fluid and electrolyte balance, reproduction, growth and development, and adaptation to stress and metabolism.
    (D) influence humoral immunity by destroying antibodies.

18. Human growth hormone is also known as
    (A) chemiosin.
    (B) erythropoietin.
    (C) osteoclastin.
    (D) somatotropin.

19. The hormone antagonist to insulin is
    (A) calcitonin.
    (B) digestive enzymes.
    (C) glucagon.
    (D) mineralocorticoids.

20. The parathyroid hormone and calcitonin work together to control the level of
    (A) androgens in the blood.
    (B) calcium in the blood.
    (C) pepsin in the blood.
    (D) progesterone in the blood.

The Endocrine System Sample Test Answer Key

1. **C**	5. **A**	9. **D**	13. **C**	17. **C**
2. **C**	6. **A**	10. **D**	14. **B**	18. **D**
3. **B**	7. **A**	11. **D**	15. **B**	19. **C**
4. **D**	8. **A**	12. **A**	16. **A**	20. **B**

THE ENDOCRINE SYSTEM SAMPLE TEST ANSWERS EXPLAINED

1. **(C)** Hormones, produced by the endocrine system, are crucial in maintaining homeo-stasis and the regulation of reproduction and development. Hormones are chemical messengers produced by a cell that results in specific changes in the activity of other cells.

2. **(C)** Review the location and function of the pineal gland on page 226.

3. **(B)** Cholesterol is the precursor to all steroid hormones which includes those that con-trol blood sugar (glucocorticoids), those that maintain blood pressure and mineral equilibrium (mineral corticoids), and those that are the male and female sex hormones.

4. **(D)** The follicle-stimulating hormone (FSH) stimulates the maturation of seminiferous tubules and sperm production. FSH originates in the pituitary and is regulated by the hypothalamus.

5. **(A)** Vasopressin is another common name for the antidiuretic hormone (ADH).

6. **(A)** The adrenal gland is located on the upper surface of the kidneys, and it is made up of two types of tissues: the adrenal medulla and the adrenal cortex.

7. **(A)** The medulla of the adrenal glands, positioned on the superior borders of the kid-neys, exudes amine hormones known as catecholamines that include epinephrine or norepinephrine. These two hormones prepare the body for greater physical functioning (the "fight or flight" response).

8. **(A)** Prolactin, a hormone created in the pituitary gland, is so named because of its function in lactation. It has other functions in the body from acting on the reproductive system to affecting behavior and controlling the immune system.

9. **(D)** Growth hormones, synthesized in the anterior lobe of the pituitary gland, influence growth in tissues, bones, and muscles.

10. **(D)** Being able to recognize that *andro-* is a prefix meaning *male* or *masculine* is the key to answering this question.

11. **(D)** The pancreas is a large, flattened, glandular organ lying in the fold of the mesentery beneath the stomach in the abdominal cavity, and serves as two glands in one—a diges-tive exocrine gland and a hormone-producing endocrine gland. Functioning as an exocrine gland, the pancreas excretes enzymes to break down the proteins, lipids, carbohydrates, and nucleic acids in food. Functioning as an endocrine gland, the pan-creas secretes the hormones insulin and glucagon to control blood sugar levels through-out the day. Both of these functions are vital to the body's survival.

12. **(A)** Calcium is the most plentiful mineral in the human body. It is necessary for the development and maintenance of strong bones and teeth, where around 99% of the body's calcium is found. Calcium also facilitates the heart, nerves, muscles, and other body systems to work properly.

13. **(C)** Primary sex characteristics allow us to physically tell males from females. Secondary sex characteristics, which appear during puberty, start when the hypothalamus releases a hormone called the gonadotropin-releasing hormone. The gonadotropin-releasing hormone tells the pituitary gland to release two more hormones: the follicle-stimulating hormone and the luteinizing hormone. These hormones signal the start of sexual development in both boys and girls.

14. **(B)** Review the section on the pancreas on page 228 for more information about the Islets of Langerhans.

15. **(B)** Feedback is part of a cause-and-effect loop or circuit where information about a system is returned to the controller of the system to adjust its performance. The positive or negative naming of the mechanisms does not signify whether the feedback is good or bad.

16. **(A)** The adrenal medulla is the inner part of the adrenal gland (one sits atop each kidney). It manufactures the hormone adrenaline that supports the body's response to stress.

17. **(C)** Review the functions of hormones and the different types of hormones on page 226.

18. **(D)** Somatotropin is commonly referred to as the human growth hormone. It promotes growth, specifically targeting the tissues, cones, and muscles of the body.

19. **(C)** Synonyms for the word *antagonist* are rival, adversary, and competitor. Glucagon is a rival, adversary, or competitor for insulin.

20. **(B)** Review the section on the parathyroid gland on page 228 if you missed this question.

OVERVIEW

- Fluid and Electrolytes
  - Involve configuration and passage
  - Body fluids are solutions made up of water and solutes of body fluids.
    - ➤ Solutions enter the body by food, drink, and intravenous fluids.
  - Solutions are classified according to their **tonicity (concentration)**.
    - ➤ Hypotonic
      - – Solutions that cause cells to **swell**
    - ➤ Isotonic
      - – Have the same concentration of solutes in the blood
    - ➤ Hypertonic
      - – Solutions that cause cells to **shrink**
  - Electrolytes have **four** essential body functions:
    1. Advance neuromuscular irritability
    2. Regulate/correct acid-base balance
    3. Regulate distribution of body fluids among body fluid compartments
    4. Maintain body fluid osmolality
- Acid-Base Balance
  - Management of hydrogen ions
    - ➤ Measured as pH
    - ➤ Maintained at 7.4 +/− 0.05
  - Three mechanisms (differing effective intervals)
    - ➤ Buffering systems in plasma
    - ➤ Ventilator changes for CO_2 excretion
    - ➤ Renal tubular excretion of hydrogen ions

HOMEOSTASIS

- The state of **equilibrium** within the body when all body systems are **balanced**
  - Includes acid-base balance, fluids, and electrolytes
- Water and solutes are in constant movement to assist in maintaining homeostasis

WATER

- **Body fluid is primarily water.**
- All solutes in the body are dissolved or suspended in water.
- Contained in major body fluid compartments
  - Extracellular fluid (ECF)
    - ➤ Any fluid not contained within cells, which includes plasma, interstitial fluid, and any fluid contained within a natural cavity (e.g., joint fluid, cerebral spinal fluid (CSF), pleural fluid, pericardial fluid, etc.)
    - ➤ Around 16–20% of body weight
    - ➤ Intravascular compartment
    - ➤ Interstitial compartment
    - ➤ Transcellular compartment

- ○ Intracellular fluid (ICF)
  - ➤ Fluid within the tissue cells
  - ➤ Around 30–40% of body weight
- ■ Fluid balance exists when water in equals water out.
- ■ The primary sources of water are eating and drinking.

SOLUTES

- ■ Substances dissolved in a solution
- ■ Classified as electrolytes or nonelectrolytes

ELECTROLYTES

- ■ Sodium—Na^+
  - ○ Major cation in ECF
  - ○ Controlled by ADH and aldosterone
  - ○ Primary controller of fluid balance in the body
  - ○ Excreted by the kidneys, which regulate absorption and excretion based on sodium intake
  - ○ Maintains ECF osmolality
  - ○ Maintains ECF volume and, with CL, influences body water distribution
  - ○ Combines with HCO_3 and CL in acid-base regulation
  - ○ Primary role in the transmission of neuromuscular impulses and the maintenance of cellular membrane potential
  - ○ **Water follows sodium**
- ■ Potassium—K^+
  - ○ Major cation in ICF
  - ○ Must be ingested daily—**Is not stored**
  - ○ Maintains cell electroneutrality and cell osmolality
  - ○ Directly impacts cardiac muscle contractions and electrical conductivity
  - ○ Regulated by kidney tubules
    - ➤ K and Na have a reciprocal relationship
  - ○ Aldosterone controls the amount of K in ECF
  - ○ Maintains intracellular homeostasis
    - ➤ Controls ICF volume
  - ○ Determines cell's resting potential
- ■ Hydrogen—H^+
  - ○ Exists in small quantities in the body
  - ○ Maintains acid-base balance at a ratio of 20:1 (bicarbonate to carbonic acid)
    - ➤ ⇑ **H ions = acidosis**
    - ➤ ⇓ **H ions = alkalosis**
- ■ Calcium—Ca
  - ○ Most abundant electrolyte in the body
  - ○ 1% in ECF
  - ○ Necessary for the strength and rigidity of bones
  - ○ Activates the enzymes necessary for blood clotting
  - ○ Ca and P have an inverse relationship

- ○ Necessary for myocardial stimulation
- ○ Extracellular Ca is affected by acid-base balance
- ■ Magnesium—Mg^+
  - ○ Second only to K in abundance in ICF
  - ○ Needed for enzymatic cellular activation
  - ○ Activates Na K pump
  - ○ Needed to maintain Ca within cells
- ■ Phosphorus—P^+
  - ○ Major anion in ICF
  - ○ Essential component (with Ca) of bones and teeth
  - ○ Assists in maintaining cell membrane integrity
  - ○ Necessary for protein, fat, and carbohydrate metabolism
  - ○ Needed for muscle and nerve function
  - ○ Assists in maintaining acid-base balance
- ■ Chloride—Cl^-
  - ○ Major anion in ECF
  - ○ Maintains serum osmolality with Na
  - ○ Cl balance tied most closely to Na balance
    - ➤ Levels usually change in direct proportion to each other

NONELECTROLYTES

- ■ Organic acids
- ■ Proteins
- ■ Glucose
- ■ Oxygen
- ■ Carbon dioxide

ACID-BASE BALANCE

- ■ Homeostasis is maintained by **equalization** between the acidity and alkalinity of body fluids.
  - ○ Acids are hydrogen ions.
    - ➤ Acids have H ions which are given up to neutralize or decrease the strength of a base.
  - ○ Bases (alkali) are H ion acceptors.
  - ○ The chemical unit of measurement of the degree of acidity or alkalinity of a substance is the potential of hydrogen or pH.
    - ➤ Scale ranges from 0 (acid) to 14 (alkaline)
      - – Neutral is pH of 7.0
      - – Acidosis is pH < 7.35
      - – Alkaline (base) is pH > 7.45
      - – **Plasma pH is 7.35–7.45**
      - – Plasma pH < 6.80 or > 7.80 cannot sustain life
- ■ Buffer Systems
  - ○ Buffer is a substance that sustains the body's acid-base balance by controlling the hydrogen ion concentration

- Carbonic Acid-Bicarbonate Buffer System
  - ➤ **Exists in ECF compartment**
  - ➤ Operates in the lungs and kidneys
  - ➤ To keep pH at 7.40, a balance ratio of 1 part carbonic acid to 20 parts bicarbonate is needed.
  - ➤ Carbonic acid is regulated by the **respiratory system**.
    - Lungs regulate H ion concentration by eliminating CO_2 (combines with water to form H_2CO_3)
    - Too much H_2CO_3 is reduced to H_2O and CO_2 that is eliminated when breathing
    - Has the ability to bring about change within minutes
  - ➤ The **renal system** fine-tunes the pH by sustaining the respiratory system control of acid-base balance.
    - Kidneys counter balance respiratory imbalances by excreting or retaining H and HCO_3.
    - May take up to 72 hours to re-establish pH balance
  - ➤ **Protein Buffer System**
    - Largest and strongest buffer system
    - Exists in ECF and ICF
    - Mainly a mechanism of intracellular fluid
    - Maintains balance because proteins carry numerous negative charges that have the ability to buffer positively charged H ions

If there is too much H_2CO_3, the kidneys expel H and keep HCO_3 to restore balance. If there is too little H_2CO_3, the kidneys keep H and expel HCO_3 to restore balance.

ANSWER SHEET
Fluid, Electrolytes, and Acid-Base Balance
Sample Test

1. Ⓐ Ⓑ Ⓒ Ⓓ
2. Ⓐ Ⓑ Ⓒ Ⓓ
3. Ⓐ Ⓑ Ⓒ Ⓓ
4. Ⓐ Ⓑ Ⓒ Ⓓ
5. Ⓐ Ⓑ Ⓒ Ⓓ
6. Ⓐ Ⓑ Ⓒ Ⓓ
7. Ⓐ Ⓑ Ⓒ Ⓓ

8. Ⓐ Ⓑ Ⓒ Ⓓ
9. Ⓐ Ⓑ Ⓒ Ⓓ
10. Ⓐ Ⓑ Ⓒ Ⓓ
11. Ⓐ Ⓑ Ⓒ Ⓓ
12. Ⓐ Ⓑ Ⓒ Ⓓ
13. Ⓐ Ⓑ Ⓒ Ⓓ
14. Ⓐ Ⓑ Ⓒ Ⓓ

15. Ⓐ Ⓑ Ⓒ Ⓓ
16. Ⓐ Ⓑ Ⓒ Ⓓ
17. Ⓐ Ⓑ Ⓒ Ⓓ
18. Ⓐ Ⓑ Ⓒ Ⓓ
19. Ⓐ Ⓑ Ⓒ Ⓓ
20. Ⓐ Ⓑ Ⓒ Ⓓ

For Questions 1–20, select the letter (A, B, C, or D) that best answers the question. Record your answers on the Fluid, Electrolytes, and Acid-Base Balance Sample Test Answer Sheet on page 239.

1. Water is used by the body to do all of the following EXCEPT

   (A) act as a friction-inducing substance between cells.
   (B) aid in body temperature regulation through perspiration.
   (C) assist with nutrient transport to cells.
   (D) assist with waste excretion.

2. The major cation in the ECF is

   (A) calcium.
   (B) magnesium.
   (C) potassium.
   (D) sodium.

3. Renal and hormonal systems are regulators of

   (A) base buffers.
   (B) electrolytes.
   (C) water-based solutes.
   (D) oxygen in the blood.

4. Sensible fluid loss occurs from which of the following?

   (A) kidneys
   (B) lungs
   (C) skin
   (D) small intestine

5. Which of the following stimulates the hypothalamus to initiate the thirst sensation?

   (A) decreased serum osmolality
   (B) intracellular dehydration
   (C) decrease in circulating blood volume
   (D) inhibition of ADH

6. Water balance and sodium balance are closely related.

   (A) This is a false statement if water losses are insensible.
   (B) This is a false statement if water losses are sensible.
   (C) This is a true statement because water follows sodium.
   (D) This is a true statement because sodium follows water.

7. A _____ solution contains fewer dissolved particles than are found in normal cells and blood.

   (A) hypertonic
   (B) hypotonic
   (C) permeable
   (D) semipermeable

8. Water and solutes are in constant movement and exchange to assist in maintaining

   (A) allocation of body fluids.
   (B) inhibition of acid-base balance.
   (C) interstitial compartments.
   (D) homeostasis of the body.

9. The primary controller of fluid balance in the body is

   (A) chloride.
   (B) magnesium.
   (C) potassium.
   (D) sodium.

10. Which of the following is necessary for myocardial stimulation?

    (A) calcium
    (B) bicarbonate
    (C) hydrogen
    (D) magnesium

11. A (An) _____ is a molecule that tends to either bind or release hydrogen ions in order to maintain a particular pH.

    (A) acid
    (B) base
    (C) buffer
    (D) nonelectrolyte

12. Which of the following electrolytes must be ingested on a daily basis, and is not stored in the body?

    (A) chloride
    (B) potassium
    (C) hydrogen
    (D) phosphorus

13. Roughly one-third of body weight is in the

    (A) intracellular fluid compartment.
    (B) extracellular fluid compartment.
    (C) kidneys.
    (D) plasma.

14. Approximately 90% of the cations in the extracellular fluid are

    (A) calcium ions.
    (B) chloride ions.
    (C) phosphorus ions.
    (D) sodium ions.

15. An increase in serum osmolality results in increased secretion of _____ from the pituitary gland, ultimately resulting in _____.

    (A) the adrenocorticotropic hormone, less urinary output
    (B) prolactin, greater urinary output
    (C) the somatotropic hormone, greater urinary elimination
    (D) vasopressin, less urinary elimination

16. Which of the following hormones regulates the level of sodium and potassium?

    (A) aldosterone
    (B) calcitonin
    (C) epinephrine
    (D) melatonin

17. Calcium ions are regulated by hormones of the _____ gland.

    (A) adrenal
    (B) parathyroid
    (C) pineal
    (D) pituitary

18. What substance is released from the juxtaglomerular apparatus in the nephron when the concentration of sodium in the blood is low?

    (A) angiotensin I
    (B) angiotensin II
    (C) renin
    (D) sodium

19. Appetite, regulation of body weight, body temperature, and water balance are associated with which of the following glands?

    (A) adrenal
    (B) hypothalamus
    (C) parathyroid
    (D) posterior lobe of the pituitary

20. A commonly used diagnostic test for evaluating acid-base balance is the arterial blood gas (ABG) that

    (A) assesses the efficiency of the renal system.
    (B) evaluates pulmonary gas exchange efficiency.
    (C) evaluates serum osmolality.
    (D) None of the above

Fluid, Electrolytes, and Acid-Base Balance Sample Test Answer Key

1. **A**		5. **C**		9. **D**		13. **A**		17. **B**
2. **D**		6. **C**		10. **A**		14. **D**		18. **C**
3. **B**		7. **B**		11. **C**		15. **B**		19. **B**
4. **A**		8. **D**		12. **B**		16. **A**		20. **B**

FLUID, ELECTROLYTES, AND ACID-BASE BALANCE SAMPLE TEST ANSWERS EXPLAINED

1. **(A)** Water acts as a lubricant between cells to allow friction-free movement.

2. **(D)** Review the definition of sodium (Na^+) on page 236.

3. **(B)** Electrolytes regulate nerve and muscle function, hydration, blood pH, blood pressure, and the rebuilding of damaged tissues. Diverse mechanisms are present and keep concentrations of different electrolytes under control. Electrolyte levels are kept constant by the kidneys and several hormones, even when the body elicits changes.

4. **(A)** Sensible loss can be perceived and measured. Urine, manufactured by the kidneys, is sensible loss. Individuals are normally aware of urination, and it can be measured.

5. **(C)** A decrease in plasma volume and an increase in plasma osmolarity produces dry mouth, stimulating the hypothalamic thirst centers. Dry mouth results from a decrease in water filtered from the bloodstream (therefore increased osmolarity) and the salivary gland receives less water, in turn producing less saliva. Hypothalamic stimulation occurs when water moves (due to hypertonic ECF) out of thirst center osmoreceptors by osmosis, causing osmoreceptors to become irritable and depolarize, causing the sensation of thirst.

6. **(C)** This is a true statement because water follows sodium. Sodium is most often found in the plasma of the bloodstream. It is a significant part of water regulation in the body. Water goes where the sodium goes. If there is too much sodium in the body, the kidney excretes it and water follows.

7. **(B)** Hypotonic solutions have a lower solute concentration. Hypertonic solutions have a higher solute concentration, and isotonic solutions have the same concentration as another solution, such as blood.

8. **(D)** Homeostasis occurs when fluid, electrolytes, and acid-balance are maintained. Water and solutes are a part of this.

9. **(D)** Review the functions of sodium as outlined on page 236.

10. **(A)** Calcium has an effect on the activation, contraction, and excitation of the cardiac and skeletal muscle.

11. **(C)** The stem of the question provides the definition of a buffer.

12. **(B)** Potassium must be ingested daily since the body does not store it. The daily dietary requirement of potassium is around 40 mEq. The average intake is 60 to 100 mEq daily. Around 20 to 40% of ingested calcium is lost via the kidneys with the remaining 5 to 10% excreted in feces.

13. **(A)** Intracellular fluid makes up around 30–40%, or approximately one-third, of body weight, whereas extracellular fluid only makes up around 16–20% of body weight.

14. **(D)** Sodium cations in the extracellular fluid are approximately 142–145 mEq with the remaining 9–12 mEq composed of potassium, magnesium, and calcium.

15. **(B)** Water balance is coordinated by the inhibition or secretion of ADH, the adrenal cortex, the aldosterone renin angiotensin system, the kidneys, and the thirst mechanism.

16. **(A)** Aldosterone helps with kidney regulation and has three important effects. It stimulates the reabsorption of sodium, stimulates the reabsorption of water, and stimulates potassium secretion from the blood.

17. **(B)** The parathyroid hormone promotes calcium transferal from bone to plasma and facilitates in intestinal and renal calcium absorption.

18. **(C)** Renin initiates the creation of angiotensin I and II by the liver, which in turn, triggers the brain to increase the thirst sensation. The **renin**-angiotensin system (RAS) is an indispensible regulator of sodium balance, extracellular fluid volume, vascular resistance, and, ultimately blood pressure.

19. **(B)** Review the purpose and functions of the hypothalamus on page 228 if you missed this question. It is important to remember that all of the systems in the body are inter-related, and you need to know how one influences the other.

20. **(B)** An arterial blood gas (ABG) measures the acidity (pH) and the levels of oxygen and carbon dioxide from an arterial blood sample. The test is used to assess how well your lungs are moving oxygen into the blood and removing carbon dioxide from the blood.

THE GASTROINTESTINAL SYSTEM

OVERVIEW

- Basically a nonsterile, open-ended, muscular tube approximately 30 feet in length in adults
  - Extends from the mouth to the anus
- Consists of gastrointestinal tract and accessory organs
  - The gastrointestinal tract is composed of the mouth, esophagus, stomach, small and large intestines, and anus.
  - The accessory organs are the liver, pancreas, gallbladder, and salivary glands.
  - The primary functions are digestion, absorption of nutrients, and elimination.

ORAL CAVITY

- The digestive process begins with mechanical chewing of food in the mouth.
  - The salivary gland secretes saliva containing amylase.
    - ➤ Chemical digestion begins.
    - ➤ Saliva production is approximately 1 liter of saliva/24 hours.
- Esophagus
  - Hollow tube or passageway that passes food from the pharynx to the stomach
    - ➤ Deglutition is the process of swallowing.
    - ➤ Approximately 10 inches long
  - **Involuntary** peristaltic activity
  - No digestion or absorption

STOMACH

- Begins at lower esophageal sphincter (connects the esophagus to the stomach) and ends at the pyloric sphincter (connects the lower stomach to the duodenum)
- The stomach is a storage organ or pouch for food and chemical breakdown.
  - Divided into four regions: cardia, fundus, body, and pylorus
  - Rugae are folds that cover the inner surface of the stomach.
  - Secretion of gastric juices is regulated by the sympathetic and parasympathetic nervous system, hormonal control
    - ➤ Three phases—cephalic, gastric, and intestinal
  - Components of gastric juices
    - ➤ Hydrochloric acid (HCl)
      - Principal cells of the gastric gland
      - Strong acid produced by parietal cells
      - Converts pepsinogen to pepsin
      - Necessary for protein digestion
      - Acts as a bactericidal agent
    - ➤ Intrinsic factor
      - Source is parietal cells of gastric glands
      - Essential for absorption of vitamin B_{12} in the small intestine

- ➤ Mucus
    - – Source is goblet cells and mucous glands
    - – Provides gelatinous, alkaline protection of stomach wall from acidic gastric juice
  - ○ Mechanical churning (peristalsis) helps digestion.
    - ➤ Chyme is partially digested food and gastric juice.
    - ➤ Four to six hours are needed for gastric emptying.
  - ○ Chyme is pushed into the small intestine via the pyloric sphincter.

SMALL INTESTINE

- ■ Begins at the pyloric sphincter and ends at the ileocecal valve at the large intestine
  - ○ Approximately 20 feet long
    - ➤ Composed of duodenum (approximately 10 inches), jejunum (approximately 8 feet), and ileum (approximately 12 feet)
  - ○ The majority of digestion and absorption takes place in the small intestine.
- ■ Duodenum
  - ○ Begins at the pyloric sphincter
  - ○ Pancreatic enzymes and bile enter in response to cholecystokinin and secretin.
    - ➤ Pancreatic enzymes: amylase, chymotrypsin, lipase, trypsin

LARGE INTESTINE

- ■ The large intestine may be referred to as the colon.
- ■ The primary function is to take in salts, vitamins, and water made by bacteria in the large intestine and defecate indigestible food and residue from the body.
- ■ Five areas
  1. Cecum
  2. Appendix
  3. Colon
     - ➤ Ascending
     - ➤ Transverse
     - ➤ Descending
  4. Rectum
     - ➤ Container for feces
     - ➤ Approximately 12 cm in length
  5. Anus
     - ➤ Terminal end of digestive tract
     - ➤ Defecation regulated through defecation reflex (spinal cord reflex)

ACCESSORY ORGANS

- ■ Support activities of the digestive tract
- ■ Liver and Hepatic system
  - ○ The liver is the largest glandular organ in the body.
    - ➤ Occupies most of the right upper quadrant; lies under the diaphragm
    - ➤ Divided into four lobes: right, left, caudate, and quadratic
      - – can be further subdivided into lobules

➤ Cell types include:
  – Kupffer's cells (reticuloendothelial cells)
  – Hepatocytes (liver cells)
➤ Functions
  – Activation of enzymes
  – Production and excretion of bile
  – Excretion of bilirubin, cholesterol
  – Carbohydrate, fats, and protein metabolism
  – Glycogen, mineral, and vitamin storage
  – Regulates blood glucose levels
  – Affects drug metabolism and detoxification
○ Biliary system
➤ Produces, carries, stores, and releases bile into duodenum to aid in the digestion of food
➤ The gallbladder is a small pouch located under, and attached to, the liver.
  – Stores bile, releasing it into the duodenum
  – Regulated by cholecystokinin (hormone)
■ Pancreas
○ Long slender organ located posterior to the stomach, extending approximately from the duodenum to the spleen
○ The head and body of the pancreas produce digestive enzymes and bicarbonate.
○ The Islets of Langerhans, in the tail of the pancreas, secrete insulin and glucagon.

ANSWER SHEET
The Gastrointestinal System Sample Test

1. Ⓐ Ⓑ Ⓒ Ⓓ
2. Ⓐ Ⓑ Ⓒ Ⓓ
3. Ⓐ Ⓑ Ⓒ Ⓓ
4. Ⓐ Ⓑ Ⓒ Ⓓ
5. Ⓐ Ⓑ Ⓒ Ⓓ
6. Ⓐ Ⓑ Ⓒ Ⓓ
7. Ⓐ Ⓑ Ⓒ Ⓓ

8. Ⓐ Ⓑ Ⓒ Ⓓ
9. Ⓐ Ⓑ Ⓒ Ⓓ
10. Ⓐ Ⓑ Ⓒ Ⓓ
11. Ⓐ Ⓑ Ⓒ Ⓓ
12. Ⓐ Ⓑ Ⓒ Ⓓ
13. Ⓐ Ⓑ Ⓒ Ⓓ
14. Ⓐ Ⓑ Ⓒ Ⓓ

15. Ⓐ Ⓑ Ⓒ Ⓓ
16. Ⓐ Ⓑ Ⓒ Ⓓ
17. Ⓐ Ⓑ Ⓒ Ⓓ
18. Ⓐ Ⓑ Ⓒ Ⓓ
19. Ⓐ Ⓑ Ⓒ Ⓓ
20. Ⓐ Ⓑ Ⓒ Ⓓ

For Questions 1–20, select the letter (A, B, C, or D) that best answers the question. Record your answers on The Gastrointestinal System Sample Test Answer Sheet on page 249.

1. Included in the components of bile are

   (A) bilirubin, bile salts, cholesterol, and lecithin.
   (B) ketone bodies, bilirubin, trace minerals, and glycerol.
   (C) proteolytic enzymes, bile salts, trypsin, and water.
   (D) synthesized hormones, bilirubin, bile salts, and pyruvic acid.

2. Select the true statement regarding the digestive process.

   (A) mouth ⇒ esophagus ⇒ stomach ⇒ small intestine ⇔ large intestine ⇒ anus
   (B) mouth ⇒ esophagus ⇒ stomach ⇒ small intestine ⇒ large intestine ⇒ anus
   (C) mouth ⇒ pharnyx ⇒ stomach ⇒ small intestine ⇒ large intestine ⇒ ⇒ anus
   (D) mouth ⇒ esophagus ⇒ stomach ⇒ small intestine ⇒ appendix ⇒ large intestine ⇒ anus

3. Accessory organs of digestion include all of the following EXCEPT

   (A) esophagus.
   (B) gallbladder.
   (C) liver.
   (D) salivary glands.

4. Which structure stores feces for elimination?

   (A) appendix
   (B) lower gastrointestinal tract
   (C) pylorus
   (D) rectum

5. Chemical digestion of food begins in the

   (A) esophagus.
   (B) mouth.
   (C) pharynx.
   (D) stomach.

6. Deglutition is the process of

   (A) absorption of nutrients.
   (B) elimination of indigestible food.
   (C) swallowing partially digested food.
   (D) None of the above

7. What valve prevents the return of feces to the small intestine?

   (A) appendix
   (B) ileocecal
   (C) lower sphincter
   (D) sigmoid

8. What percentage of digestion occurs in the esophagus?

   (A) 0%
   (B) 5–8%
   (C) 9–11%
   (D) depends upon the fiber content of the partially digested food

9. Secretion of gastric juices is regulated by all of the following EXCEPT

   (A) cholecystokinin, peptide, and secretin.
   (B) gastrin.
   (C) the parasympathetic nervous system.
   (D) the sympathetic nervous system.

10. Where does the majority of digestion and absorption take place?

    (A) ascending colon
    (B) pylorus
    (C) small intestine
    (D) stomach

11. Partially digested food and gastric juice is referred to as

    (A) agglutination.
    (B) chyme.
    (C) fasciculation.
    (D) malabsorption.

12. The stomach begins at the _____ and ends at the _____.

    (A) esophagus, duodenum
    (B) pharynx, ceccal sphincter
    (C) lower esophageal sphincter, pyloric sphincter
    (D) veriform appendix, jejunic sphincter

13. One function of the _____ is to take in salts, vitamins, and water.

    (A) accessory organs
    (B) large intestine
    (C) stomach
    (D) transverse colon

14. All of the following are digestive enzymes EXCEPT

    (A) salivary amylase.
    (B) bile.
    (C) trypsin.
    (D) sucrase.

15. One purpose of Kupffer's cells is to

    (A) destroy bacteria.
    (B) regulate digestion.
    (C) stimulate metabolism.
    (D) withhold bile secretion.

16. Which system produces, carries, stores, and releases bile?

    (A) biliary
    (B) pancreatic
    (C) hepatic
    (D) None of the above

17. The gallbladder is located in the

    (A) lower left quadrant.
    (B) lower right quadrant.
    (C) upper left quadrant.
    (D) upper right quadrant.

18. The liver has all of the following functions in digestion EXCEPT

    (A) activation of enzymes.
    (B) combines blood clotting factors.
    (C) excretion of cholesterol.
    (D) protein metabolism.

19. Specialized cells in the head and body of the pancreas produce

    (A) bicarbonate.
    (B) cystokinin.
    (C) insulin.
    (D) amino acids.

20. An individual has a disorder of carbohydrate metabolism related to dysfunction of the beta cells of the pancreas. You would expect the blood glucose levels of this individual to

    (A) drop below normal range.
    (B) remain within normal range.
    (C) rise above normal range.
    (D) All of the above

The Gastrointestinal System Sample Test Answer Key

1. **A**	5. **B**	9. **A**	13. **B**	17. **D**
2. **B**	6. **C**	10. **C**	14. **B**	18. **B**
3. **A**	7. **B**	11. **B**	15. **A**	19. **A**
4. **D**	8. **A**	12. **C**	16. **A**	20. **C**

THE GASTROINTESTINAL SYSTEM SAMPLE TEST ANSWERS EXPLAINED

1. **(A)** Bile is a yellow-green liquid manufactured in the liver and held in the gallbladder. When released, it passes through the common bile duct into the duodenum where it facilitates fat digestion. The principal constituents of bile are cholesterol, bile salts, and the pigment bilirubin.

2. **(B)** Choice B is the correct pathway for the digestive system in the human body. If you missed this question, review each part of the anatomy of the gastrointestinal system on pages 245–247.

3. **(A)** The esophagus is a hollow tube in which food passes from the mouth to the stomach.

4. **(D)** Review the areas of the large intestine on page 246 if you had difficulty answering this question.

5. **(B)** The mouth, or the oral cavity, is the initial site of digestion where food particles are broken down by mechanical chewing.

6. **(C)** Deglutination is the process of swallowing food that has been partially digested following mechanical chewing.

7. **(B)** Review the location of the ileocecal valve in relation to the small and large intestines on page 246 if you missed this question.

8. **(A)** Food is not digested in the esophagus. It is a hollow tube that allows the passage of food from the mouth to the stomach. The type of content of the food does not matter.

9. **(A)** Cholecystokinin, peptide, and secretin inhibit the production of gastric acid.

10. **(C)** The majority of digestion and absorption takes place in the small intestine. Review the description of the small intestine on page 246 for more information.

11. **(B)** Chyme is partially digested food and gastric juice.

12. **(C)** The stomach begins at the lower esophageal sphincter and ends at the pyloric sphincter.

13. **(B)** This is the primary function of the large intestine. The large intestine then defecates any indigestible food and/or residue from the body.

14. **(B)** Bile is a greenish-yellow fluid produced in the liver, stored in the gallbladder, and released into the small intestine. While bile is an important component of the digestive process, it is not an enzyme.

15. **(A)** Kupffer *cells* are a type of macrophage that capture and destroy bacteria, and break down old, worn-out red blood cells passing through the sinusoids of the liver. The Kupffer cells are phagocytic. They also store hemosiderin that is available for the production of hemoglobin. Hemosiderin is an iron-containing pigment that is formed from the hemoglobin of red blood cells that have disintegrated. Expended white blood cells are also broken down.

16. **(A)** The biliary system manufactures, transfers, masses, and releases bile into the duodenum to aid in digestion. The biliary system includes the gallbladder, bile ducts, and certain cells inside the liver and bile ducts outside the liver.

17. **(D)** Knowing where organs are located in the abdomen is the key to selecting the correct answer. The abdomen is frequently divided into four quadrants.

18. **(B)** The liver plays a role in more than one system. Coagulation factors released into the blood assist with hemostasis or the cessation of bleeding.

19. **(A)** The specialized cells in the head and body of the pancreas produce digestive enzymes and bicarbonate, about 1,500–2,000 ml of digestive solution/day. The Islets of Langerhans, in the tail of the pancreas, secrete glucagon and insulin.

20. **(C)** The endocrine functions of the pancreas are accomplished by alpha and beta cells that compose the Islets of Langerhans. Alpha cells secrete glucagon, and beta cells secrete insulin. Both are essential for carbohydrate metabolism. When beta cells are affected by disease, blood levels rise.

OVERVIEW

- The primary purpose is to transport oxygen from the lungs and nutrients from the gastrointestinal tract to body cells for cellular metabolism and transport cell and tissue waste products to excretory organs.
- Constituents of whole blood
  - Total blood volume is approximately 5 liters or 7 to 8% total body weight in adults.
  - Plasma is the liquid portion of whole blood **with** clotting factors.
  - Serum is the liquid portion **without** clotting factors or blood cells.
  - Blood cells are erythrocytes, leukocytes, platelets, and proteins.
    - ➤ Erythrocytes, leukocytes, and platelets develop from stem cells and differentiate into mature blood cells (see Figure 6.6).
    - ➤ Each type of blood cell has its own structure, function, and life span.
  - Plasma proteins (fibrinogen, prothrombin, and thromboplastin)
- The formation of blood or blood cells in the living body is called **hematopoiesis**.
- The number of blood cells in the body is constant because production and destruction is balanced.

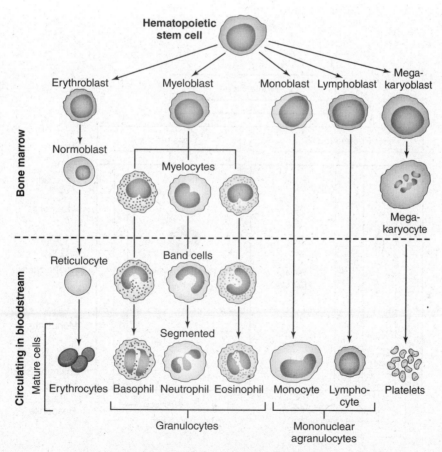

Figure 6.6. Hematopoietic Stem Cell

BONE MARROW

- Spongy center of bones where hematologic and immunologic cell lines arise and mature prior to being released into circulation
- Most cells are produced in the red marrow of the vertebrae, skull, ribs, pelvis, and proximal epiphyses of the humerus and femur.
- Pluripotent stem cell
    - A self-renewing cell from which all differentiated bone marrow cell lines derive
    - Erythrocytes, leukocytes, and platelets develop from stem cells and differentiate into mature blood cells.

LIVER

- Functions as part of the hematological system
    - Synthesizes plasma factors including albumin and clotting factors
    - Clears damaged and nonfunctioning RBCs from circulation
    - Synthesizes coagulation factors VII, IX, X, and prothrombin

COMPONENTS OF WHOLE BLOOD

- See Figure 6.7
- Plasma
    - **Extracellular** fluid
    - Majority is located in circulation
    - Provides circulation for blood cells

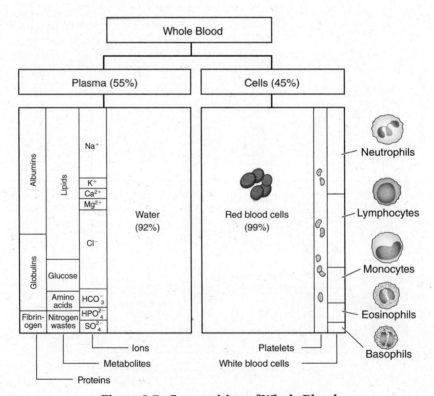

Figure 6.7. Composition of Whole Blood

- Slightly cloudy yellowish fluid of whole blood composed of water (approximately 90%), proteins, electrolytes, hormones, nutrients, enzymes, antibodies, coagulation factors, waste products, oxygen, and carbon dioxide
  - ➤ Contains all of the components of blood except RBCs, WBCs, and thrombocytes
  - ➤ Approximately 55% of a blood sample
- **Serum**
  - Fluid remaining when plasma is allowed to clot
- **Red Blood Cells (Erythrocytes, RBCs)**
  - Most abundant type of blood cell
  - Approximately 99% of blood cells
  - Biconcave, disk-like shape provides wider surface for diffusion of oxygen
  - Erythropoesis
    - ➤ Tissue hypoxia $\Rightarrow$ kidneys release **erythropoietin** $\Rightarrow$ red bone marrow $\Rightarrow$ erythrocytes (RBCs) production
    - ➤ Requires numerous substances
      - – Folic acid
      - – Vitamin B complex
      - – Vitamin D
      - – Iron
    - ➤ Released into circulation as reticulocytes and become RBCs in around 24 hours
    - ➤ The function of RBCs is to carry hemoglobin via circulation to cells and carbon dioxide to the lungs.
    - ➤ RBCs have around a 3-month (120-day) life span.
      - – Old RBCs are removed from circulation by the spleen and liver.
      - – RBC destruction = RBC production
    - ➤ Phagocytic cells identify, absorb, and destroy biologically aged RBCs.
      - – Cells come from bone marrow, lymph nodes, the liver, and the spleen.
      - – Heme in the RBC is converted to bilirubin and transported to the liver.
    - ➤ Glucose and the glycolytic pathways provide metabolic needs.
    - ➤ $\Downarrow$ RBCs = Early RBC death
- **Leukocytes**
  - Also known as white blood cells
  - Provide immunity and protection from contagion by phagocytosis
  - Short life span and require constant replenishing
  - Three types of granulocytes:
    1. Basophils
       - – Less effective at phagocytosis than eosinophils and neutrophils
       - – Similar to mast cells
       - – Releases heparin, histamine, and serotonin
       - – Seen in allergic and inflammatory reactions
    2. Eosinophils
       - – Less of an effect at phagocytosis than neutrophils
       - – Capacity to overwhelm antigen–antibody complexes from allergic reactions
       - – Capacity to shield from parasitic infections
    3. Neutrophils
       - – Phagocytes
       - – Evolve from metamyelocytes to bands (less mature neutrophils)

- Lymphocytes
  - ➤ Originate in lymph nodes and bone marrow
  - ➤ Immune system cells
  - ➤ B-cells are directly **cytotoxic** and involved in **humoral immunity**.
  - ➤ T-cells originate in the thymus, produce antibodies, and are involved in **cell-mediated immunity**.
- Platelets
  - May be referred to as thrombocytes
  - They are small blood components that help the clotting process by:
    - ➤ Platelet **adherence** (sticking to the lining of injured blood vessels)
    - ➤ Platelet **aggregation** (attaching to other platelets to enlarge the forming plug)
    - ➤ Providing support for the clotting cascade
  - **Platelets are not cells**, but rather they are fragments of cytoplasm enclosed in membranes.
  - Platelets are made in the bone marrow and survive in the circulatory system for approximately 10 days.
- Hemostasis (Clotting Process)
  - See Figure 6.8
  - A dynamic process by which the body prevents blood loss
    - ➤ Involves the formation of a blood clot or thrombus that prevents further loss from damaged tissues, blood vessels, or organs
  - Involves three mechanisms
    - ➤ Vascular spasm
    - ➤ Injured vessel constricts; stops capillary bleeding
  - Formation of platelet plug
    - ➤ Platelets aggregate the site of injury and form loose plugs; they stop bleeding in larger injuries
  - Activation of clotting factors
    - ➤ Via intrinsic or extrinsic pathways
  - Clotting factors
    - ➤ Compromised of proteins and other substances
    - ➤ Numbered I to XII that are involved in forming a fibrin clot at the site of tissue or endothelial damage
    - ➤ Common factors
      - – Factor I (fibrinogen)
      - – Factor II (prothrombin)
      - – Factor III (thromboplastin)
      - – Factor IV (calcium)
      - – Factor VIII (antihemophilic factor)
  - Clotting cascade
    - ➤ Comprised of intrinsic and extrinsic pathways that merge, forming a common pathway
    - ➤ Intrinsic pathway
      - – Activated after **endothelial damage** when factor XII (Hageman factor), circulating in the blood, comes in contact with collagen

Intrinsic and Extrinsic Coagulation Cascades

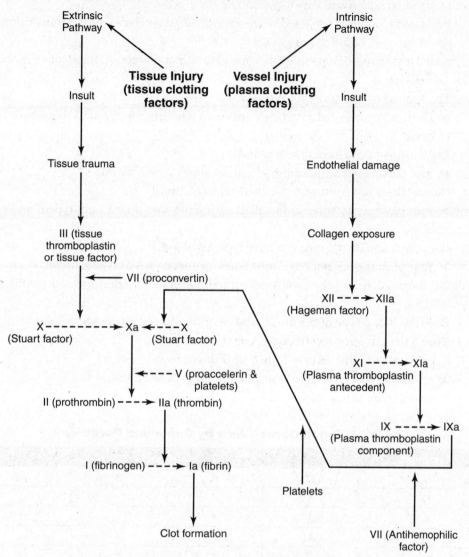

Figure 6.8. Intrinsic and Extrinsic Coagulation Cascade

➤ Extrinsic pathway
  – Activated after tissue trauma when factor III, released from **damaged tissues,** comes in contact with factor VII (Proconvertin) circulating in the blood
➤ The last step in the clotting cascade is the conversion from factor I (fibrinogen) to factor 1a (fibrin), forming a stable clot.
➤ The fibrin clot is eventually removed by the enzyme plasmin.

ABO BLOOD GROUP SYSTEM

■ Blood type or group is determined by two specific types of **antigen**, or protein, found on the red cell **membrane**
  ○ Antigens are inherited from parents.
  ○ Designated "A" (Type A) or "B" (Type B) antigen

- Two natural **antibodies** are found in the **plasma** that trigger the immune response.
    - Designated anti-A and anti-B antibodies
    - Immune response is triggered when an individual receives a blood transfusion with blood carrying **non-self antigens**.
- The ABO test shows that people have one of four blood types: A, B, AB, or O. If your red blood cells have:
    - The A antigen, you have **type A blood**.
        - ➤ The liquid portion of your blood (plasma) has anti-B antibodies that attack type B blood.
    - The B antigen, you have **type B blood**.
        - ➤ Your plasma has anti-A antibodies that attack type A blood.
    - Neither the A nor B antigen, you have **type O blood**.
        - ➤ Your plasma has anti-A and anti-B antibodies that attack both type A and type B blood.
    - Both the A and B antigens, you have **type AB blood**.
        - ➤ Your plasma does not have antibodies against type A or type B blood.
- Blood transfusions can be fatal if incompatible blood is administered to the wrong individual.
    - **Both the blood type of the donor and recipient must be considered**. See Table 6.1.
    - **Type A** patient must receive **Type A or O** donor blood.
    - **Type B** patient must receive **Type B or O** donor blood.
    - **Type AB** patient can receive **Type A, B, AB, or O** donor blood.
    - **Type O** patient can receive **Type O** donor blood only.

Table 6.1. Blood Donor Types by Donor and Recipient

Recipient	Donor			
	O	A	B	AB
O	X			
A	X	X		
B	X		X	
AB	X	X	X	X

RH FACTOR

- Rhesus (Rh) factor is an inherited trait that refers to a specific protein found on the surface of red blood cells.
    - If your blood has the protein, you're Rh positive.
    - If your blood lacks the protein, you're Rh negative.
    - A negative or positive sign after the blood type indicates Rh status (A−, AB+, O+).
    - Although Rh factor doesn't affect your health, it can affect pregnancy. Pregnancy requires special attention if one parent is Rh negative and the other is Rh positive.

ANSWER SHEET
The Hematologic System Sample Test

1. Ⓐ Ⓑ Ⓒ Ⓓ
2. Ⓐ Ⓑ Ⓒ Ⓓ
3. Ⓐ Ⓑ Ⓒ Ⓓ
4. Ⓐ Ⓑ Ⓒ Ⓓ
5. Ⓐ Ⓑ Ⓒ Ⓓ
6. Ⓐ Ⓑ Ⓒ Ⓓ
7. Ⓐ Ⓑ Ⓒ Ⓓ

8. Ⓐ Ⓑ Ⓒ Ⓓ
9. Ⓐ Ⓑ Ⓒ Ⓓ
10. Ⓐ Ⓑ Ⓒ Ⓓ
11. Ⓐ Ⓑ Ⓒ Ⓓ
12. Ⓐ Ⓑ Ⓒ Ⓓ
13. Ⓐ Ⓑ Ⓒ Ⓓ
14. Ⓐ Ⓑ Ⓒ Ⓓ

15. Ⓐ Ⓑ Ⓒ Ⓓ
16. Ⓐ Ⓑ Ⓒ Ⓓ
17. Ⓐ Ⓑ Ⓒ Ⓓ
18. Ⓐ Ⓑ Ⓒ Ⓓ
19. Ⓐ Ⓑ Ⓒ Ⓓ
20. Ⓐ Ⓑ Ⓒ Ⓓ

For Questions 1–20, select the letter (A, B, C, or D) that best answers the question. Record your answers on The Hematologic System Sample Test Answer Sheet on page 261.

1. The primary purpose of the hematologic system is
   (A) the removal of damaged/nonfunctioning RBCs.
   (B) the promotion of hematopoiesis.
   (C) the synthesizing erythrocytes and plasma proteins.
   (D) transportation.

2. Plasma is categorized as _____ fluid.
   (A) extracellular
   (B) hematopopoetic
   (C) intracellular
   (D) None of the above

3. Erythropoesis requires all of the following EXCEPT
   (A) factor IV.
   (B) folic acid.
   (C) iron.
   (D) vitamin B_{12}.

4. Which of the following provides passive immunity and protection from contagion by phagocytosis?
   (A) basophils
   (B) eosinophils
   (C) leukocytes
   (D) lymphocytes

5. A fibrin clot is eventually removed by plasmin, which is a(an)
   (A) enzyme.
   (B) hormone.
   (C) humoralytic factor.
   (D) lymphocyte.

6. An individual has elevated basophils. His problem could be caused by
   (A) antibody factors.
   (B) an inflammatory reaction.
   (C) overgrowth of phagocytes.
   (D) a parasitic infestation.

7. Which of the following has its origin in the hematopoietic stem cell?
   (A) albumin
   (B) bone marrow
   (C) plasma proteins
   (D) platelets

8. Plasma contains what percentage of erythrocytes?
   (A) 0%
   (B) 45%
   (C) 55%
   (D) 99%

9. Fluid that remains when plasma is allowed to clot is called
   (A) albumin.
   (B) packed red blood cells.
   (C) serum.
   (D) T-cell antibodies.

10. Cells that defend against micro-organisms and some types of malignant cells are called
    (A) B-lymphocytes.
    (B) natural killer cells.
    (C) neutrophils.
    (D) T-lymphocytes.

11. All blood cells are produced in the

    (A) intracellular fluid.
    (B) liver.
    (C) marrow of the bone.
    (D) spleen

12. Red blood cells circulate in the bloodstream
    for approximately

    (A) 10 days.
    (B) 120 days.
    (C) 2 months.
    (D) 4 months.

13. Liquid that has no clotting factors is (are)

    (A) globulins.
    (B) plasma.
    (C) platelets.
    (D) serum.

14. Which of the following is a true statement? Red
    blood cells

    (A) are less viscous than water.
    (B) are shaped like biconcave disks.
    (C) may be referred to as lymphocytes.
    (D) transport nutrients.

15. Bilirubin, a bile pigment, is formed from the
    breakdown of

    (A) fibrin.
    (B) hemoglobin.
    (C) leukocytes.
    (D) thrombin.

16. Prothrombin, a clotting factor, is
    manufactured in the

    (A) bone marrow.
    (B) kidney.
    (C) liver.
    (D) plasma.

17. An individual with blood type O negative is
    considered a(an)

    (A) antibody AB carrier.
    (B) antibody A carrier.
    (C) universal donor.
    (D) universal recipient.

18. All of the following are involved in hemostasis
    EXCEPT

    (A) activation of coagulation cascade.
    (B) activation of plasmin.
    (C) formation of platelet plug.
    (D) vascular spasm/constriction.

19. The extrinsic pathway of the coagulation
    cascade is activated

    (A) after tissue trauma.
    (B) before thrombin activation.
    (C) when factor XII comes in contact with
        collagen.
    (D) when fibrin is converted to fibrinogen.

20. Which of the following would you expect to be
    elevated in an individual with bacterial
    pneumonia?

    (A) liver enzymes
    (B) leukocytes
    (C) red blood cells
    (D) vitamin C

The Hematologic System Sample Test Answer Key

1.	**D**	5.	**A**	9.	**C**	13.	**D**	17.	**C**
2.	**A**	6.	**B**	10.	**B**	14.	**B**	18.	**B**
3.	**A**	7.	**D**	11.	**C**	15.	**B**	19.	**A**
4.	**C**	8.	**A**	12.	**B**	16.	**C**	20.	**B**

THE HEMATOLOGIC SYSTEM SAMPLE TEST ANSWERS EXPLAINED

1. **(D)** Blood transports oxygen from the lung to the cells and carbon dioxide from the cells to the lungs. Other blood constituents transport metabolic waste from the cells to the kidneys. Others transport nutritional components from the digestive system to the cells and hormones throughout the body.

2. **(A)** Plasma is the liquid portion of blood. Plasma, which is 92 percent water, constitutes 55% of blood volume, and contains albumin, fibrinogen, and globulins. Furthermore, plasma is straw colored and is collected from whole blood after blood cells are removed.

3. **(A)** The production of red blood cells, or erythropoiesis, takes place in the bone marrow where the pluripotent stem cells beget the erythrocyte lineage. Erythropoiesis is controlled by erythropoietin that is produced predominantly in the kidneys. Diminished blood oxygen levels stimulate the kidneys to manufacture additional erythropoietin that acts on the bone marrow to increase and accelerate erythropoiesis. Folic acid, iron, and vitamin B_{12} are needed for the manufacture of blood cells. Factor IV is calcium required in many stages of blood clotting.

4. **(C)** Also called white blood cells, leukocytes are vital blood components that perform the key roles of providing immunity and protection from contagion by phagocytosis. There are different types of leukocytes, each having a clear-cut purpose in the body.

5. **(A)** Plasmin is the active primary or chief enzyme of the fibrinolytic system. It has an affinity for fibrin and has the particular ability to dissolve fibrin clots formed by the coagulation cascade.

6. **(B)** Basophils are a type of leukocyte and granulocyte. They are immune cells that have granules with enzymes that are released during allergic reactions and asthma.

7. **(D)** Hematopoietic Stem Cells (HSCs) have the property of self-renewal and, through cell division and differentiation, form populations of progenitor cells which are committed to the main marrow cell lines: Erythroid, Granulocytic and Monocytic, Megakaryocytic and Lymphocytic. They differentiate into erythrocytes, leukocytes, and platelets.

8. **(A)** Whole blood is divided into the components of plasma (55%) and cells (45%). Plasma is over 90% water plus ions, metabolites, and proteins. The cell component is almost 100% red blood cells (erythrocytes) plus platelets and white blood cells. See Figure 6.7. Composition of Whole Blood on page 256.

9. **(C)** Albumin is the most common protein in the blood. Produced by the liver, albumin regulates osmotic pressure between blood and tissue. Serum is the fluid remaining when plasma is allowed to clot.

10. **(B)** Natural killer cells have the ability to attack and destroy other cells without prior sensitization. They are small leukocytes that develop in the bone marrow and are the body's first line of defense against cancer and virus infected cells.

11. **(C)** The two types of bone marrow are "red marrow," which comprises primarily hematopoietic tissue, and "yellow marrow," which is primarily fat cells. Erythrocytes, platelets, and most leukocytes are in red marrow. Both types of bone marrow are extremely vascular. All bone marrow is red at birth. As an individual ages, more and more of the red marrow is converted to the yellow type. Red marrow is found mainly in the flat bones, (cranium, pelvis, ribs, scapulae, sternum, and vertebrae) and in the cancellous material at the epiphyseal ends of bones (femur and humerus). Yellow marrow is located in the hollow center of the middle segment of long bones. Yellow marrow has the ability to change back to red marrow in instances of severe blood loss. This increases blood cell production.

12. **(B)** Erythrocytes (red blood cells), produced through erythropoiesis, develop from committed stem cells to mature erythrocytes in around seven days. Erythrocytes live in the circulation for approximately 100 to 120 days. Erythrocytes age during this time and are removed from circulation when they are no longer useful.

13. **(D)** Serum is clear fluid that can be separated from clotted blood. Serum, as opposed to plasma, is the liquid portion of normal, unclotted blood containing erythrocytes, leukocytes, and platelets.

14. **(B)** Eyrthrocytes are biconcave shaped disks. The shape allows the erythrocyte to carry more oxygen.

15. **(B)** The bile pigment, bilirubin, is from the normal breakdown of hemoglobin, the oxygen-carrying substance in red blood cells. These processes occur naturally as old red blood cells wear out and are replaced in the body. Bilirubin is then carried in the bloodstream to the liver, where it is combined with bile. Bile, also called gall, gets its greenish-yellow color from bilirubin. Bile is a fluid secreted by the liver to aid in the digestion of dietary fat. Bile is stored in the gallbladder. When it is needed for digestion, the gallbladder pushes it out into the small intestine through a tube called a bile duct.

16. **(C)** Prothrombin is manufactured in the liver, as are numerous other clotting mechanisms.

17. **(C)** Individuals with O negative blood are considered universal donors. The red blood cells in O blood have no other antigens. The lack of antigens means individuals with other blood types will not react to O negative blood. Around 7% of the population has O negative blood. The universal recipient is AB blood type. They can receive blood from a person with any blood type.

18. **(B)** Plasmin, an enzyme, ultimately removes the fibrin clots. Damaged endothelial cells secrete a protein that converts the inactive plasmin to its active form, plasminogen, so that degradation of the fibrin clot can begin.

19. **(A)** The extrinsic pathway is stimulated after tissue trauma or damage when factor III (thromboplastin) is released from the site of injury and comes in contact with factor VII (proconvertin) circulating in the blood. The intrinsic pathway is stimulated after endothelial damage.

20. **(B)** Leukocytes (white blood cells) circulate throughout the body, detecting and destroying bacteria, fungi, parasites, viruses, and other proteins identified as foreign to the body. An elevated white blood cell count usually indicates increased production to fight an infection, or reactions to a drug, diseases of the bone marrow, or immune system disorders.

OVERVIEW

- Composed of many interdependent cell types that collectively protect the body from bacterial, parasitic, fungal, and viral infections as well as growth of tumor cells
- Cells of the immune system
  - Engulf bacteria
  - Kill parasites and/or tumor cells
  - Kill viral-infected cells
- Function is to phagocytize foreign material and remove old or damaged cells from circulation

LYMPH SYSTEM

- Composed of lymphatic vessels and lymph nodes
  - Lymph fluid transported toward the heart is filtered through lymph nodes clustered around vessels.
- Large clusters of nodes are found in inguinal, axillary, and cervical regions of the body.
- Organs of the lymphoid system are the thymus gland, areas of the spleen, tonsils, and Peyer's patches.

MONONUCLEAR PHAGOCYTE SYSTEM

- Also known as the reticuloendothelial system (RAS)
- Composed of monocytes that migrated to various tissues and transformed into macrophages
  - Large phagocytic cells destroy bacteria, viruses, and other foreign substances in the lymph before they are returned to the blood.
- Tissues include connective tissue, lungs, liver (Kupffer's cells), spleen, lymph nodes, and microglial cells of the central nervous system.

WHITE CELLS

- Some white cells differentiate into lymphocytes.
- B-cells produce antibodies.
- T-cells attack antigens directly.
  - Specificity
  - Memory
  - Self-recognition
  - Natural killer cells

THE IMMUNE RESPONSE

Immunity is a state of responsiveness to foreign substances such as microorganisms and tumor proteins.

- Immune responses serve three functions:
  1. Defense
  2. Homeostasis
  3. Surveillance

- Properties of the immune response:
  - Specificity
  - Memory
  - Self-recognition
  - Self-limitation
  - Specialization

ANTIBODY-MEDIATED IMMUNITY

- Also called humoral immunity
  - Initiated by the B-cell
- Primary immune response
  - Exposure to antigen
  - Latent period
    - ➤ Mature B-cells produce no detectable antibodies
    - ➤ Latent 5–6 days, IgM found in the circulation
    - ➤ IgG detected but in smaller amounts than IgM
  - With no further exposure, antibody levels fall.
- Secondary immune response
  - Exposure to antigen
  - Rapid production of antibodies
    - ➤ Presence of memory cells left from first exposure to antigens
    - ➤ IgM levels same as with first exposure
    - ➤ IgG in much higher levels than in primary exposure
- Classes of immunoglobins
  - IgG—75% of total antiviral, antitoxin, antibacterial (only maternal antibody that passes placenta)
  - IgA—15%, predominant in body secretions
  - IgM—10%, largest, first antibody produced in primary immune response to an antigen
  - IgD—0.2%, function unclear
  - IgE—0.004%, primary antibody in allergic responses
- Functions of antibodies
  - Neutralization of bacterial toxins
    - ➤ Formulation of toxin–antibody complexes
    - ➤ Prevents toxins from binding to tissue cells
    - ➤ Complexes removed from body to phagocytosis or through body fluids
  - Neutralization of viruses
    - ➤ Prevent the attachment and entrance of viruses to body cells
    - ➤ Neutralized virus may be ingested and removed by phagocytosis.
  - Opsonization of bacteria
    - ➤ Opsonin: a substance that makes bacteria easier to be phagocytized
    - ➤ Necessary since bacteria have capsules that resist phagocytosis
- Memory cells to the specific antigen are also formed with antibody–antigen binding.

CELL-MEDIATED IMMUNITY

- Initiated by the T-cells; 60–70% of the circulating lymphocytes
- Types of T-cells
  1. T_c—cytotoxic T-cells, killer cells
  2. T_h—helper cells, control cell-mediated and humoral responses, augment antibody production
  3. T_s—suppressor cells, control cell-mediated and humoral responses, inhibit antibody production
  4. Memory cells
  5. Lymphokine-producing cells (lymphokines stimulate other cells to participate in the immune response)

MONOCLONAL ACTIVITY

- Acts against a specific antigen
- Produced by clone of B-cell
- Can be made in a laboratory
- Used in treatment of cancer and viral infections
- May be related to species, race, or genetic tendency

ACQUIRED IMMUNITY

- Produced by the immune system itself
- Active acquired immunity
  - Results from exposure to the antigen and subsequent development of antibodies
    - ➤ Memory cells are formed and reinvasion of the antigen will result in a more rapid and vigorous response.
  - Acquired from having the disease
    - ➤ Body develops antibodies, which takes some time.
    - ➤ Long lasting, sometimes for life
  - Acquired by inoculation with a form of the disease (vaccination)
    - ➤ May not last as long, may require "boosters"
- Passive acquired immunity
  - Results from administration of antibodies produced by another source
    - ➤ May be of a natural source (through breastfeeding)
  - Primarily through injection of antibodies as with gamma globulin or immune serum globulin
    - ➤ Short-lived, since individual does manufacture antibodies, and therefore no memory cells

ANSWER SHEET
The Immune System Sample Test

1. Ⓐ Ⓑ Ⓒ Ⓓ
2. Ⓐ Ⓑ Ⓒ Ⓓ
3. Ⓐ Ⓑ Ⓒ Ⓓ
4. Ⓐ Ⓑ Ⓒ Ⓓ
5. Ⓐ Ⓑ Ⓒ Ⓓ
6. Ⓐ Ⓑ Ⓒ Ⓓ
7. Ⓐ Ⓑ Ⓒ Ⓓ

8. Ⓐ Ⓑ Ⓒ Ⓓ
9. Ⓐ Ⓑ Ⓒ Ⓓ
10. Ⓐ Ⓑ Ⓒ Ⓓ
11. Ⓐ Ⓑ Ⓒ Ⓓ
12. Ⓐ Ⓑ Ⓒ Ⓓ
13. Ⓐ Ⓑ Ⓒ Ⓓ
14. Ⓐ Ⓑ Ⓒ Ⓓ

15. Ⓐ Ⓑ Ⓒ Ⓓ
16. Ⓐ Ⓑ Ⓒ Ⓓ
17. Ⓐ Ⓑ Ⓒ Ⓓ
18. Ⓐ Ⓑ Ⓒ Ⓓ
19. Ⓐ Ⓑ Ⓒ Ⓓ
20. Ⓐ Ⓑ Ⓒ Ⓓ

For Questions 1–20, select the letter (A, B, C, or D) that best answers the question. Record your answers on The Immune System Sample Test Answer Sheet on page 271.

1. The immune system is composed of

   (A) many dependent cell types that collectively protect the body.
   (B) many dependent cell types that individually protect the body.
   (C) many interdependent cell types that collectively protect the body.
   (D) many interdependent cell types that individually protect the body.

2. A bacteriostatic solution is a biological or chemical agent that

   (A) complements the immune system.
   (B) inhibits the growth and reproduction of bacteria.
   (C) interacts with bacteria.
   (D) offers maximum protection from bacteria.

3. Large clusters of lymph nodes are found in all of the following areas of the body EXCEPT

   (A) axillary.
   (B) cervical.
   (C) inguinal.
   (D) pharyngeal.

4. Peyer's patches are located in the

   (A) beginning of the large intestine.
   (B) mucous membranes that line the respiratory tract.
   (C) pharynx at the entrance of the auditory tubes.
   (D) mucosa that line the ileum of the small intestine.

5. One function of the immune system is to eradicate old or damaged cells from the circulation. Which lymphatic organ is responsible for this action?

   (A) The bone marrow
   (B) The kidneys
   (C) The lymph nodes
   (D) The spleen

6. Humoral immunity is initiated by the

   (A) B-cells.
   (B) IgE cells.
   (C) lymphokine cells.
   (D) recognition cells.

7. The type of immunity that is inborn

   (A) is actively acquired.
   (B) is passively acquired.
   (C) requires "booster" shots.
   (D) results from genetic constitution.

8. All of the following are included in the lymph system EXCEPT

   (A) the kidneys.
   (B) the spleen.
   (C) the thymus.
   (D) the tonsils.

9. In order for the immune system to mount a successful defense against specific antigens, it must accomplish five (5) tasks. Identify these tasks in their order of occurrence.

1. Antigen mutation	2. Costimulation
3. Destruction of foreign substance	4. Genetic decomposition
5. Lymphatic activation	6. Lymphatic selection
7. Memorization	8. Osmotic response
9. Recognition	

   (A) 2, 8, 5, 4, 1
   (B) 5, 2, 7, 4, 1
   (C) 8, 6, 9, 5, 3
   (D) 9, 6, 5, 3, 7

10. A bacteriocidal solution is a drug or chemical that

    (A) inhibits bacteria.

    (B) kills bacteria.

    (C) stops bacterial reaction.

    (D) transmutates bacteria.

11. Blood enters the spleen via the

    (A) hepatic artery.

    (B) palatine artery.

    (C) splenic artery.

    (D) transhepatic artery.

12. All antibody molecules are composed of

    (A) carbohydrates.

    (B) glycogen.

    (C) adenine monophosphate.

    (D) protein.

13. The thymus gland is the largest gland

    (A) in the fetal stage.

    (B) in the senior years.

    (C) in the teen years.

    (D) in the young child.

14. Movement of fluid through the lymphatic system is helped by

    (A) contraction of skeletal muscles.

    (B) microphage stimulation.

    (C) RBC movement.

    (D) right ventricular pressure.

15. The spleen is located in the

    (A) abdominal cavity.

    (B) cranial cavity.

    (C) thoracic cavity.

    (D) None of these cavities

16. Lymph nodes found in the neck are referred to as _____ nodes.

    (A) cranial

    (B) cervical

    (C) inguinal

    (D) thoracic

17. Antigens are chemical molecules the body identifies as

    (A) antibodies.

    (B) lacteals.

    (C) non-self.

    (D) self.

18. The presence of _____ may cause a white milky consistency in the lymph.

    (A) fats

    (B) nutrients

    (C) wound drainage

    (D) waste materials

19. Cytotoxic T-cells are also referred to as

    (A) cloned cells.

    (B) killer cells.

    (C) memory cells.

    (D) passive cells.

20. A young man comes to your clinic with a cut on his thigh. The wound and the surrounding skin are red, painful, swollen, and warm to the touch. This set of symptoms is referred to as the

    (A) natural killer cell response.

    (B) chemical alarm or response.

    (C) complement response.

    (D) inflammatory response.

The Immune System Sample Test Answer Key

1. **C**	5. **D**	9. **D**	13. **D**	17. **C**
2. **B**	6. **A**	10. **B**	14. **A**	18. **A**
3. **D**	7. **D**	11. **C**	15. **A**	19. **B**
4. **D**	8. **A**	12. **D**	16. **B**	20. **D**

THE IMMUNE SYSTEM SAMPLE TEST ANSWERS EXPLAINED

1. **(C)** The human body, as a system, is composed of numerous subsystems, such as the immune system, which is a system unto itself. All systems of the body work together for the "good" of the body. Two words in Choice C give away the correct answer— "interdependent" and "collectively."

2. **(B)** The key to selecting the correct answer is being able to break down the word into "bacterio-" and "-static." Bacterio- is a prefix meaning "of bacteria or bacterial things." Static is something that lacks development. Bacteriostatic agents inhibit the growth, reproduction, or development of bacteria.

3. **(D)** Review the lymph system, and the locations of lymph nodes, on page 268.

4. **(D)** Peyer's patches are collections of numerous lymphoid follicles closely packed together on the mucous membrane of the small intestine.

5. **(D)** The spleen is similar in structure to a lymph node, and the spleen is the largest lymphatic organ in the body. Spleenic functions include removing old/damaged blood cells from circulation and storing approximately one-third of the body's supply of platelets. The spleen is not requisite for life—other organs such as the bone marrow and liver can assume many of its functions.

6. **(A)** The humoral response may be referred to as the antibody-mediated response. It is initiated by B-lymphocytes that recognize antigens (autoantigen or heteroantigen). Daughter cells of the B-lymphocytes that are involved in the response are plasma cells and memory cells.

7. **(D)** Inborn immunity may be referred to as genetic, inherent, native, and natural immunity. Such immunity occurs as a result of an individual's genetic make-up or physiology. It does not develop from a previous infection or vaccination.

8. **(A)** The kidneys are part of the renal system, not the lymph system.

9. **(D)** The correct order is recognition (9), lymphatic selection (6), lymphatic activation (5), destruction of foreign substance (3), and memorization (7).

10. **(B)** As with question 2, selecting the correct answer has to do with breaking down the word. "Cidal" means the capability to kill or killing. A bacteriocidal agent kills bacteria.

11. **(C)** Aorta ⇨ splenic artery ⇨ spleen ⇨ splenic vein ⇨ inferior vena cava

12. **(D)** Antibodies are recognition proteins located in the serum and other body fluids. They react with specific antigens that provoke their creation. Antibodies are members of a family of globular proteins termed immunoglobins.

13. **(D)** The thymus gland is largest in the young child and grows until puberty when it weighs approximately 40 grams. It slowly decreases in size until around the age of 65 when it weighs approximately 6 grams.

14. **(A)** Review the description of the lymph system on page 268 if you missed this question.

15. **(A)** The spleen is located in the abdominal cavity, and it is an important part of both the lymph system and the mononuclear phagocyte system.

16. **(B)** The key to answering this question correctly is being able to define *cervical* which means relating to the neck.

17. **(C)** The body identifies antigens as non-self. Antigens are substances that, as a consequence of coming into contact with certain body tissues, induce a state sensitivity.

18. **(A)** Chyle is produced in the digestive system as lymph absorbs triglycerides from the intestinal villi. The presence of triglycerides turns the chyle a milky white color.

19. **(B)** Cytotoxic T-cells are lymphocytes toxic to specific antigens. Antigens that are exposed to cytotoxic T-lymphocytes can respond in a number of ways by undergoing necrosis, stopping growth and division, or activating a genetic program of regulated cell death.

20. **(D)** The inflammatory response is the body's normal response to injury and/or infection. Redness, pain, swelling, and heat are hallmarks of this response. Depending on the injury and/or infection, disability may also be present. The inflammatory response is classified as part of the second line of defense.

OVERVIEW

- Regarded as an organ because it comprises two tissues, connective and epithelial
  - Largest body organ composed of three layers
  - Accessory organs are nails, hair, and glands
    - ➤ May be referred to as epidermal appendages

EPIDERMIS

- Top-most layer composed of stratified squamous epithelium
- Skin covering of four layers of the entire body except for the palms of hands and the soles of feet, which have five layers
  - Has four cell types
    1. Keratinocytes
       - Produce keratin
       - Waterproof skin
    2. Langerhans cells
       - Phagocytic microphages
    3. Melanocytes
       - Produce melanin
       - Protect from UV light
    4. Merkel cells
       - Sensory function

DERMIS

- Middle layer directly underneath epidermis, composed of connective tissue
  - Provides strength, elasticity, and extensibility
- Composed of blood vessels, hair follicles, lymphatics, nerves, sebaceous, and sweat glands
- Consists of two layers
  - Papillary layer
    - ➤ Combination of loose connective tissue, small elastic fibers, and network of capillaries
  - Reticular layer
    - ➤ Complex bed of vascular connective tissues containing lymphatic tissue and nerves

HYPODERMIS

- Deepest layer that provides a bolster between skin layers and muscles and bones
- Depending upon the location in the body, it is composed of loose connective tissue or adipose tissue.

ACCESSORY ORGANS

- Hair
- Nails
- Sebaceous glands (also known as oil glands)
- Sudoriferous glands
  - Apocrine glands
  - Ceruminous glands
  - Eccrine glands
  - Mammary glands

INTEGUMENTARY FUNCTIONS

- Aesthetic
- Circulatory
- Immunologic
- Protective
- Sensory
- Thermoregulatory
- Vitamin D production
- Water balance

ANSWER SHEET
The Integumentary System Sample Test

1. Ⓐ Ⓑ Ⓒ Ⓓ
2. Ⓐ Ⓑ Ⓒ Ⓓ
3. Ⓐ Ⓑ Ⓒ Ⓓ
4. Ⓐ Ⓑ Ⓒ Ⓓ
5. Ⓐ Ⓑ Ⓒ Ⓓ
6. Ⓐ Ⓑ Ⓒ Ⓓ
7. Ⓐ Ⓑ Ⓒ Ⓓ

8. Ⓐ Ⓑ Ⓒ Ⓓ
9. Ⓐ Ⓑ Ⓒ Ⓓ
10. Ⓐ Ⓑ Ⓒ Ⓓ
11. Ⓐ Ⓑ Ⓒ Ⓓ
12. Ⓐ Ⓑ Ⓒ Ⓓ
13. Ⓐ Ⓑ Ⓒ Ⓓ
14. Ⓐ Ⓑ Ⓒ Ⓓ

15. Ⓐ Ⓑ Ⓒ Ⓓ
16. Ⓐ Ⓑ Ⓒ Ⓓ
17. Ⓐ Ⓑ Ⓒ Ⓓ
18. Ⓐ Ⓑ Ⓒ Ⓓ
19. Ⓐ Ⓑ Ⓒ Ⓓ
20. Ⓐ Ⓑ Ⓒ Ⓓ

For Questions 1–20, select the letter (A, B, C, or D) that best answers the question. Record your answers on The Integumentary System Sample Test Answer Sheet on page 279.

1. The rate of sweat secretion is controlled by
   (A) the anterior pituitary system.
   (B) apocrine glands.
   (C) eccrine glands.
   (D) the sympathetic nervous system.

2. A sebaceous gland is also known as a(an)
   (A) adipose gland.
   (B) hormonal gland.
   (C) oil gland.
   (D) pore gland.

3. The _____ is the middle layer of skin.
   (A) epidermis
   (B) dermis
   (C) hypodermis
   (D) None of the above

4. The cell types in the epidermis responsible for waterproofing are
   (A) keratinocytes.
   (B) Langerhans cells.
   (C) melanocytes.
   (D) Merkel cells

5. The skin allows approximately _____ milliliters of insensible water loss during a normal day.
   (A) 100–300
   (B) 400–600
   (C) 700–900
   (D) 1,000

6. Melanin protects the skin from
   (A) endogenous production of vitamin D.
   (B) excessive heat and cold.
   (C) invasion of bacteria.
   (D) ultraviolet rays.

7. Sweat glands are also known as
   (A) chemical glands.
   (B) lymphatic glands.
   (C) growing glands.
   (D) sudoriferous glands.

8. Which of the following provides mechanical/ perfunctory strength to the skin?
   (A) dermal layer
   (B) epidermal layer
   (C) hypodermal layer
   (D) subcutaneous layer

9. Sebum
   (A) encourages oiliness of hair.
   (B) inhibits bacterial growth.
   (C) stimulates acne growth.
   (D) stimulates pore opening.

10. Earwax is secreted by the
    (A) ceruminous glands.
    (B) epocrine glands.
    (C) Langerhans cells.
    (D) Merkel cells.

11. What parts of the body have five layers of skin instead of four?
    (A) elbows and knees
    (B) legs and arms
    (C) palms of hands and soles of feet
    (D) pubic regions and genitalia

12. The type of skin that covers the body is _____ tissue.
    (A) connective
    (B) dermal
    (C) epidermal
    (D) epithelial

13. The skin conserves heat by

    (A) halting mitosis.

    (B) increasing hormone production.

    (C) producing heat-resistant enzymes.

    (D) moderating sweat secretions.

14. What protein is readily hydrated, demonstrating swelling of skin on submersion in water and dryness of skin likely from a lack of water?

    (A) keratin

    (B) melanin

    (C) sebum

    (D) valine

15. "Goose bumps" are produced when

    (A) the arrector pili muscle contracts and the hair becomes erect.

    (B) the cardiac cycle is stimulated.

    (C) the myometrium is momentarily depressed.

    (D) the sympathetic nervous system abruptly responds to stimuli.

16. Skin temperature depends chiefly on the

    (A) amount of oxygenated blood in the arterial system.

    (B) release of histamine into the skin.

    (C) rate of blood flow through the skin.

    (D) tissue hydration in superficial tissues.

17. All of the following are considered epidermal appendages EXCEPT

    (A) hair.

    (B) nails.

    (C) papilla.

    (D) sebaceous glands.

18. Adipose cells are found in the

    (A) dermis.

    (B) hypodermis.

    (C) stratum corneum.

    (D) stratum germinativum.

19. The major functions of the skin are all of the following EXCEPT

    (A) assists in regulating body temperature.

    (B) protects underlying body tissues.

    (C) receives stimuli from the external environment.

    (D) synthesizes vitamin C.

20. Human scalp hair grows at a rate of approximately

    (A) 0.4 cm per month.

    (B) 1.0 cm per month.

    (C) 1.3 cm per month.

    (D) 2.0 cm per month.

THE INTEGUMENTARY SYSTEM SAMPLE TEST ANSWERS EXPLAINED

1. **(D)** The sympathetic nervous system influences body functioning in many ways, such as stimulating sweat glands, increasing blood to skeletal muscles, bronchodilation, reducing blood flow to the abdomen, releasing glucose stores from the liver, constricting the peripheral vessels, increasing the chronotropic and inotropic effect in the heart, decreasing digestive activity, and others. Sympathetic stimulation releases norepinephrine, which releases adrenalin and noradrenalin. These are released into the body to prolong the effects of sympathetic stimulation.

2. **(C)** Sebaceous glands are cutaneous glands located in the derma. They produce and secrete sebum, an oily substance that lubricates the hair and skin.

3. **(B)** The skin is composed of three layers. The top layer is the epidermis, the middle layer is the dermis, and the third, or bottom, layer is the hypodermis.

4. **(A)** All of the options are cell types found in the epidermis that consists of stratified squamous epithelium. Keratinocytes produce the protein, keratin, which waterproofs the skin. Langerhans cells network with white blood cells during the immune response by processing antigens. Melanocytes produce keratinocytes that protect from ultraviolet rays and gives skin its color. Merkel cells perform the sensory function of touch reception.

5. **(B)** Insensible water loss from the skin, also known as transepidermal water loss, is water loss that an individual is not aware of—it is not seen or felt. It is not sweat. An adult loses from 400–600 ml/24 hrs.

6. **(D)** Melanin is a pigment that determines hair, eye, and skin color. Melanin also protects the skin from UV sunrays. Dark skinned individuals have greater amounts of melanin in the skin and do not sunburn as easily as light skinned individuals sunburn because of lesser amounts of melanin in the skin.

7. **(D)** Sudoriferous glands, located in the subcutaneous tissues, secrete perspiration (sweat).

8. **(A)** The dermis, the second layer of skin, is composed of connective tissues that provide elasticity, extensibility, and strength.

9. **(A)** Sebum, produced by the sebaceous glands, is an oily substance that keeps the hair and skin moisturized.

10. **(A)** Earwax, or cerumen, is a yellowish, waxy substance found in the ears of mammals. It is part of the ear's defense system and protects, lubricates, and slows bacterial growth.

11. **(C)** The palms of the hands and soles of the feet each have five layers of skin because of the unique tasks they perform, such as picking up things and walking.

12. **(D)** Epithelial tissue is a sheet or lining of cells that cover the body surface and line hollow organs and body cavities. They are also the predominant tissue in glands. Epithelial tissues serve to absorb, diffuse, filter, protect, secrete, and excrete.

13. **(D)** Sweating is the primary mechanism in the body's regulation of temperature. Heat, nervous, emotion, and gustatory stimuli will cause sweat glands to secrete.

14. **(A)** Keratin is the only option that is a protein. Valine is an amino acid. Amino acids are organic compounds that combine to form proteins. They are considered the building blocks of protein.

15. **(A)** The arrector pili are a microscopic band of muscle tissue connected to a hair follicle on the dermis. When stimulated, the arrector pili will contract and cause the hair to become more perpendicular to the skin surface (stand on end). Their common name is "goose bumps."

16. **(C)** The temperature of the skin is determined by the amount of heat brought to it by the blood stream and upon the quantity of heat loss from the surface. The rate of blood flow is the chief determinant of skin temperature. Other factors are contraction or dilation of the various structures of the skin, temperature, humidity, and movement of the surrounding air. All come together to determine the temperature of the skin.

17. **(C)** A papilla is a small, nipple-like projection, such as a protrusion on the skin, at the source or root of a hair or feather, or at the base of a developing tooth. An easily understood example is the small, round protuberances on the top of the tongue containing taste buds.

18. **(B)** Adipose cells are specialized connective tissue cells that synthesize and contain large fat globules. The hypodermis lies inferior to the dermis and superior to tissues and organs, and consists mainly of adipose tissue. The majority of body fat is stored in the hypodermis.

19. **(D)** The skin synthesizes vitamin D, not C.

20. **(C)** Hair grows at approximately 1.3 centimeters, or one-half inch, per month.

OVERVIEW

- Consists of 206 bones that comprise the skeleton
  - ○ Provides the internal framework for muscle attachment
  - ○ Protects organs from injury
  - ○ Supports body tissues
  - ○ Assists with movement by acting as levers
  - ○ Provides the site for hematopoiesis
  - ○ Provides for mineral storage
  - ○ Provides for energy storage
- Consists of 600+ muscles under voluntary or purposeful control
  - ○ Produces or prevents movement through **contraction** and **relaxation** of striated fibers
  - ○ Muscle tissue is rich in blood supply.
  - ○ Requires chemical energy for muscle action
    - ➤ Adenosine triphosphate (ATP) is produced and stored in muscle.
  - ○ Metabolism of muscle generates heat that is essential for upholding body temperature.

NOTE

Striated muscle is the only muscle in the body with voluntary control.

THE SKELETON

- Composed of two groups
  1. Axial skeleton
     - ➤ Bones focused around the vertical axis of the skeleton
     - ➤ Cranium
     - ➤ Facial bones
     - ➤ Hyoid bone
     - ➤ Ear ossicles
     - ➤ Vertebral column
     - ➤ Thoracic cage
  2. Appendicular skeleton
     - ➤ Limbs that are attached to the axial skeleton
     - ➤ Shoulder girdle
     - ➤ Upper limbs
     - ➤ Pelvic girdle
     - ➤ Lower limbs

BONES

- Structure
  - ○ Compact bones are dense, smooth, and homogenous
    - ➤ Alternate name is **lamellar** bone
  - ○ Spongy bone consists of small, lattice-like, irregular-shaped bone pieces with open spaces.

- Types
  - Long bones
    - ➤ Longer than they are wide
    - ➤ Arms, legs, fingers, and toes
  - Short bones
    - ➤ Irregular block shape
    - ➤ Weight bearers
    - ➤ Wrists and ankles
  - Flat bones
    - ➤ Two thin pieces of compact bone enclosing a middle region of spongy bone
    - ➤ Provide for tendon attachment
    - ➤ Shoulder blades, ribs, breast bone, pelvic bones, skull
  - Irregular bones
    - ➤ Different shapes
    - ➤ Provide for attachment of muscle tendons and ligaments
    - ➤ Wormian bones, mandible, kneecap, sesmoid bones, vertebrae
- Features of long bones
  - Diaphysis
  - Epiphysis
  - Metaphysis
  - Marrow cavity
    - ➤ Stores **yellow marrow**
  - Periosteum
  - Endosteum
- Features of short, flat, and irregular bones
  - Spongy and irregular bones are encircled by a thin layer of compact bone.
  - **Red marrow** is found in flat bones of the ribs, vertebrae, sternum, and hip bones.
- Bone formation (Ossification)
  - Intramembranous ossification
    - ➤ Occurs in flat bones of the skull
    - ➤ **Osteoblasts form bone, osteocytes maintain bone, osteoclasts dissolve bone.**
  - Endochrondral ossification
    - ➤ Occurs when hyaline cartilage is replaced by bone tissues
    - ➤ Occurs in long bones

JOINTS

- Movement
  - Amphiarthroses
    - ➤ Cartilaginous
    - ➤ No joint cavity
    - ➤ **Slightly movable joints**
    - ➤ Vertebral joints
  - Diarthroses
    - ➤ Synovial
    - ➤ **Freely movable joints**
    - ➤ Mandible, vertebrae

- ○ Synthroses
  - ➤ Fibrous
  - ➤ **Fixed joints**
- ■ Types of Diarthroses
  - ○ Articulations
    - ➤ Hold bones together but allow for mobility of rigid skeleton
    - ➤ Ball and socket
      - – Hip and shoulder joints
    - ➤ Condyloid
      - – Wrist joint
    - ➤ Gliding
      - – Between sacrum and ilium
    - ➤ Hinge
      - – Elbow, knee, ankle, interphalangeal joints
    - ➤ Pivot
      - – Between axis and atlas
    - ➤ Saddle
      - – Thumb
- ■ Joint movements
  - ○ Abduction/adduction
  - ○ Circumrotation/rotation
  - ○ Dorsiflexion/Plantar flexion
  - ○ Elevation/depression
  - ○ Extension/flexion
  - ○ Inversion/eversion
  - ○ Medial rotation/lateral rotation
  - ○ Protraction/retraction
  - ○ Supination/pronation

MUSCLES

- ■ Tissue
  - ○ Differentiated from other tissues by its capacity to contract and perform mechanical or power-driven work
  - ○ Structural unit is the muscle cell or muscle fiber
- ■ Characterization
  - ○ **Smooth muscle**
    - ➤ Located in the walls of vessels and intestines
    - ➤ Slow contraction speed
    - ➤ Involuntary control
    - ➤ Fibers are extended and rod- or pin-shaped and pointed at the ends
    - ➤ No striations
  - ○ **Cardiac muscle**
    - ➤ Located in the walls of the heart
    - ➤ Intermediate contraction speed (between fast and slow speed)
    - ➤ Involuntary control
    - ➤ Long, cylindrical, branching fibers
    - ➤ Striations present

- Skeletal muscles
  - ➤ Connected to the skeleton
  - ➤ Rapid speed of contraction
  - ➤ Voluntary control
  - ➤ Long, cylindrical, nonbranching fibers with blunt ends
  - ➤ Striations present
- Skeletal Muscle Function
  - Muscle fiber **contraction** occurs as slender filaments are pulled toward each other, increasing the overlay of thick filaments in the muscle fiber.
  - **Relaxation** of muscle fibers occurs when there are no nerve impulses to stimulate contraction.
- Functional Components
  - Cartilage
    - ➤ Absorbs weight, stress, shock, and strain
    - ➤ Nonvascular, connective tissue
  - Ligament
    - ➤ Strong fibrous tissue
    - ➤ Provides joint stability
    - ➤ Binds bone
  - Muscle
    - ➤ Enables body movement
    - ➤ Creates body heat for maintenance of body temperature
    - ➤ Upholds body position
  - Tendon
    - ➤ Connects muscle to bone
    - ➤ Nonelastic connective tissue extending from muscle sheath

ANSWER SHEET
The Musculoskeletal System Sample Test

1. Ⓐ Ⓑ Ⓒ Ⓓ   8. Ⓐ Ⓑ Ⓒ Ⓓ   15. Ⓐ Ⓑ Ⓒ Ⓓ

2. Ⓐ Ⓑ Ⓒ Ⓓ   9. Ⓐ Ⓑ Ⓒ Ⓓ   16. Ⓐ Ⓑ Ⓒ Ⓓ

3. Ⓐ Ⓑ Ⓒ Ⓓ   10. Ⓐ Ⓑ Ⓒ Ⓓ   17. Ⓐ Ⓑ Ⓒ Ⓓ

4. Ⓐ Ⓑ Ⓒ Ⓓ   11. Ⓐ Ⓑ Ⓒ Ⓓ   18. Ⓐ Ⓑ Ⓒ Ⓓ

5. Ⓐ Ⓑ Ⓒ Ⓓ   12. Ⓐ Ⓑ Ⓒ Ⓓ   19. Ⓐ Ⓑ Ⓒ Ⓓ

6. Ⓐ Ⓑ Ⓒ Ⓓ   13. Ⓐ Ⓑ Ⓒ Ⓓ   20. Ⓐ Ⓑ Ⓒ Ⓓ

7. Ⓐ Ⓑ Ⓒ Ⓓ   14. Ⓐ Ⓑ Ⓒ Ⓓ

For Questions 1–20, select the letter (A, B, C, or D) that best answers the question. Record your answers on The Musculoskeletal System Sample Test Answer Sheet on page 289.

1. All of the following are components of the axial skeleton EXCEPT

   (A) the coccyx.
   (B) the nasal bone.
   (C) the sternum.
   (D) the ulna.

2. The ear ossicles contain all of the following EXCEPT

   (A) incus.
   (B) malleus.
   (C) palatine.
   (D) stapes.

3. A functional capability of muscles is

   (A) absorbing weight.
   (B) involuntary control.
   (C) joint stability.
   (D) upholding body position.

4. All of the following are joint movements EXCEPT

   (A) extension/reduction.
   (B) inversion/eversion.
   (C) medial rotation/lateral rotation.
   (D) protraction/retraction.

5. Striated muscle is composed of

   (A) endometria.
   (B) involuntary fibers.
   (C) sarcomeres.
   (D) synovial membranes.

6. Cardiac muscle is almost completely reliant on _____ to function.

   (A) cardiac enzymes
   (B) oxygen
   (C) pH of blood
   (D) pneumotasis

7. Adenosine triphosphate (ATP) is stored in

   (A) flat bones.
   (B) muscle.
   (C) pineal gland.
   (D) plasma.

8. Muscles found in the heart wall are

   (A) long, cylindrical, branching fibers with striations present.
   (B) long, cylindrical, nonbranching fibers without striations.
   (C) short, nontubular, branching fibers with striations present.
   (D) short, nontubular, nonbranching fibers without striations.

9. Lamellar bone is an alternate name for

   (A) spongy bone.
   (B) compact bone.
   (C) long bones.
   (D) short bones.

10. The shoulder girdle, pelvic girdle, and upper and lower limbs make up the

    (A) appendage skeleton.
    (B) appendicular skeleton.
    (C) diarthrotic skeleton.
    (D) lateral skeleton.

11. The thumb is an example of a

    (A) condyloid joint.
    (B) gliding.
    (C) pivot.
    (D) saddle.

12. One way in which muscle tissues are differentiated from each other is by their capacity to

    (A) absorb shock.
    (B) act as levers.
    (C) create heat for the body.
    (D) perform power driven work.

13. All of the following are characteristics of smooth muscle EXCEPT

    (A) located in the walls of the intestines.
    (B) short, rod-shaped fibers with no points at the ends.
    (C) slow speed of contraction.
    (D) striations are absent.

14. Hip and shoulder joints are _____ joints.

    (A) ball and socket
    (B) condyloid
    (C) hinge and gliding
    (D) pivot

15. Endochrondral ossification occurs in the _____ bones.

    (A) fibrous
    (B) long
    (C) rearticulated
    (D) short

16. The _____ is(are) an example of a diarthrotic joint.

    (A) ankle
    (B) periosteum
    (C) pubic synthesis
    (D) sutures of the skull

17. _____ is the major protein of the bone matrix.

    (A) Albumin
    (B) Collagen
    (C) Glutamic acid
    (D) Trytophan

18. Flexion is movement at a joint to _____ the angle between two bones.

    (A) rotate
    (B) reduce
    (C) pronate
    (D) supinate

19. The ends of a long bone are known as the

    (A) epiphysis.
    (B) periosteal plates.
    (C) synovial cavities.
    (D) wormian epiphyses.

20. The function of synovial fluid is to lubricate a (an) _____ joint.

    (A) amphiarthrotic
    (B) diarthrotic
    (C) gomphotic
    (D) synarthrotic

The Musculoskeletal System Sample Test Answer Key

1. **D**		5. **C**		9. **B**		13. **B**		17. **B**
2. **C**		6. **B**		10. **B**		14. **A**		18. **B**
3. **D**		7. **B**		11. **D**		15. **B**		19. **A**
4. **A**		8. **A**		12. **D**		16. **A**		20. **B**

THE MUSCULOSKELETAL SYSTEM SAMPLE TEST ANSWERS EXPLAINED

1. **(D)** The axial skeleton provides support and protection for the brain, spinal cord, and the organs in the ventral body cavity. It also provides a surface for the attachment of muscles, directs respiratory movements, and stabilizes portions of the appendicular skeleton. It consists of the cranium, facial bones, hyoid, ear ossicles, vertebral column, and the thoracic cage, and revolves around the vertical axis of the skeleton. The ulna is a part of the appendicular skeleton.

2. **(C)** The palatine bone is located behind the maxilla. It is not in the ear.

3. **(D)** The purpose of skeletal muscles is to move bones of the body to maintain position and create movement. Skeletal muscles need bones to pull against to allow muscles to contract or relax as needed to accomplish the particular function the body is performing at the time.

4. **(A)** The joint action is extension/flexion, not extension/reduction. Extension is movement where the angle between two bones increases. Extension is also known as straightening. Flexion is movement where the angle between two bones decreases. It is commonly known as bending. An example is bending and straightening the elbow.

5. **(C)** Skeletal, cardiac, and striated muscles are alternate terms for the same type of muscle. These muscles are made up of elongated, multinucleated, transversely striated muscle fibers (or sarcomeres).

6. **(B)** In order for the heart to function to meet the body's needs, it requires oxygen and fuel. Heart muscles receive oxygen via the coronary arteries. The amount of oxygen required by the heart depends on the body's level of activity. At rest, cardiac muscles extract around 80% of the oxygen from the coronary arteries. As activity increases, a greater amount of oxygen is required. ATP is the fuel or energy needed.

7. **(B)** Mitochondria are the powerhouses of the cell. They produce ATP as the energy supply for life processes. It is stored in the liver and muscles. ATP production by the mitochondria is done by the process of cellular respiration. Oxygen is used in a process that generates energy. Glucose from food intake is broken down into ATP.

8. **(A)** Cardiac muscles are unique in the body— they are found only in the heart. Cardiac muscles are self-contracting, autonomically regulated, and must continue to contract in rhythmic fashion to sustain life. Cardiac muscle cells have a branched shape so that each cell is in contact with three of four other cardiac muscle cells. Together all of the cardiac muscle cells in the heart form a giant network connected end to end. At the ends of each cell is a region of overlapping, finger-like extensions of the cell membrane known as intercalated disks.

9. **(B)** Lamellar or compact bone is the dense bone that exhibits osteons when viewed under a microscope. Compact bone is the hard material that makes up the shaft of long bones and the outside surfaces of other bones. It is comprised of cylindrical units called osteons.

10. **(B)** The appendicular skeleton, composed of the shoulder girdle, pelvic girdle, and upper and lower limbs, is one of the two groups that comprise the human skeleton. The other group is the axial skeleton.

11. **(D)** Review the examples of the types of joint articulations (places of union) on page 287.

12. **(D)** The basic function of a muscle is to generate force or physical power. Thicker muscles can produce greater amounts of force whereas smaller, thinner muscles, such as those around the eye, produce smaller amounts of force.

13. **(B)** Smooth muscles do have points at the ends of the short, rod-shaped fibers.

14. **(A)** Review the examples of the types of joint articulations (places of union) on page 287.

15. **(B)** The process of bone ossification begins around 6 weeks after fetal development. The skeleton develops from fibrous membranes and hyaline cartilage. Bone formation is called ossification. Endochrondral ossification occurs in the long bones when hyaline cartilage is replaced by bone tissue.

16. **(A)** Review the examples of the types of joint articulations (places of union) on page 287.

17. **(B)** Collagen is the most abundant protein in the body. Collagen is a type of protein fiber found in great numbers throughout the body. It provides strength and cushioning to many different areas of the body, including the skin. Collagen is found in various types of connective tissue, such as cartilage, tendons, bones, and ligaments.

18. **(B)** Flexion reduces the angle between two bones.

19. **(A)** The epiphyses are located at the ends of the bone where it articulates with another bone. The diaphysis is the shaft of the bone located between the epiphyses. The articular cartilage covers the ends of the bone and the periosteum covers the entire bone.

20. **(B)** Diarthrotic joints are freely movable joints, as opposed to immovable joints and somewhat movable joints. All diarthrotic joints are synovial, and include most of the joints of the body. Each contains a fluid-filled joint cavity. Diarthrotic joints are composed of hyaline cartilage and have sponge that absorbs compression. They also protect the ends of bones from being crushed. Diarthrotic joints have nerves detecting pain and a rich blood supply.

THE NERVOUS SYSTEM

OVERVIEW

- Communication network of neurons that allows the organism to interact with the external and internal environment
- The main task is the regulation of body functions.
- Purpose is adaptation to changes and maintenance of homeostasis and survival
- The autonomic nervous system is divided into two systems:
  1. Central Nervous System (CNS)
  2. Peripheral Nervous System (PNS)

CELLS OF THE NERVOUS SYSTEM

- Cell components
  - Nucleus
  - Nucleolus
  - Nissl bodies
  - Endoplasmic reticulum
  - Golgi Apparatus
  - Microfilaments/Neurotubules
  - Mitochondria
- Neurons (nerve cells)
  - Neurons are similar to other cells in the body, and
    - Are surrounded by a cell membrane
    - Have a nucleus that contains genes
    - Contain cytoplasm, mitochondria, and other organelles
    - Carry out basic cellular processes such as protein synthesis and energy production
  - Neurons differ from other cells in the body, and
    - Have specialized cell parts called dendrites and axons
      - Dendrites bring electrical signals **to the cell body**
      - Axons take information **away from the cell body** and many are covered by an insulating substance, myelin, which speeds the conduction time along nerve fibers.
    - Communicate with each other through an electrochemical process
    - Contain some specialized structures and chemicals
  - Organized by the **direction** they send information
    - Sensory (afferent) neurons
      - Send information from sensory receptors **toward** the central nervous system
    - Motor (efferent) neurons
      - Send information **away from** the central nervous system to muscles or glands
    - Interneurons
      - Send information **between** sensory neurons and motor neurons
      - Most found in the CNS
  - Upper motor neurons are located in the motor cortex.
  - Lower motor neurons are located in the anterior horn of the spinal cord.

- ○ Reflex arc
  - ➤ Rapid, predictable, and involuntary response to stimuli
  - ➤ Action resulting from passing a nerve impulse over a reflex arc
  - ➤ Basic circuit
    - – Sensory receptor (gathers stimuli) ⇒ Afferent nervous fibers ⇒ Reflex center (processes information) ⇒ Efferent nerve fibers (transduction of response) ⇒ Effector (Response to stimuli)
  - ➤ Autonomic reflexes regulate activity of smooth muscles.
  - ➤ Somatic reflexes stimulate skeletal muscles.
- ■ Other cell types
  - ○ Glial cells
    - ➤ Astrocytes
    - ➤ Oligodendrocytes
  - ○ Schwann cells
- ■ Neurotransmitters
  - ○ Chemical messenger that carries, modulates, and boosts signals from one neuron to the next via synapses
    - ➤ Also located at the axon endings of motor neurons
      - – Stimulate muscle fibers
  - ○ The effect of the given neurotransmitter may be inhibitory or excitatory and may do both in different parts of the brain.
  - ○ Types
    - ➤ Acetylcholine
    - ➤ Amino acids (aspartate, gamma aminobutyric acid (GABA), glycine, glutamate)
    - ➤ Lipids (cannabinoids, nitric oxide)
    - ➤ Monoamines (dopamine, epinephrine, histamine, norepinephrine, serotonin)
    - ➤ Neuropeptides (endorphins, oxytocin, vasopressin)
    - ➤ Purines (adenosine, adenosine triphosphate)

CENTRAL NERVOUS SYSTEM

- ■ Involuntary System
- ■ **You do not have to initiate it or think about it in order for it to work.**
- ■ Consists of the brain and spinal cord
- ■ Process of information
  - ○ Emotions
  - ○ Integration
  - ○ Motor commands
  - ○ Learning and thinking
  - ○ Observation
  - ○ Memory
- ■ Interpretation center for the body
  - ○ Responsible for integrating and reacting to sensory information
- ■ Two types of tissue
  1. Gray matter consists of:
    - ➤ Nerve cell bodies
    - ➤ Dendrites
    - ➤ Axons

2. White matter consists of:
   ➤ Axons
     – Looks **white** due to the myelin sheathing of the axons
- Commonalities of brain and spinal cord
  ○ Living nervous tissue has jelly-like consistency.
    ➤ Requires special protection from bodily damage
      – The entire CNS is encased in bone.
      – The brain is encased within the cranium.
      – The spinal cord runs inside a canal in the vertebrae.
    ➤ The CNS is washed in a cerebrospinal fluid (CSF).
      – CSF provides a unique chemical environment for nervous tissue and protection against bodily damage.
  ○ Blood brain barrier is the relatively impermeable membranes of capillaries in the CNS that maintain a special chemical environment of nervous tissue.
- Brain
  ○ Encased in skull composed of frontal bone, parietal bones (2), temporal bones (2), sphenoid bone, ethmoid bone, and occipital bone
  ○ Organizing and processing center of the nervous system
    ➤ **Consumes around 25% of all the oxygen used by the body**
    ➤ Exceedingly **sensitive** to low amounts of glucose and/or oxygen
  ○ Site of consciousness, sensation, coordination, memory, and **regulation of homeostasis**
  ○ Four major divisions
    1. Cerebrum
      – Largest part of the brain; consists of two hemispheres; has nerve centers for sensory and motor activities
      – Each hemisphere is divided into four lobes (see Figure 6.9). Those four lobes are the frontal lobe, parietal lobe, temporal lobe, and occipital lobe.
      – Cross-section shows three layers of nervous tissue (cerebral cortex, cerebral white matter, and basil ganglia)
    2. Diencephalon
      – Connects cerebrum to the brainstem
      – The thalamus is a relay station for sensory nerve impulses traveling from the spinal cord to the cerebrum and contains the pineal gland (in epithalamus), which produces melatonin (the hormone that helps regulate the biological clock).
      – Hypothalamus: controls the autonomic nervous system and regulates behavior, body temperature, the biological clock, emotions, hunger, and thirst; also produces ADH and oxytocin, and controls hormone production in the anterior pituitary gland
    3. Brain stem
      – Connects diencephalon to the spinal cord
      – Contains four regions: midbrain, pons, medulla oblongata, and reticular formation
      – Reticular formation contains the reticular activation system (RAS), which is responsible for maintaining wakefulness and alertness and filters out unimportant sensory information.

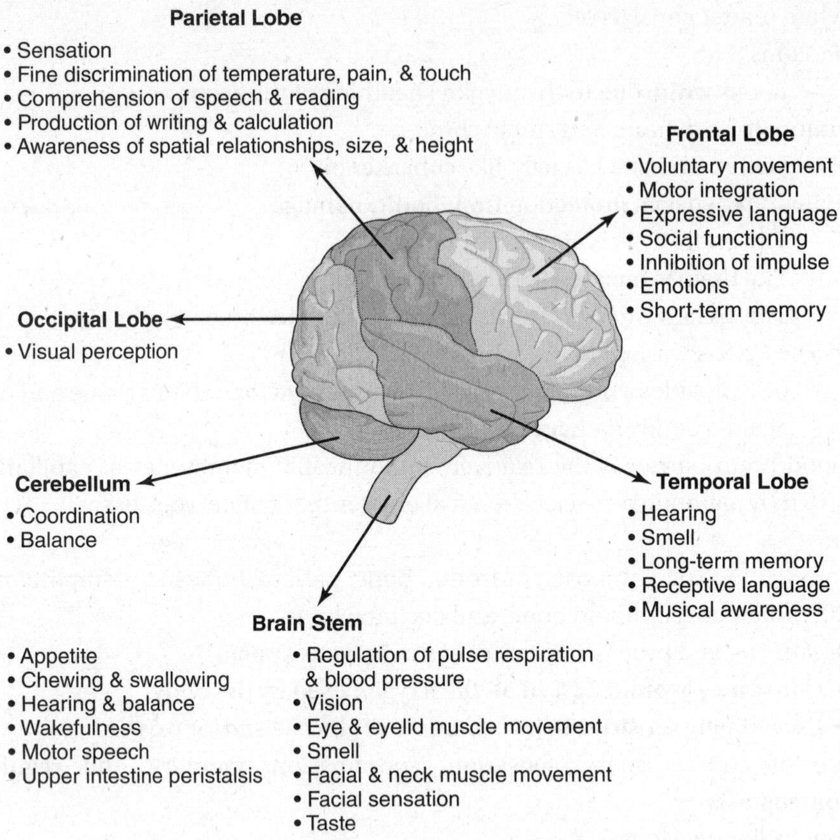

Parietal Lobe

• Sensation
• Fine discrimination of temperature, pain, & touch
• Comprehension of speech & reading
• Production of writing & calculation
• Awareness of spatial relationships, size, & height

Frontal Lobe

• Voluntary movement
• Motor integration
• Expressive language
• Social functioning
• Inhibition of impulse
• Emotions
• Short-term memory

Occipital Lobe

• Visual perception

Cerebellum

• Coordination
• Balance

Temporal Lobe

• Hearing
• Smell
• Long-term memory
• Receptive language
• Musical awareness

Brain Stem

• Appetite
• Chewing & swallowing
• Hearing & balance
• Wakefulness
• Motor speech
• Upper intestine peristalsis

• Regulation of pulse respiration & blood pressure
• Vision
• Eye & eyelid muscle movement
• Smell
• Facial & neck muscle movement
• Facial sensation
• Taste

Figure 6.9. Brain Lobes with Functions

4. Cerebellum

   – Large mass of gray and white matter

   – Serves as a reflex center for the coordination of the skeletal muscle (helps maintain posture and produce a smooth gait)

   – Evaluates and coordinates motor movement by comparing actual skeletal movements to movement that was intended

○ Limbic system

➤ Involved in **survival emotions**

➤ Associated with emotions, such as fear, pleasure, anger, and sorrow

■ Cerebrospinal Fluid and Ventricles

○ The brain has four ventricles or cavities filled with cerebrospinal fluid (CSF).

➤ Each cerebral hemisphere has a lateral ventricle.

➤ The third ventricle is attached to the lateral ventricles by the interventricular foramen.

➤ The fourth ventricle is attached to the third ventricle via the vertebral aqueduct, and to the central canal of the spinal cord.

   – Allows CSF to flow into the subarachnoid space

○ Cerebrospinal fluid is found in:

➤ Subarachnoid space

➤ The central canal of the spinal cord

➤ Ventricles in the brain

- CSF is clear, watery, lymph-like fluid that:
  - ➤ Services the nutritional and waste needs of nerve cells in the CNS
  - ➤ Provides a chemically balanced environment
  - ➤ Absorbs physical shocks to the brain
- Spinal Cord and Meninges
  - The spinal cord serves as a conduit for signals between the brain and the rest of the body.
    - ➤ Controls simple musculoskeletal reflexes without input from the brain
    - ➤ Encased in vertebral column consisting of seven cervical vertebrae, twelve thoracic vertebrae, five lumbar vertebrae, one sacrum (five fused sacral vertebrae), and one coccyx (four fused coccygeal vertebrae)
  - Coordinating center for the reflex arc
    - ➤ The **Reflex Arc** is a simple example of nerve activity.
      - – Examples are knee-jerk reflex and withdrawal reflex
  - Meninges surround and protect the spinal cord and the brain.
    - ➤ Composed of three layers
      1. Dura mater (outermost layer)
      2. Arachnoid mater (middle layer)—subarachnoid space contains cerebrospinal fluid
      3. Pia mater (lowermost layer)

PERIPHERAL NERVOUS SYSTEM (PNS)

- Responsible for voluntary nerve action
  - May be referred to as the visceral system
  - **You have to consciously and voluntarily make the system move or work.**
  - Consists of nerves that exit from the spinal cord at different levels of the spinal column as well as their offshoots
    - ➤ Includes cranial nerves
  - Acts as a communication relay between the brain and the extremities
    - ➤ Detection and transmission of sensory stimuli
    - ➤ Determination of response and transmission to motor effectors
  - Proteins serve as molecular machines that are responsible for all transactions between the neuron and its environment.
- Composed of
  - Twelve pairs of cranial nerves (see Table 6.2)
  - Thirty-one pairs of spinal nerves and their branches to the body
  - Sensory nerves
    - ➤ Sensory (afferent) neurons
      - – Send impulses to CNS ⇒ brain for interpretation
    - ➤ Motor (efferent) neurons
      - – After interpretation ⇒ motor neurons in the brain ⇒ spinal cord directs specific organ cells to respond to the sensory neuron impulse
- PNS splits into two divisions
  1. Somatic nervous system
     - ➤ Voluntary system
     - ➤ Controls skeletal muscles

Table 6.2. Cranial Nerves

Nerve		Type	Function
I.	Olfactory	Sensory	Smell
II.	Optic	Sensory	Vision
III.	Oculomotor	Motor	Eyelid and eyeball movement, lens shape
IV.	Trochlear	Motor	Eyeball movement; proprioception
V.	Trigeminal	Sensory Motor	Scalp skin, eye, mouth, and face Jaw muscles
VI.	Abducens	Motor	Lateral deviation of eye
VII.	Facial	Sensory Motor	Taste (salt, sweet, sour) on front of tongue Facial expression, salivation
VIII.	Vestibulocochlear	Sensory	Equilibrium, hearing
IX.	Glossopharyngeal	Sensory Motor	Taste (bitter) on back of tongue Pharyngeal muscle movement
X.	Vagus	Sensory Motor	Parasympathetic sensations, motor control of smooth muscles associated with digestive enzymes, heart, lungs, and viscera. Gag reflex
XI.	Accessory	Motor	Shoulder and head movement
XII.	Hypoglossal	Motor	Tongue and throat muscle movement

2. Autonomic nervous system splits into two additional divisions
  ➤ Parasympathetic nervous system
    – Returns organs to a quiet, calm state
    – "Rest and digestion"
  ➤ Sympathetic nervous system
    – Carries impulses to body organs and mobilizes the response to stress ("fight or flight")
■ PNS involuntarily regulates smooth muscles and glands including:
  ○ Bladder
  ○ Eyes
  ○ Gastrointestinal system
  ○ Heart
  ○ Peristalsis (digestion)
  ○ Respiratory system

ANSWER SHEET
The Nervous System Sample Test

1. Ⓐ Ⓑ Ⓒ Ⓓ
2. Ⓐ Ⓑ Ⓒ Ⓓ
3. Ⓐ Ⓑ Ⓒ Ⓓ
4. Ⓐ Ⓑ Ⓒ Ⓓ
5. Ⓐ Ⓑ Ⓒ Ⓓ
6. Ⓐ Ⓑ Ⓒ Ⓓ
7. Ⓐ Ⓑ Ⓒ Ⓓ

8. Ⓐ Ⓑ Ⓒ Ⓓ
9. Ⓐ Ⓑ Ⓒ Ⓓ
10. Ⓐ Ⓑ Ⓒ Ⓓ
11. Ⓐ Ⓑ Ⓒ Ⓓ
12. Ⓐ Ⓑ Ⓒ Ⓓ
13. Ⓐ Ⓑ Ⓒ Ⓓ
14. Ⓐ Ⓑ Ⓒ Ⓓ

15. Ⓐ Ⓑ Ⓒ Ⓓ
16. Ⓐ Ⓑ Ⓒ Ⓓ
17. Ⓐ Ⓑ Ⓒ Ⓓ
18. Ⓐ Ⓑ Ⓒ Ⓓ
19. Ⓐ Ⓑ Ⓒ Ⓓ
20. Ⓐ Ⓑ Ⓒ Ⓓ

For Questions 1–20, select the letter (A, B, C, or D) that best answers the question. Record your answers on The Nervous System Sample Test Answer Sheet on page 301.

1. All of the following are components of a neuron EXCEPT

   (A) axons.
   (B) endoplasmic reticulum.
   (C) masseter.
   (D) mitochrondria.

2. The main function of the nervous system is

   (A) adaptation to changes, maintenance of homeostasis, and survival.
   (B) deregulation of body functions and regulation of cells of the nervous system.
   (C) to provide rapid, predictable, and involuntary responses to stimuli.
   (D) to send information from afferent neurons away from the CNS to muscles and glands.

3. Astrocytes and oligodendrocytes are examples of

   (A) cerebral white matter.
   (B) glial cells.
   (C) neurotransmitters.
   (D) Schwann cells.

4. The autonomic nervous systems contain which of the following two systems?

   (A) central and peripheral
   (B) limbic and somatic
   (C) parasympathetic and sympathetic
   (D) voluntary and involuntary

5. The brainstem connects the _____ to the _____.

   (A) cerebral cortex, basal ganglia
   (B) limbic system, medulla oblongata
   (C) midbrain, infundibulum
   (D) spinal cord, diencephalon

6. The coordinating center for the reflex arc is the

   (A) cerebellum.
   (B) cerebrum.
   (C) spinal cord.
   (D) vagus nerve.

7. The _____, located in the _____, regulates coughing, sneezing, swallowing, and vomiting.

   (A) central sulcus, frontal lobe
   (B) medulla oblongata, brain stem
   (C) occipital lobe, cerebellum
   (D) parietal network, temporal lobe

8. Impulses cross over to the opposite sides of the brain via

   (A) cranial nerves.
   (B) decussation of pyramids.
   (C) diencephalon.
   (D) meninges.

9. The parasympathetic nervous system is active during periods of

   (A) bronchiole dilation.
   (B) embarrassment.
   (C) rest.
   (D) sweating.

10. Blood is supplied to the brain via all of the following EXCEPT the

    (A) autonomic artery.
    (B) basilar arteries.
    (C) Circle of Willis.
    (D) internal carotid arteries.

11. The central nervous system is made up of the

    (A) autonomic and somatic nervous systems.
    (B) brain and spinal cord.
    (C) cranial nerves and spinal nerves.
    (D) motor and sensory systems.

12. The sympathetic nervous system is also known as the

    (A) fight or flight response.
    (B) involuntary skeletal response.
    (C) rest and digest response.
    (D) somatic response.

13. Select the correct circuit for the reflex arc.

    (A) Sensory receptor (gathers stimuli) ⇔ Afferent nervous fibers ⇒ Reflex center (processes information) ⇒ Efferent nerve fibers (transduction of response) ⇔ Effector (Response to stimuli)
    (B) Sensory receptor (gathers stimuli) ⇒ Afferent nervous fibers ⇔ Reflex center (processes information) ⇔ Efferent nerve fibers (transduction of response) ⇒ Effector (Response to stimuli)
    (C) Sensory receptor (gathers stimuli) ⇐ Afferent nervous fibers ⇐ Reflex center (processes information) ⇐ Efferent nerve fibers (transduction of response) ⇐ Effector (Response to stimuli)
    (D) Sensory receptor (gathers stimuli) ⇒ Afferent nervous fibers ⇒ Reflex center (processes information) ⇒ Efferent nerve fibers (transduction of response) ⇒ Effector (Response to stimuli)

14. An individual has had a stroke (disruption of cerebral circulation resulting in sensory and motor deficits) in the parietal lobe. You would expect her to have which of the following deficits?

    (A) coordination and balance
    (B) receptive language and musical awareness
    (C) social functioning and inhibition of impulses
    (D) understanding speech and reading

15. Neurotransmitters are

    (A) afferent messengers.
    (B) autonomic messengers.
    (C) chemical messengers.
    (D) efferent messengers.

16. The central nervous system is the

    (A) interpretation center for the body.
    (B) largest part of the brain.
    (C) relay station for motor nerve impulses traveling from the spinal cord to the cerebrum.
    (D) reflex center for cardiac and respiratory rates.

17. Several weeks after sustaining a severe head injury, an individual has difficulty maintaining posture and walks with a jerking and awkward gait. You would suspect that his head injury affected his

    (A) brain stem.
    (B) cerebellum.
    (C) limbic system.
    (D) ventricles.

18. Aside from carbon, oxygen, and hydrogen, which of the following elements is contained in all proteins?

    (A) copper
    (B) nitrogen
    (C) rhodium
    (D) sulfur

19. Proprioception is defined as

    (A) age-related changes of the ear that affect hearing.
    (B) sensation about the body's position in space that is transferred to the brain after changes in body posture.
    (C) the ability of Schwann cells to wrap myelin sheaths around dendrites to form a multilayered insulation.
    (D) widening of a cerebral blood vessel.

20. Which of the following systems is voluntary and controls skeletal muscles?

    (A) afferent system
    (B) motor system
    (C) peripheral nervous system
    (D) somatic nervous system

The Nervous System Sample Test Answer Key

1. **C**	5. **D**	9. **C**	13. **D**	17. **B**
2. **A**	6. **C**	10. **A**	14. **D**	18. **B**
3. **B**	7. **B**	11. **B**	15. **C**	19. **B**
4. **C**	8. **B**	12. **A**	16. **A**	20. **D**

THE NERVOUS SYSTEM SAMPLE TEST ANSWERS EXPLAINED

1. **(C)** The masseter muscle is one of the facial muscles. It is one of the muscles that closes the jaw.

2. **(A)** The nervous system is responsible for transmitting, receiving, and translating data from the body and the external environment. It oversees and synchronizes internal organ function and responds to changes in the internal and external environment. These functions allow the body to adapt to changes, maintain homeostasis, and survive.

3. **(B)** Glial cells provide support for neurons. Astrocytes help form the blood brain barrier and help seal off damaged nerve tissue. Oligodendrocytes form the myelin sheaths around neurons.

4. **(C)** The autonomic nervous system is a subsystem of the peripheral nervous system. It contains the parasympathetic and sympathetic systems and regulates key involuntary functions of the body.

5. **(D)** The brain stem provides many of the basic survival and reflex functions for the body. Life is unsustainable with brain stem damage. The brain stem forms the connections between the brain (specifically the diencephalon) and the body via the spinal cord. Ten of the brain's twelve cranial nerves originate in the brain stem.

6. **(C)** The spinal cord is the coordinating center for the reflex arc.

7. **(B)** The medulla oblongata is located in the lower half of the brain stem. It contains the cardiac, respiratory, vomiting, and vasomotor centers and deals with autonomic, involuntary functions, such as coughing, sneezing, breathing, swallowing, heart rate, and blood pressure.

8. **(B)** Decussation means "crossing" and "pyramids" refers to the main motor nerve tracts descending within the CNS. These main motor or pyramidal tracts consist of bundles of nerve fibers descending the CNS. The triangular shaped bundles are referred to as "pyramidal tracts." The main motor tracts cross from right to left or from left to right in the medulla. This explains why an injury to one side of the brain (as with a stroke) usually brings about paralysis on the contralateral side of the body.

9. **(C)** The parasympathetic system returns the body functions to normal after they have been altered by sympathetic stimulation. In times of danger, the sympathetic system prepares the body for violent activity. The parasympathetic system reverses these changes when the danger is over.

10. **(A)** The autonomic artery does not exist. Be careful when selecting an option that you've never heard of before.

11. **(B)** The brain and spinal cord comprise the central nervous system. The remaining options are parts of the peripheral nervous system.

12. **(A)** The sympathetic system is activated when the body experiences actual or imagined danger. It is often referred to as the "fight or flight" response.

13. **(D)** The reflex arc is a basic circuit that begins with sensory receptors (gathering of stimuli) and ends with the effector (response to stimuli). The circuit runs in one direction only.

14. **(D)** The parietal lobe has several purposes. These include sensation, perception, and spatial reasoning. The parietal is accountable for processing sensory information from various parts of the body. Functions of the parietal lobe include: feeling pain, pressure, and touch; controlling and processing the five senses of the body; movement; visual orientation, perception, and recognition; speech; and cognition and information processing. Impairment of the parietal lobe can result in difficulties with spatial reasoning, reading, writing, and understanding symbols and language.

15. **(C)** Neurotransmitters use chemicals that modify or enable transmission of nerve impulses from a neuron to a muscle, gland, or another neuron. Adrenergic neurotransmitters include dopamine, epinephrine, norepinephrine, and serotonin. Cholinergic neurotransmitters use acetylcholine.

16. **(A)** The central nervous system consists of the brain and the spinal cord and serves as the interpretation center for the body.

17. **(B)** The cerebellum has to do with the coordination of muscle movement and the maintenance of balance and muscle tone.

18. **(B)** All proteins contain the elements of nitrogen, oxygen, hydrogen, and carbon. In some instances, proteins contain sulfur or phosphorus. Proteins are constructed from amino acids.

19. **(B)** Proprioception is determined by assessing the fourth cranial nerve. Choice B is the definition of proprioception.

20. **(D)** The somatic nervous system, part of the peripheral nervous system, is linked with the voluntary control of body movements via the skeletal muscles and facilitation of involuntary reflex arcs.

OVERVIEW

- May be referred to as the urinary system
- The primary function is to control the composition and concentration of the extracellular fluids surrounding the body cells.
- Contains the kidneys, ureters, bladder, urethra, and urinary meatus
- The body's drainage system
  - Assists in maintaining homeostasis
  - Regulates water balance
  - Filters harmful/toxic substances from the circulating blood
  - **In order for normal urination to occur, all parts of the urinary tract need to work together in the correct order.**
- Urine formation occurs in the nephrons.
  - Involves four processes:
    1. Filtration
    2. Reabsorption
    3. Secretion
    4. Excretion
  - Urine contains water, toxic substances, and waste products.

THE KIDNEYS

- **External Kidney**
  - Two dark red, bean-shaped organs surrounded by an adipose layer
    - ➤ Adrenal gland sits atop each kidney
  - Located in the posterior abdomen behind the peritoneum on either side of the vertebral column between the 12th thoracic vertebrae and the 3rd lumbar vertebrae
  - Blood supply, nerves, lymphatic vessels, and ureter enter and exit the kidney at the hilum.
  - Surrounded by three layers
    1. Renal fascia
       - Thin, outermost layer of fibrous, connective tissue surrounds each kidney
       - **Fastens** the kidney to surrounding structures
    2. Adipose capsule
       - The middle layer **cushions** the kidney.
    3. Renal capsule
       - The inner layer **protects** the kidney from trauma and infection.
- **Internal Kidney**
  - Renal cortex
    - ➤ Outer part of convex side of the kidney
    - ➤ Metabolically functioning area where **aerobic** metabolism occurs and ammonia and glucose are formed
    - ➤ Has **extensive** oxygen supply
    - ➤ Contains glomeruli, tubules, and part of Loop of Henle

- Renal medulla
  - ➤ Middle portion of the kidney is adjacent to the renal cortex
  - ➤ Region of glycolytic metabolism
  - ➤ Area of **high** oxygen consumption that supplies energy for active transport but has limited oxygen supply
  - ➤ Contains 6 to 10 renal pyramids formed by collecting ducts
    - – Papillae are apices of pyramids. Urine flows through the papillae to the renal pelvis.
  - ➤ Contains collecting ducts and part of Loop of Henle
- Renal sinus
  - ➤ Innermost portion where urine is collected
  - ➤ Narrowest portion becomes the proximal end of the ureter.
  - ➤ Major calix channels urine from the renal sinus to the renal pelvis.
  - ➤ Minor calix collects urine from the collecting ducts.
  - ➤ Contains the renal pelvis and calyces
- Blood and Nerve Supply
  - Each kidney receives rich blood supply via the large renal artery.
    - ➤ Normal kidneys receive approximately one-quarter of the heart's blood output, or approximately 1.2 L of blood each minute
    - ➤ Arterial flow
      - – Abdominal aorta ⇒ renal artery ⇒ segmental arteries ⇒ lobar arteries ⇒ interlobar arteries ⇒ arcuate arteries ⇒ efferent arterioles ⇒ glomeruli of nephrons
    - ➤ Venous flow
      - – Blood flow back to the heart is the reverse of arterial flow. Renal vein joins the inferior vena cava.
    - ➤ Autonomic nerves from the renal plexus follow the renal artery into the kidney.
      - – Nerve fibers regulate blood flow.

- Nephrons
  - Functional unit of the kidneys
    - ➤ Filtering and excreting of the kidneys
    - ➤ Consists of the glomeruli, tubules, and collecting bodies
  - Glomeruli
    - ➤ Filters blood and produces glomerular filtrate
      - – Filtrate contains water, glucose, salts, and urea. Large molecules, such as protein, are too large to fit through the blood capillary walls.
    - ➤ Supplied by afferent arterioles and drained by afferent arterioles, both in Bowman's capsule
      - – The Bowman's capsule collects the filtrate, and it enters the tubules. All glucose is reabsorbed immediately into the blood capillaries. As the remaining filtrate travels through the tubules, water and salts that are needed by the body are reabsorbed into the blood capillaries.
    - ➤ The waste, consisting of excess water, excess salts, and urea, is urine.
    - ➤ The collecting duct collects the urine, which is then transported via the ureters to the bladder.
    - ➤ The bladder stores urine until the body is ready to expel it through the urethra.
  - Neurological control is supplied by the sympathetic and parasympathetic nerves.

ANSWER SHEET
The Renal System Sample Test

1. Ⓐ Ⓑ Ⓒ Ⓓ
2. Ⓐ Ⓑ Ⓒ Ⓓ
3. Ⓐ Ⓑ Ⓒ Ⓓ
4. Ⓐ Ⓑ Ⓒ Ⓓ
5. Ⓐ Ⓑ Ⓒ Ⓓ
6. Ⓐ Ⓑ Ⓒ Ⓓ
7. Ⓐ Ⓑ Ⓒ Ⓓ

8. Ⓐ Ⓑ Ⓒ Ⓓ
9. Ⓐ Ⓑ Ⓒ Ⓓ
10. Ⓐ Ⓑ Ⓒ Ⓓ
11. Ⓐ Ⓑ Ⓒ Ⓓ
12. Ⓐ Ⓑ Ⓒ Ⓓ
13. Ⓐ Ⓑ Ⓒ Ⓓ
14. Ⓐ Ⓑ Ⓒ Ⓓ

15. Ⓐ Ⓑ Ⓒ Ⓓ
16. Ⓐ Ⓑ Ⓒ Ⓓ
17. Ⓐ Ⓑ Ⓒ Ⓓ
18. Ⓐ Ⓑ Ⓒ Ⓓ
19. Ⓐ Ⓑ Ⓒ Ⓓ
20. Ⓐ Ⓑ Ⓒ Ⓓ

For Questions 1–20, select the letter (A, B, C, or D) that best answers the question. Record your answers on The Renal System Sample Test Answer Sheet on page 309.

1. The purpose of the glomeruli is
    (A) excretion of excess sodium.
    (B) filtration of blood.
    (C) protection of the kidneys.
    (D) reabsorption of waste products.

2. The Loop of Henle
    (A) has ascending afferent and descending efferent tubules.
    (B) has ascending and descending limbs.
    (C) collects and, along with ADH, determines the pH of urine.
    (D) has proximal nonconvoluted tubules.

3. Filtrate leaving the proximal tubule is
    (A) homostatic.
    (B) hypertonic.
    (C) hypotonic.
    (D) isotonic.

4. One process used in the formation of urine is
    (A) concentration.
    (B) filtration.
    (C) costimulation.
    (D) uremic metabolism.

5. Venous blood flow back to the heart is the reverse of arterial flow. Leaving the kidney, the renal vein joins with the _____ vein.
    (A) abdominal aorta
    (B) inferior vena cava
    (C) superior mesenteric
    (D) suprarenal

6. Kidneys receive blood via the
    (A) aorta.
    (B) lobar artery.
    (C) renal artery.
    (D) segmental artery.

7. Select the correct blood flow.
    (A) Abdominal aorta ⇒ renal artery ⇒ lobar arteries ⇒ segmental arteries ⇒ interlobar arteries ⇒ inarcuate arteries ⇒ afferent arterioles ⇔ glomeruli of nephrons
    (B) Abdominal aorta ⇒ renal artery ⇒ segmental arteries ⇒ interlobar arteries ⇒ lobar arteries ⇒ arcuate arteries ⇒ afferent arterioles ⇒ glomeruli of nephrons
    (C) Abdominal aorta ⇒ renal artery ⇒ lobar arteries ⇒ segmental arteries ⇒ interlobar arteries ⇐ inarcuate arteries ⇒ efferent arterioles ⇒ glomeruli of nephrons
    (D) Abdominal aorta ⇒ renal artery ⇒ segmental arteries ⇒ lobar arteries ⇒ interlobar arteries ⇒ arcuate arteries ⇒ efferent arterioles ⇒ glomeruli of nephrons

8. Which of the following is supplied by afferent arterioles and drained by efferent arterioles?
    (A) fenestrae of the adrenal glands
    (B) the glomeruli in the Bowman's capsule
    (C) major calix of the adrenal medulla
    (D) papillae of the Loop of Henle

9. Within the _____, the descending limb allows for the reabsorption of water through _____ , whereas the ascending limb allows for the _____ transport of salts, such as sodium, to move out of the tubules and be reabsorbed.
    (A) basement membrane, fenestration, interstitial
    (B) filtration slits, endothelial pores, low and/or high pressure
    (C) Loop of Henle, osmosis, active and passive
    (D) renal plexus, reduction, absorption

10. Filtration, reabsorption, and secretion determine the

    (A) amount of urine collected in the Bowman's capsule.
    (B) quantity and quality of the urine.
    (C) speed of movement of the waste materials out of the tubules.
    (D) water and solute transport regulated by hormones.

11. Nerve fibers regulate blood flow to the kidneys. Stimulation of parasympathetic fibers would

    (A) decrease urinary output.
    (B) increase urinary output.
    (C) maintain an approximately constant urinary output.
    (D) Not enough information is given to answer the question.

12. Which of the following is NOT a part of the renal system?

    (A) accessory duct
    (B) collecting duct
    (C) proximal convoluted tubule
    (D) ureter

13. Extracellular fluids surrounding the cells of the body are called _____ fluids.

    (A) hydrolytic
    (B) intracellular
    (C) interstitial
    (D) isotonic

14. The hormone that controls the reabsorption of water from the distal convoluted tubules and collecting is

    (A) aldosterone.
    (B) antidiuretic.
    (C) epinephrine (adrenalin).
    (D) renin.

15. The kidneys' regulation of blood volume is a factor in the regulation of _____.

    (A) functioning of the Loop of Henle
    (B) blood pressure
    (C) chemicals in the body
    (D) facilitation of negative feedback

16. The urinary system handles the major work of _____.

    (A) excretion
    (B) removing bacteria from the hematologic system
    (C) supporting the adrenal glands
    (D) vacuation

17. The amount of blood flowing through the glomeruli is approximately _____ per hour.

    (A) 1.50 L
    (B) 3.75 L
    (C) 5.25 L
    (D) 7.50 L

18. The length of the urethra

    (A) depends upon developmental age.
    (B) is longest in the adult female.
    (C) is longest in the adult male.
    (D) may decrease with atrophy in old age.

19. The release of antidiuretic hormone (ADH) is regulated by the

    (A) adrenal cortex.
    (B) anterior lobe of the pituitary.
    (C) hypothalamus.
    (D) plasma calcium levels.

20. Which of the following is found in urine when fat is being used as the primary energy source?

    (A) calcium biphosphate
    (B) ketones
    (C) potassium
    (D) sodium and chloride ions

The Renal System Sample Test Answer Key

1. **B**		5. **B**		9. **C**		13. **C**		17. **D**
2. **B**		6. **C**		10. **B**		14. **B**		18. **C**
3. **D**		7. **D**		11. **B**		15. **B**		19. **C**
4. **B**		8. **B**		12. **A**		16. **A**		20. **B**

THE RENAL SYSTEM SAMPLE TEST ANSWERS EXPLAINED

1. **(B)** The primary function of the kidney is the filtration of blood. The glomeruli is a part of this filtration system.

2. **(B)** The Loop of Henle is involved with the regulation of urine concentration and has an ascending limb or tubule and a descending limb or tubule.

3. **(D)** The fluid is isotonic because as ions are reabsorbed by the gradient time system, water is also reabsorbed, maintaining the osmolarity of the fluid in the PCT.

4. **(B)** Filtration of blood is a primary kidney function with urine formation as the end result. While concentration of urine is one function of the kidney, urine cannot be concentrated until it is formed. The key word is *formation*.

5. **(B)** Blood leaving the heart travels via the aorta. Blood returning to the heart travels via the superior or inferior vena cava. As the renal vein leaves the kidney, it joins with the inferior vena cava.

6. **(C)** Arterial blood leaves the heart via the aorta. Arterial blood destined for the kidneys does so via the renal artery that branches off the aorta.

7. **(D)** The flow of arterial blood from the heart is in one direction. This automatically excludes choices A and C as answers. Review arterial flow on page 308.

8. **(B)** Blood enters the kidney via the renal artery. Arteries supplying the glomeruli in the Bowman's capsule have been subdivided into microscopic vessels called afferent arterioles. As blood leaves the glomeruli, it flows into the efferent arterioles.

9. **(C)** This question may require additional thought because it involves many elements both in the stem and the options. The key to selecting the correct answer is understanding that the Loop of Henle has ascending and descending limbs or tubules.

10. **(B)** Glomerular filtration, tubular reabsorption, and tubular secretion occur within the nephron and determine the quality and quantity of urine.

11. **(B)** Stimulation of the sympathetic fibers decreases urinary output. Stimulation of the parasympathetic fibers increases urinary output.

12. **(A)** The accessory duct does not exist.

13. **(C)** Interstitial fluid is the extracellular fluid immersing the cells in the majority of tissues. It excludes fluid in the lymph and blood vessels.

14. **(B)** The antidiuretic hormone, or vasopressin, is secreted by the posterior lobe of the pituitary gland. It constricts blood vessels, increases blood pressure, promotes intestinal motility, and reduces the elimination of urine.

15. **(B)** One of the mechanisms for renal regulation of blood pressure is the maintenance of volume and composition of extracellular fluid. A normal plasma volume is essential for the control of blood pressure. A change in plasma volume eventually affects blood pressure. An increase in plasma volume escalates the cardiac workload, eventually raising blood pressure. A decrease in plasma volume lowers arterial pressure.

16. **(A)** Urine is formed in the nephrons and contains water, toxic substances, and waste products. The urinary system excretes these substances.

17. **(D)** The glomerular filtration rate is approximately 7.50 liters/hour or 180 liters/day.

18. **(C)** The length of the urethra does not depend upon developmental age, and it does not atrophy with age. Consider the location of the bladder in both sexes, and then consider the length of the urethra needed to excrete urine in both sexes.

19. **(C)** The hypothalamus oversees the amount of water in the body by discerning the electrolyte concentration in the blood. A high concentration of electrolytes indicates a low water level in the body. ADH, produced by the hypothalamus and released by the posterior pituitary, increases the amount of water withheld by the kidneys when the water level is low.

20. **(B)** Ketones are produced when the body burns fat for energy. They are also produced when you lose weight or if there is not enough insulin to help your body use sugar for energy.

OVERVIEW

- Reproduction has to do with the independent production of sperm and eggs, and the actions leading to fertilization.
- Unlike other body systems, there are marked differences between male and female reproductive systems.
  - **Two systems are separate, but interdependent.**
    - ➤ Male system
      - Consists of scrotum with testes and penis
      - Sperm production
    - ➤ Female system
      - Consists of fallopian tubes, uterus, vagina, and ovaries
      - Egg production
- Basic purposes of the reproductive system
  - Perpetuation of the species
  - Female system involves development from conception to shortly after birth.
  - Sexual delectation

MALE REPRODUCTIVE SYSTEM

- External genitalia
  - Penis
    - ➤ Surrounds the urethra with erectile tissue
  - Scrotum
    - ➤ Divided into two halves with each scrotal sac containing:
      - One testicle
      - Epididymis
      - Vas deferens (ejaculatory ducts and spermatic cord)
- Internal genitalia
  - Testes
    - ➤ Two ovoid-shaped glands containing:
      - Seminiferous tubules where **spermatogenesis** occurs (production of spermatozoa—male gametes or reproductive cells)
      - Secretion of hormones—Testosterone is necessary for the development and maintenance of male sex organs and secondary sex characteristics. (Androgen or masculinizing hormone by Leydig cells)
  - Epididymis
    - ➤ Duct of the testes
    - ➤ Conducts sperm from the testes to vas deferens
  - Vas deferens
    - ➤ Conducts sperm to the ejaculatory duct in the prostate gland and into the urethra
  - Seminal vesicles
  - Spermatic cord
    - ➤ Contains vas deferens, arteries, veins, and lymphatic tissues that supply testes
  - Ejaculatory duct

- Prostate gland
  - Lies below the bladder and is shaped like a donut
  - Urethra passes through the center of the prostate
  - Thin alkaline substance that makes up the largest part of seminal fluid
- Urethra
- Bulbourethral glands (Cowper's glands)
  - Located behind the urethra and secrete mucous into the semen
- Sexual identity/development
  - Begins at conception
  - Gender is determined by the XY chromosomes of the male.
  - Puberty
    - Achievement of sexual maturity
- Sexual response pattern
  - Male and female sexual responses are characterized by vasocongestion and myotonia.
  - Sexual desire is controlled by the limbic system of the brain and mediated by the ratio of testosterone.
  - Four phases (excitement, plateau, orgasm, and resolution)

FEMALE REPRODUCTIVE SYSTEM

- External genitalia
  - Mons pubis protects the pubic bone from trauma
  - Clitoris
    - Small organ composed of erectile tissue
    - Located behind the junction of the labia minora
    - Homologous to the corpora cavernosa and gland of the penis
  - Labia majora
  - Labia minora
  - Bartholin glands (greater vestibular gland)
    - Two bean-shaped glands, one located on each side of the vaginal orifice
    - Homologous to the bulbourethral glands in the male
  - Skene's glands
  - Urethral meatus
  - Perineum
    - Region between the vaginal orifice and the anus
  - Hymen
    - A fold of the mucous membrane that forms a border around the external opening of the vagina, partially closing the orifice
- Internal genitalia
  - Vagina
    - Situated between the rectum and urethra and bladder
    - Organ that receives seminal fluid from the male
    - Excretory duct for uterine secretions and menstrual flow
    - Lower part of the birth canal

- Uterus
  - Walls
    - Inner wall has lining of mucosa called endometrium
    - Myometrium is a thick, middle coat of muscle
    - Outer layer is peritoneum
  - Has rich blood supply from the uterine arteries
  - Functions
    - Menstruation
    - Pregnancy
    - Labor and expulsion of fetus
- Ovaries
  - Located behind and below the uterine tubes
  - Large almond size and shape
  - Functions
    - Oogenesis—formation of mature female gametes (ova)
    - Secretion of estrogens and progesterone
- Fallopian tubes
- The Pelvis
  - Bony ring formed by four united bones
    - Two innominate
    - Coccyx
    - Sacrum
- The Breasts
  - Found under skin over the pectoral muscles
  - Size depends on the deposits of adipose tissue
  - Divided into lobes and lobules
  - Function
    - Secretes milk for infants

THE FEMALE REPRODUCTIVE CYCLE

- **Recurring** cycles
- Menstruation
  - Ovarian cycle
  - Menstrual cycle
    - Menstrual phase
    - Proliferative phase
    - Secretory phase
  - Gestation
    - The time in which a fetus develops, beginning with fertilization and ending at birth
    - Normal human pregnancy ranges from 38 to 42 weeks.
  - Lactation
    - Secretion of milk from the mammary glands
    - Period of time a mother lactates to feed her young

- ○ Menopause
  - ➤ Begins when menses cease for at least one year
  - ➤ Usually between the ages of 40 and 55
  - ➤ With menopause
    - – Ovaries atrophy
    - – Estrogen levels fall
    - – Changes in the vagina as well as the cardiovascular, skeletal, and integumentary systems

ANSWER SHEET
The Reproductive System Sample Test

1. Ⓐ Ⓑ Ⓒ Ⓓ

2. Ⓐ Ⓑ Ⓒ Ⓓ

3. Ⓐ Ⓑ Ⓒ Ⓓ

4. Ⓐ Ⓑ Ⓒ Ⓓ

5. Ⓐ Ⓑ Ⓒ Ⓓ

6. Ⓐ Ⓑ Ⓒ Ⓓ

7. Ⓐ Ⓑ Ⓒ Ⓓ

8. Ⓐ Ⓑ Ⓒ Ⓓ

9. Ⓐ Ⓑ Ⓒ Ⓓ

10. Ⓐ Ⓑ Ⓒ Ⓓ

11. Ⓐ Ⓑ Ⓒ Ⓓ

12. Ⓐ Ⓑ Ⓒ Ⓓ

13. Ⓐ Ⓑ Ⓒ Ⓓ

14. Ⓐ Ⓑ Ⓒ Ⓓ

15. Ⓐ Ⓑ Ⓒ Ⓓ

16. Ⓐ Ⓑ Ⓒ Ⓓ

17. Ⓐ Ⓑ Ⓒ Ⓓ

18. Ⓐ Ⓑ Ⓒ Ⓓ

19. Ⓐ Ⓑ Ⓒ Ⓓ

20. Ⓐ Ⓑ Ⓒ Ⓓ

For Questions 1–20, select the letter (A, B, C, or D) that best answers the question. Record your answers on The Reproductive System Sample Test Answer Sheet on page 319.

1. All of the following are basic purposes of the reproductive system EXCEPT

   (A) female system involved from conception to shortly after birth.
   (B) monthly egg production in the female.
   (C) perpetuation of the species.
   (D) sexual delectation.

2. The male reproductive system is responsible for _____ , whereas the female reproductive system is responsible for _____ .

   (A) egg production, sperm production
   (B) female gender, male gender
   (C) male gender, female gender
   (D) sperm production, egg production

3. Which of the following describes menarche?

   (A) cessation of menses
   (B) completion of puberty
   (C) preparation of endometrium for pregnancy
   (D) onset of menses

4. The _____ serves as one of the ducts through which sperm pass in their journey from the testes to the exterior.

   (A) ductus deferens
   (B) epididymis
   (C) ovaducts
   (D) spermatic cord

5. All of the following male reproductive structures are paired EXCEPT

   (A) ejaculatory duct.
   (B) oviduct.
   (C) seminal vesicle.
   (D) urethra.

6. All of the following are female sex organs EXCEPT

   (A) fallopian tubes.
   (B) mons veneris.
   (C) ovaries.
   (D) vagina.

7. The innermost wall or lining of the uterus is the

   (A) endometrium.
   (B) mesovarium.
   (C) myometrium.
   (D) parietal peritoneum.

8. The _____ is external female genitalia.

   (A) labia
   (B) mons pubis
   (C) vaginal orifice
   (D) vulva

9. The lactation nurse at the community clinic is preparing a lesson on "breasts and pregnancy" for women early into their pregnancy. It is important the attendees leave the meeting understanding that

   (A) the development of the pectoral muscles during pregnancy influences the functional ability of the breast.
   (B) the follicle-stimulating hormone (FSH) dominates the functional ability of the breast.
   (C) the size and color of the areola and nipple are directly related to the functional ability of the breast.
   (D) the size of the breast does not relate to its functional ability.

10. Rupture of the mature follicle with the expulsion of its ripe ovum is known as

    (A) inhibition.
    (B) menstruation.
    (C) luteinization.
    (D) ovulation.

11. Which of the following systems DOES NOT undergo changes with menopause?

    (A) cardiovascular system
    (B) nervous system
    (C) reproductive system
    (D) skeletal system

12. Secretion of milk from the mammary glands is known as

    (A) cleavage.
    (B) excretion.
    (C) gestation.
    (D) lactation.

13. _____ depends chiefly on large numbers of normal-sized and normal-shaped sperm being ejaculated.

    (A) Conception
    (B) Histogenesis
    (C) Male fertility
    (D) Spermatogenesis

14. The clitoris in the female is _____ to the corpora cavernosa and gland of the penis.

    (A) autologous
    (B) heterologous
    (C) homologous
    (D) tautologous

15. A normal human pregnancy lasts from

    (A) 38 to 42 weeks
    (B) 43 to 48 weeks
    (C) depends on the age of the female
    (D) depends on the number of previous pregnancies

16. The fleshy pouch suspended below the perineum containing the testes is called the

    (A) glans penis.
    (B) prepuce.
    (C) prostate gland.
    (D) scrotum.

17. During the process of meiosis, a spermatocyte with 46 chromosomes will produce spermatid having chromosomes that number

    (A) 23
    (B) 46
    (C) 92
    (D) depends on whether the sperm have the ability to produce male or female offspring

18. Androgens are also known as

    (A) female sex hormones.
    (B) lactation inhibitors.
    (C) male sex hormones.
    (D) spermatic lubricators.

19. During pregnancy, the female reproductive tract produces the hormones estrogen and

    (A) androgen.
    (B) beta-estrogen.
    (C) progesterone.
    (D) testosterone.

20. The _____ is a muscular tube extending between the uterus and the external genitalia.

    (A) mammary extension
    (B) suspensory ligament
    (C) urethra
    (D) vagina

The Reproductive System Sample Test Answer Key

1. **D**	5. **D**	9. **D**	13. **A**	17. **A**
2. **D**	6. **B**	10. **D**	14. **C**	18. **C**
3. **D**	7. **A**	11. **B**	15. **A**	19. **C**
4. **A**	8. **B**	12. **D**	16. **D**	20. **D**

THE REPRODUCTIVE SYSTEM SAMPLE TEST ANSWERS EXPLAINED

1. **(D)** Sexual delectation is sexual enjoyment or pleasure and has nothing to do with the basic purposes of the reproductive system.

2. **(D)** If you missed this question, review the Reproductive System Overview on page 315.

3. **(D)** Menarche is the onset of menses in the female. Menopause is the cessation of menses.

4. **(A)** The ductus deferens is a tube in the male reproductive system that conveys sperm from the epididymis in the testes to the urethra.

5. **(D)** There are two ejaculatory ducts, oviducts, and seminal vesicles. There is one urethra.

6. **(B)** The mons veneris, or mons pubis, is a fat pad covering the pubic bone. In the female, its purpose is to provide cushioning and protection.

7. **(A)** The endometrium is a mucous membrane that lines the inside of the uterus. It changes throughout the menstrual cycle as it becomes thick with blood vessels in preparation for pregnancy. If pregnancy does not occur, the lining is cast off and menstruation occurs.

8. **(B)** The mons pubis is a rounded mound of adipose tissue covering the pubic symphysis that unites the right and left pubic bones. It is usually present in both males and females. In general, it's more pronounced in women than in men. Its primary purpose is to protect the pubic bone during sexual intercourse.

9. **(D)** Breast size has nothing to do with functionality of the breast. Regardless of breast size or shape, being able to produce breast milk lies in the breast tissue in milk producing cells.

10. **(D)** The stem of this question is the definition of ovulation.

11. **(B)** Menopause take place when menses have ceased for at least one year, and this marks the end of the menstrual cycle. Menopausal women are no longer able to have children. Most women experience menopause between the ages of 40 and 55. The ovaries' atrophy and estrogen levels fall after menopause. Changes occur in the vagina, cardiovascular system, integumentary system, and skeletal system. The nervous system does not change.

12. **(D)** The stem of this question is the definition of lactation. In this sense, the term *lactate* means to produce milk and has nothing to do with the salt or ester of lactic acid.

13. **(A)** Aside from having a healthy egg, there must be sufficient quantity, movement, and structure of sperm for conception. A deficit in any of these areas may affect male fertility.

14. **(C)** The key to determining the correct answer to this question is being able to define the terms or break them down into their parts. While there are similarities in some of the suffixes, which may lead you to believe that multiple choices are correct, choice C, homologous, is the most correct answer.

15. **(A)** A normal pregnancy is usually 38 to 42 weeks in length.

16. **(D)** The testes are located in the scrotum of the male.

17. **(A)** Meiosis, also known as reduction division, occurs in primary sex cells. It is a type of cell division leading to the formation of viable egg and sperm cells. The purpose of meiosis is to reduce the number of chromosomes to half (23) in gametes so that upon fertilization the human chromosome number is kept constant at 46.

18. **(C)** The key to determining the correct answer is recognizing that *andro-* (prefix) has to do with masculinity or males of a species.

19. **(C)** Estrogen and progesterone are produced by the corpus luteum during early pregnancy. Around 10 weeks, the placenta assumes production.

20. **(D)** The vagina is a hollow, cylindrical organ that receives the penis during sexual intercourse, is a conduit for menstrual blood flow from the uterus, and is a birth canal during childbirth.

OVERVIEW

- Functions
  - **The respiratory system exists for the purpose of gas exchange between the blood and atmosphere.**
  - Other functions include speech production and fluid balance.
- Respiration has the following processes:
  - Pulmonary ventilation
    - ➤ The process of inspiration and expiration
  - External expiration
    - ➤ The exchange process between the blood and the lungs
  - Gas transport
    - ➤ Carried out by the cardiovascular system
  - Internal respiration
    - ➤ The process of gas exchange between interstitial fluids, blood, and the cells
    - ➤ Cellular respiration (inside the cell) generates energy (ATP) using O_2 and glucose and producing waste CO_2

RESPIRATORY STRUCTURES

- Lungs
  - The most important function is **gas exchange**.
  - Located in the thoracic cavity bounded by the ribs, vertebrae, clavicles, and diaphragm
  - Right lung > left lung
  - The major organ system in **control of body pH**
- Upper respiratory tract
  - Conducts air to lower respiratory tract
  - Composed of:
    - ➤ Nose
      - Humidifies inspired air
      - Acts as a filter
    - ➤ Sinuses
      - Air filled
      - Trap particles
    - ➤ Mouth
    - ➤ Pharynx
      - Divided into the oropharynx and nasopharynx
      - Maintains middle-ear pressure
      - Warms and humidifies inspired air
      - Pathway for digestive and respiratory tracts
    - ➤ Larynx
      - May be called the "voice box"
      - Joins the upper and lower airways
      - Initiates a cough reflex

- All structures are covered with mucus-secreting cells and cilia.
- Olfactory sensors are located in the uppermost area.
- Lower respiratory tract
  - Resembles an upside-down tree
  - Composed of:
    - Trachea
      - May be referred to as the "wind pipe"
      - Flexible hollow tube composed of smooth muscle
      - Branches into the left and right main stem bronchi
    - Bronchi
      - Right main stem bronchi is shorter, wider, and more vertical (higher risk of aspiration into right lung)
      - Right and left main stem bronchi repeatedly divide into smaller and smaller branches that end in alveoli.
    - Respiratory membrane
      - Consists of the alveolar and capillary wall
      - Gas exchanges across this membrane.
    - Alveolar types
      - Site of gas exchange
      - Type I cells alveolar walls (squamous epithelium, specific for gas exchange, susceptible to injury by inhaled agents, and are constructed to prevent fluid transudation into the alveoli)
      - Type II cells secrete surfactant (extremely active metabolically)
      - Type III cells phagocytize foreign matter.
    - Pleura
      - Encircles lungs
      - The area between the visceral and parietal pleural space is the intrapleural space.
      - The pleural fluid lubricates the pleura to decrease resistance during respiration.
- Pulmonary Vasculature
  - Pulmonary blood supply is provided by the pulmonary and bronchial arteries.
  - Provides blood supply to the lungs and pleural tissue
    - Arteries arise from thoracic aorta
    - Considered part of systemic circulation
    - **Does not participate in gas exchange**
- Respiratory muscles
  - Diaphragm
    - **Major muscle of ventilation**
    - Innervated by phrenic nerve
  - Accessory muscles of ventilation
    - **Inspiration**
      - External intercostal muscles
      - Sternocleidomastoid muscles
      - Scalene muscles
      - Pectoralis major muscles
      - Trapezius

> **Expiration**
>   – Internal intercostal muscles
>   – External abdominal obliquus muscles
>   – Internal abdominis obliquus muscles
>   – Transverse abdominis muscles
>   – Rectus abdominis muscles

GAS EXCHANGE PROCESS (FOUR STAGES)

- Ventilation
  - The process of moving air to and from the atmosphere and the lung alveoli
  - Apportionment of air within the lungs to maintain appropriate quantities of O_2 and CO_2 in the alveoli
  - The most important structures in gas exchange are the alveoli and alveolar bud.
- Diffusion
  - Movement of a substance from a region of high concentration to a region of low concentration
  - No metabolic energy is required for diffusion of gases.
    > The work of breathing is provided for by the respiratory muscles and the heart.
- Transport of gases in the circulation
  - Oxygen
    > Roughly 97% of O_2 is transported in chemical combination with the protein hemoglobin in the erythrocyte.
    > The remaining O_2 (around 3%) is transported in the plasma.
  - Carbon dioxide
    > Around 25% of CO_2 binds to hemoglobin in the red cells, forming carbaminohemoglobin (HCO_2).
    > Approximately 8% of CO_2 is transported as a gas in the plasma.
    > The majority of CO_2 (65%) is transported as dissolved bicarbonate ions (HCO_3) in plasma.
- Diffusion between the systemic capillary bed and body tissue cells
  - Pressure gradients permit the diffusion of O_2 and CO_2 between systemic, capillaries, interstitial fluid, and cells.
  - O_2 is consumed through **aerobic metabolism** in the mitochondria of each cell.
    > Produces energy bonds of ATP and waste products of O_2 and CO_2

CONTROL OF BREATHING

- Breathing is controlled by the contractions of respiratory muscles, which are controlled by nerve stimulation.
- Respiratory control centers
  - Medullary inspiratory center
    > Located in the brain stem
    >   – Includes parts of the medulla oblongata and pons
    > Stimulates contraction of the inspiratory muscles (diaphragm, external intercostal muscle)

- Pneumotaxic area
  - Located in pons (brain stem)
  - Inhibits inspiratory center
  - Prevents lungs from overinflating
- Apneustic area
  - Located in pons
  - Stimulated inspiratory center
- Respiratory control centers are influenced by stimuli from the following:
  - Central chemoreceptors
    - Located in the medulla oblongata
    - Monitors the chemistry of cerebrospinal fluid
    - Based on pH, receptors stimulate the respiratory center to increase the respiratory rate.
  - Peripheral receptors
    - Located in aortic bodies of aortic arch and carotid bodies in carotid artery walls
    - Activated when lungs expand to physical limits
    - Based on pH, pCO_2 or pO_2 stimulates the respiratory center.
  - Stretch receptors
    - Located in the walls of bronchi and bronchioles
    - Activated when lungs are stimulated to physical limits
    - Stimulation allows expiration to begin

ANSWER SHEET
The Respiratory System Sample Test

1. Ⓐ Ⓑ Ⓒ Ⓓ
2. Ⓐ Ⓑ Ⓒ Ⓓ
3. Ⓐ Ⓑ Ⓒ Ⓓ
4. Ⓐ Ⓑ Ⓒ Ⓓ
5. Ⓐ Ⓑ Ⓒ Ⓓ
6. Ⓐ Ⓑ Ⓒ Ⓓ
7. Ⓐ Ⓑ Ⓒ Ⓓ

8. Ⓐ Ⓑ Ⓒ Ⓓ
9. Ⓐ Ⓑ Ⓒ Ⓓ
10. Ⓐ Ⓑ Ⓒ Ⓓ
11. Ⓐ Ⓑ Ⓒ Ⓓ
12. Ⓐ Ⓑ Ⓒ Ⓓ
13. Ⓐ Ⓑ Ⓒ Ⓓ
14. Ⓐ Ⓑ Ⓒ Ⓓ

15. Ⓐ Ⓑ Ⓒ Ⓓ
16. Ⓐ Ⓑ Ⓒ Ⓓ
17. Ⓐ Ⓑ Ⓒ Ⓓ
18. Ⓐ Ⓑ Ⓒ Ⓓ
19. Ⓐ Ⓑ Ⓒ Ⓓ
20. Ⓐ Ⓑ Ⓒ Ⓓ

For Questions 1–20, select the letter (A, B, C, or D) that best answers the question. Record your answers on The Respiratory System Sample Test Answer Sheet on page 329.

1. All of the following are processes of respiration EXCEPT

   (A) external ventilation.
   (B) gas transport.
   (C) internal respiration.
   (D) pulmonary ventilation.

2. The major structure in control of the body pH are

   (A) the lungs.
   (B) the nonalveolar cells.
   (C) the respiratory membranes.
   (D) covered with nonmucus-secreting cells and cilia.

3. The pleura of the lungs

   (A) is extremely active metabolically.
   (B) is found between the visceral and parietal pleural spaces.
   (C) phagocytizes foreign matter.
   (D) surrounds the lungs.

4. The diaphragm is innervated by the

   (A) lumbar nerve.
   (B) phrenic nerve.
   (C) sarcolemmas nerve.
   (D) vagus nerve.

5. The pneumotaxic area in the brain stem

   (A) controls the sequence of breathing.
   (B) inhibits the inspiratory center.
   (C) regulates the ratio of inspiration and expiration.
   (D) stimulates voluntary respirations.

6. The route by which air normally enters the respiratory system is the

   (A) larynx.
   (B) mouth.
   (C) nose.
   (D) trachea.

7. You might say, "My throat is sore and burns if I drink orange juice." Your health care provider would say, "Your _____ is inflamed."

   (A) adenoids
   (B) laryngopharynx
   (C) nasopharynx
   (D) pharynx

8. Which of the following has the highest risk of aspirating or sucking foreign bodies (such as food, fluids, gum, coins, paperclips, etc.) into the lungs?

   (A) bronchial tree
   (B) left pleurobronchi
   (C) right main stem bronchi
   (D) tracheopharynx

9. The correct anatomical term for "wind pipe" is

   (A) bronchi.
   (B) larynx.
   (C) nasal cavity.
   (D) trachea.

10. The maximum volume of air that can be exhaled from the lungs after completely inhaling is the _____ of the lungs.

    (A) functional residual capacity (FRC)
    (B) residual volume (RV)
    (C) total lung capacity (TLC)
    (D) vital capacity (VC)

11. The majority of oxygen carried in the blood is bound to the protein _____ in red blood cells.

    (A) deoxyhemoglobin
    (B) hemoglobin
    (C) interleukin
    (D) ribosome

·12. All of the following cartilages support the larynx EXCEPT the

    (A) adventitia.
    (B) cuneiform.
    (C) corniculate.
    (D) cricoid.

13. Identify the major muscle of ventilation.

    (A) diaphragm
    (B) external intercostal
    (C) internal abdominis obliquus
    (D) transverse abdominis

14. Pulmonary vasculature, which provides blood supply to the lungs and pleural tissues, includes all of the following EXCEPT

    (A) Their arteries arise from the thoracic aorta.
    (B) They are considered part of systemic circulation.
    (C) They are constructed to prevent fluid transudation into the alveoli.
    (D) They participate in gas exchange.

15. What is the best description of the lower respiratory tract? It resembles

    (A) a slingshot.
    (B) an upside-down tree.
    (C) clusters of small grapes.
    (D) two elongated inflated balloons.

16. Ventilation is defined as

    (A) a process of moving air to and from the atmosphere as well as to the lungs and alveoli.
    (B) limiting contraction of the inspiratory muscles, thus preventing the lungs from overinflating.
    (C) the ability of the lungs and thoracic cavity to expand.
    (D) the movement of molecules, by passive diffusion or active transport, from the bronchioles to the alveoli.

17. Breathing is regulated by contractions of respiratory muscles, which are controlled by _____ stimulation.

    (A) enzymatic
    (B) nerve
    (C) pressure gradient
    (D) type III respiratory cell

18. Oxygen is consumed through _____ metabolism in the mitochondria of each cell.

    (A) aerobic
    (B) antimicrobial
    (C) carbaminohemoglobin
    (D) hormonal

19. All of the following are part of the respiratory processes EXCEPT

    (A) the apneustic area.
    (B) the medullary inspiratory center.
    (C) the pneumotaxic area.
    (D) the reflex area.

20. Which of the following applies to the right lung?

    (A) It has a greater number of sympathetic nerves than parasympathetic nerves.
    (B) It has a smaller inspiratory reserve than the left lung.
    (C) It is composed of three lobes.
    (D) It serves as a site for moisturizing air.

The Respiratory System Sample Test Answer Key

1. **A**		5. **B**		9. **D**		13. **A**		17. **B**
2. **A**		6. **C**		10. **D**		14. **C**		18. **A**
3. **D**		7. **D**		11. **B**		15. **B**		19. **D**
4. **B**		8. **C**		12. **A**		16. **A**		20. **C**

THE RESPIRATORY SYSTEM SAMPLE TEST ANSWERS EXPLAINED

1. **(A)** External ventilation does not exist. The processes of respiration are pulmonary ventilation, external respiration, gas transport, and internal respiration.

2. **(A)** One process used to regulate blood pH entails the release of mildly acidic carbon dioxide from the lungs. Blood carries carbon dioxide to the lungs, where it is exhaled. The brain adjusts the amount of carbon dioxide exhaled by controlling the speed and depth of breathing. By adjusting the speed and depth of breathing, the brain and lungs are able to regulate the blood pH minute by minute.

3. **(D)** The pleura are serous membranes encasing the lungs and lining the walls of the pleural cavity (where the lungs are located).

4. **(B)** The left and right phrenic nerves arising from the third through the fifth spinal nerves innervate the diaphragm.

5. **(B)** Three areas in the brain control respirations. These include the medullary inspiratory center in the medulla oblongata, the apneustic area in the pons, and the pneumotaxic area that holds the inspiratory muscles in check by restraining contraction of the inspiratory muscles and overexpanding the lungs.

6. **(C)** The key to answering this question correctly is paying attention to the phrase *normally enters.*

7. **(D)** The pharynx is part of the digestive (and respiratory) pathway. Swallowing food and fluids when the pharynx is inflamed may cause discomfort.

8. **(C)** The right main bronchus in humans is wider, shorter, and more vertical than the left main bronchus. It is approximately 2.5 centimeters long and enters the right lung nearly opposite the fifth thoracic vertebra. The left main bronchus is smaller in diameter and is longer than the right, approximately 5 centimeters long. It enters the left lung opposite the sixth thoracic vertebra. If food, liquids, or foreign bodies are aspirated, they often will lodge in the right main stem bronchus.

9. **(D)** The trachea is a hollow tube connecting the larynx and the left and right bronchi. The phrase "windpipe" is a lay term for trachea.

10. **(D)** The stem of the question is the definition for vital capacity (VC).

11. **(B)** Hemoglobin is the carrier of oxygen in the bloodstream. Its unique shape allows it to carry a greater amount of oxygen.

12. **(A)** The adventitia is the outermost connective tissue covering of an organ or structure, especially an artery or vein.

13. **(A)** Although other muscles assist the process of ventilation, the diaphragm is the major muscle.

14. **(C)** Pulmonary vasculature has to do with the flow of blood from the right ventricle through the pulmonary artery to the lungs, where carbon dioxide is exchanged for oxygen, and back through the pulmonary vein to the left atrium. The pulmonary circulation is a low-pressure, high-flow circuit. The low pressure prevents fluid moving out of the pulmonary vessels into the interstitial space and allows the right ventricle to operate at a low energy exertion. Pulmonary vasculature carries deoxygenated or oxygenated blood and does not participate in gas exchange.

15. **(B)** The lower respiratory tract consists of the trachea, the bronchial tubes, and the lungs, and their anatomical structures resemble an upside-down tree. The trachea represents the main trunk, and the bronchial system represents the branches of the tree.

16. **(A)** Choice A is the correct definition of ventilation.

17. **(B)** Muscles must be stimulated to perform an action. Nerves provide that stimulation.

18. **(A)** The aerobic phase of cellular respiration takes place inside of the mitochondria. Oxygen serves the important function as the final hydrogen carrier. These events take place during the Krebs citric acid cycle.

19. **(D)** The ventilation, or rhythmical pattern of breathing, is controlled by separate respiratory centers (in the medulla oblongata and pons) that promote the contraction of the diaphragm and intercostal muscles. These centers control respirations whether a person is awake, asleep, or engaged in physical activity. These centers are the medullary inspiratory center, the pneumotaxic area, and the apneustic center. The respiratory centers are affected by stimuli received from the following sensory neurons: central chemoreceptors of the central nervous system, peripheral chemoreceptors of the peripheral nervous system, and stretch receptors in the walls of the bronchi and bronchioles.

20. **(C)** The right lung has three lobes. The left lung has two lobes.

ANSWER SHEET
Numerical Ability Test

1. Ⓐ Ⓑ Ⓒ Ⓓ
2. Ⓐ Ⓑ Ⓒ Ⓓ
3. Ⓐ Ⓑ Ⓒ Ⓓ
4. Ⓐ Ⓑ Ⓒ Ⓓ
5. Ⓐ Ⓑ Ⓒ Ⓓ
6. Ⓐ Ⓑ Ⓒ Ⓓ
7. Ⓐ Ⓑ Ⓒ Ⓓ
8. Ⓐ Ⓑ Ⓒ Ⓓ
9. Ⓐ Ⓑ Ⓒ Ⓓ
10. Ⓐ Ⓑ Ⓒ Ⓓ
11. Ⓐ Ⓑ Ⓒ Ⓓ
12. Ⓐ Ⓑ Ⓒ Ⓓ
13. Ⓐ Ⓑ Ⓒ Ⓓ
14. Ⓐ Ⓑ Ⓒ Ⓓ
15. Ⓐ Ⓑ Ⓒ Ⓓ
16. Ⓐ Ⓑ Ⓒ Ⓓ
17. Ⓐ Ⓑ Ⓒ Ⓓ

18. Ⓐ Ⓑ Ⓒ Ⓓ
19. Ⓐ Ⓑ Ⓒ Ⓓ
20. Ⓐ Ⓑ Ⓒ Ⓓ
21. Ⓐ Ⓑ Ⓒ Ⓓ
22. Ⓐ Ⓑ Ⓒ Ⓓ
23. Ⓐ Ⓑ Ⓒ Ⓓ
24. Ⓐ Ⓑ Ⓒ Ⓓ
25. Ⓐ Ⓑ Ⓒ Ⓓ
26. Ⓐ Ⓑ Ⓒ Ⓓ
27. Ⓐ Ⓑ Ⓒ Ⓓ
28. Ⓐ Ⓑ Ⓒ Ⓓ
29. Ⓐ Ⓑ Ⓒ Ⓓ
30. Ⓐ Ⓑ Ⓒ Ⓓ
31. Ⓐ Ⓑ Ⓒ Ⓓ
32. Ⓐ Ⓑ Ⓒ Ⓓ
33. Ⓐ Ⓑ Ⓒ Ⓓ
34. Ⓐ Ⓑ Ⓒ Ⓓ

35. Ⓐ Ⓑ Ⓒ Ⓓ
36. Ⓐ Ⓑ Ⓒ Ⓓ
37. Ⓐ Ⓑ Ⓒ Ⓓ
38. Ⓐ Ⓑ Ⓒ Ⓓ
39. Ⓐ Ⓑ Ⓒ Ⓓ
40. Ⓐ Ⓑ Ⓒ Ⓓ
41. Ⓐ Ⓑ Ⓒ Ⓓ
42. Ⓐ Ⓑ Ⓒ Ⓓ
43. Ⓐ Ⓑ Ⓒ Ⓓ
44. Ⓐ Ⓑ Ⓒ Ⓓ
45. Ⓐ Ⓑ Ⓒ Ⓓ
46. Ⓐ Ⓑ Ⓒ Ⓓ
47. Ⓐ Ⓑ Ⓒ Ⓓ
48. Ⓐ Ⓑ Ⓒ Ⓓ
49. Ⓐ Ⓑ Ⓒ Ⓓ
50. Ⓐ Ⓑ Ⓒ Ⓓ

Model Examinations

NUMERICAL ABILITY TEST

50 TEST ITEMS: TIME: 100 MINUTES

Directions: For each question, select the letter (A, B, C, or D) that corresponds to your answer. Mark your answer on the Numerical Ability Answer Sheet on page 335.

1. Mary is planning a pizza party for her son. The manager of the local pizza restaurant says one of his pizzas contains 14 slices. Mary is planning on inviting 15 of her son's friends to the party. How many large pizzas will Mary need to order if she figures each child attending the party will eat four pieces?

   (A) 4
   (B) 10
   (C) 7
   (D) 5

2. A woman is diagnosed as having a bacterial infection and is given a prescription for an antibiotic. The prescription instructs the woman to take 3 tablets daily for 18 days. The pharmacist tells the woman each antibiotic tablet costs $2.58. What will the woman pay for the prescription of antibiotics?

   (A) $46.44
   (B) $139.32
   (C) $54.00
   (D) $156.74

3. Select the response in which the fractions $\frac{15}{45}$, $\frac{18}{75}$, and $\frac{45}{60}$ are written from least to greatest.

   (A) $\frac{15}{45}, \frac{18}{75}, \frac{45}{60}$
   (B) $\frac{18}{75}, \frac{15}{45}, \frac{45}{60}$
   (C) $\frac{45}{60}, \frac{18}{75}, \frac{15}{45}$
   (D) $\frac{15}{45}, \frac{45}{60}, \frac{18}{75}$

4. Jackson is considering buying an insurance policy, but he cannot afford more than $500.00 a year in annual premiums. He is considering a $15,000 policy with an annual premium of $35 per $1,000. Can Jackson afford the policy?

   (A) No, the annual premium is $25 more than Jackson can afford.
   (B) No, the annual premium is $525 more than Jackson can afford.
   (C) Yes, the annual premium is exactly $500 a year.
   (D) Yes, Jackson could afford a policy valued at $18,500.

5. Lacy owns 800 shares of Congo Gold Mines Limited stock. The stock pays a dividend of $8.50 per share semiannually. How much will Lacy receive in dividends in one year?

   (A) $6,800
   (B) $13,600
   (C) $68
   (D) $136

6. A motorist drove at a speed of 55 miles per hour for five hours before stopping for a rest. After resting, the motorist drove at a speed of 65 miles per hour for six additional hours. What was the average miles per hour driven by the motorist?

   (A) 59.75 mph
   (B) 60 mph
   (C) 66.5 mph
   (D) 60.5 mph

7. $(4 \times 13) + (15 \times 8) =$

   (A) 399
   (B) 172
   (C) 40
   (D) 158

8. A hospital is looking into how nurses spend their time. Nurses are asked to keep track of time spent in four areas: (1) direct patient care, (2) preparing and administering medications, (3) assisting other health care professionals, and (4) nonpatient care activities. Results demonstrate that nurses spend three fifths of their time performing direct patient care, one eighth of their time preparing and administering medications, and one sixth of their time assisting other health care professionals. What percentage of the nurses' time was spent performing nonpatient care activities?

   (A) 20%
   (B) 12%
   (C) 19%
   (D) 11%

9. A circle has a circumference of 8 inches. The radius of the circle is

   (A) 1.25 inches.
   (B) 2.5 inches.
   (C) 25.12 inches.
   (D) .3925 inches.

10. What is the value of $17.3 + 5.75 - 16.02$?

    (A) 7.0
    (B) 7.03
    (C) 39.1
    (D) 6.82

11. A nurse's aide makes $5.58 an hour working the 7 A.M.–3 P.M. shift. She makes $6.00 an hour working the 3 P.M.–11 P.M. shift. What amount does she earn based on the following time card?

Monday	7:00 A.M.–11:20 A.M.
	12:20 P.M.–3:00 P.M.
Tuesday	3:00 P.M.–8:00 P.M.
	8:30 P.M.–11:00 P.M.
Wednesday	7:00 A.M.–11:00 P.M.
	3:00 P.M.–11:00 P.M.

    (A) $176.70
    (B) $225.43
    (C) $170.19
    (D) $183.00

12. The normal dosage for a medication is 20 mg/kg/day. The patient weighs 50 kg. How much medication should the patient receive? Solve for x.

    (A) 1,000 mg
    (B) 200 mg
    (C) 1,500 mg
    (D) 900 mg

13. Philip has $3.00 to spend on marbles. One marble costs 37¢. How many marbles can Philip buy?

    (A) 10
    (B) 8
    (C) 5
    (D) 7

14. A man borrowed a sum of money with an interest rate of 8% annually for five years. At the end of five years, he had paid $500 in interest. What amount did the man borrow?

(A) $2,000
(B) $1,250
(C) $3,125
(D) $2,500

15. Bryan has $3,500 to pay for one semester of college. One third of his money will pay room and board, one fifth will pay for books and supplies, and one fourth will pay for tuition. Any money left will be spending money. How much will Bryan have for spending money?

(A) $657.84
(B) $758
(C) $507.55
(D) $800

16. What is the simple interest on $750 at 15% for 26 months?

(A) $158.75
(B) $4.33
(C) $1,300
(D) $244.13

17. Results of the biology exam indicated 89 students took the exam. The biology teacher told the class that one sixth of the class had failed the exam. Posted results of the exam indicated 15% of the class received above 90%. What is the difference between the number of students that failed the exam and the number of students who scored above 90% on the exam?

(A) 80
(B) 2
(C) 15
(D) 11

18. A graduate student is hired to double-check data collected by a researcher. There are 854 data sets to check. After learning the system, the graduate student can check 6 sets per hour. After 8 hours, another graduate student is enlisted to speed the process of checking data sets. The second student can check 4.5 data sets per hour. How many total hours are needed to double-check all the data sets? Round to the nearest hour.

(A) 81 hours
(B) 85 hours
(C) 77 hours
(D) 90 hours

19. John and Penny have five children. Their youngest child is 5 years old and the oldest child is 30 years old. How old are the remaining children if the second child is 5 years older than the youngest child, the third child is 15 years younger than the oldest child, and the fourth child is twice the age of the second child?

(A) 10, 15, and 20 years
(B) 10, 12, and 24 years
(C) 5, 10, and 20 years
(D) 5, 15, and 30 years

20. A grocery store has a candy bin that sells various types of candy. Jaw Lockers sell for $2.50 a pound, Sour Cherries for $3.00 a half pound, Orange Blitzes for $1.50 a pound, and Goofy Gum for 75¢ a pound. What is the average cost per pound of the candy in the bin?

(A) $2.69
(B) $1.94
(C) $3.00
(D) $1.50

21. Virginia's monthly salary is $3,514. Taxes and social security deduct 34%. Her employer deducts $150 for repayment of a loan prior to issuing Virginia's check. How much does Virginia take home each month?

    (A) $2,169.24
    (B) $1,143.76
    (C) $1,245.76
    (D) $1,898.43

22. In April, 950 graduates of nursing programs took the licensure examination. Of these, 843 passed the examination. How many graduates were unsuccessful on the licensure examination?

    (A) 112
    (B) 68
    (C) 843
    (D) 107

23. Find the sum of 8 – 2 + (–10).

    (A) –4
    (B) 0
    (C) 20
    (D) 12

24. In ΔDEF, the measure of $\angle D$ is four times the measure of $\angle F$. The measure of $\angle E$ is 2.5 times the measure of $\angle F$. What is the measure of $\angle F$?

    (A) 24°
    (B) 48°
    (C) 60°
    (D) 96°

25. Your monthly grocery bill increases from $157.65 to $298.60 when your son comes home from college. The percentage of increase is

    (A) 47.2%.
    (B) 141%.
    (C) 89.4%.
    (D) 57.7%.

26. A researcher is developing a new trail mix. The recipe contains 8 ounces of raisins, 6 ounces of pecans, 4 ounces of peanuts, and 5 ounces of dried fruit. How many more ounces of dried fruit must be added to make the trail mix 25% dried fruit in weight?

    (A) 3 ounces
    (B) 2.5 ounces
    (C) 4 ounces
    (D) 1 ounce

27. A patient is taking a medication ordered at 45 milliequivalents (meq) by mouth 4-times-per-day (qid) with juice. The medication is available as 30 meq/20 mL. How many mL of medication should be administered per dose?

    (A) 15 mL
    (B) 25 mL
    (C) 30 mL
    (D) 35 mL

28. A patient taking a blood pressure medication is not responding to therapy. The physician increases the blood pressure medication from 300 mg a day to 650 mg a day. What is the percentage of increase in blood pressure medication?

    (A) 117%
    (B) 100%
    (C) 46%
    (D) 216%

29. A hospital's central supply has 596 winter blankets on hand when an early snowstorm strikes the area. Based on hospital census, one third of the blankets go to medical-surgical floors, one fifth of the blankets go to critical care areas, and three sevenths of the blankets go to surgery. What fraction of the blankets will be left in central supply?

    (A) two thirds
    (B) one third
    (C) one twenty-fifth
    (D) one fourth

30. Bill bought 25 shares of Ski Copper Mountain stock at $5.85 a share. He sold the shares five years later at $46.50 a share. What is Bill's profit?

    (A) $1,162.50
    (B) $146.25
    (C) $1,016.25
    (D) $1,308.75

31. A telephone company needs to install a new antenna on the top of a building. The manager of the company does not know what height antenna to purchase because the original antenna records were lost. Installation records for the original antenna indicate that guide wires were placed 12 feet from the base of the antenna, and a total of 80 feet of wire was used for four supports. How tall an antenna does the manager need to order?

    (A) 8 feet
    (B) 12 feet
    (C) 16 feet
    (D) 32 feet

32. The student nurses' club is having their annual bake sale. They plan to sell 75 cupcakes for 50¢ apiece, 250 cookies for 25¢ apiece, 150 donuts for 60¢ apiece, and 150 donut holes for 15¢ apiece. If all the bake goods are sold, how much will the club make?

    (A) $212.50
    (B) $215.46
    (C) $208.40
    (D) $200.50

33. $75.84 + 6.02 + 100.877 + 41.0 - 87.471 =$

    Round the answer to the nearest whole number.

    (A) 136
    (B) 137
    (C) 223
    (D) 224

34. $10 + 8 \times 15 + 10 \div 2 =$

    (A) 140
    (B) 170
    (C) 135
    (D) 157

35. A physician's order reads, "Give 1 gram of Penicillin before breakfast." The pharmacy is out of 1 gram tablets and sends tablets containing 125 mg of Penicillin per tablet. How many Penicillin tablets will the nurse administer before breakfast?

    (A) 12.5
    (B) 8
    (C) 10
    (D) 7

36. Select one-sixth written as a decimal.

    (A) 0.167
    (B) 0.06
    (C) 0.6
    (D) 1.67

37. Ordered: Talcot gr X by mouth. One dose only.

    Available: Talcot 600 mg tablets

    How many tablets will the nurse administer?

    (A) 0.5
    (B) 1
    (C) 10
    (D) Not enough information is given to calculate the problem.

38. Solve for x.

    $15x + 6x - 3x + 18 = 36x$

    (A) 1.0
    (B) 2.25
    (C) 3.0
    (D) 4.15

39. A student makes the following grades on homework assignments: 78, 84, 56, 96, 78, 85, 85, 95, 0, 73. What is the student's average grade on the assignments?

    (A) 85
    (B) 73
    (C) 81
    (D) 96

40. $18 + 7(2 \times 6) - (6 + 3) =$

    (A) 93
    (B) 291
    (C) 192
    (D) 35

41. When five times a number is increased by 14, the result is 54. What is the number?

    (A) 13.6
    (B) 68
    (C) 8
    (D) 4

42. A newly married couple bought an old house in need of repair for $35,000. They spent $20,000 refurbishing the house. After living in the house for many years, they sell the house for $65,000. How much profit did the couple make on the house?

    (A) $30,000
    (B) $45,000
    (C) $10,000
    (D) $15,000

43. A train is traveling at 86 miles per hour. How long will it take the train to reach a city 400 miles away?

    (A) 4 hours 42 minutes
    (B) 6 hours
    (C) 5 hours 4 minutes
    (D) 8 hours

44. What percent of 15 is 8?

    (A) 53%
    (B) 120%
    (C) 7%
    (D) 23%

45. Which of the following is the lowest common factor of 15, 48, and 63?

    (A) 5
    (B) 3
    (C) 4
    (D) 7

46. Central supply has the following items in stock:

    17 boxes of abdominal pads at $15 a box
    6 boxes of Band-Aids at $7.50 a box
    43 boxes of alcohol pads at $4 a box
    150 boxes of tissues at $1.50 a box
    11 boxes of cloth tape at $8.40 a box

    Issued to the nursing units during one day were:

    10 boxes of abdominal pads
    5 boxes of Band-Aids
    18 boxes of alcohol pads
    10 boxes of tissues
    3 boxes of cloth tape

    What is the dollar amount of supplies issued to the nursing units?

    (A) $299.70
    (B) $354.32
    (C) $158.07
    (D) $340.85

47. Marcia works as a freelance writer and sells her stories to the highest bidder. She recently wrote a story on the return of the buffalo herds to the Goodnight Ranch in Texas. Four magazines have made offers to purchase her story. Magazine A offered $458 minus 3% for editing, Magazine B offered $450 minus 2% for editing, Magazine C offered $480 minus 5% for editing, and Magazine D offered a flat $440 for the story. Which magazine will pay Marcia the greatest amount for her story?

    (A) Magazine A
    (B) Magazine B
    (C) Magazine C
    (D) Magazine D

48. The number following 20 in the series 5, 12, 9, 16, 13, 20 is

    (A) 15
    (B) 17
    (C) 21
    (D) 24

49. How many total inches are in 7 feet 4 inches and 4 feet 10 inches?

(A) 257 inches
(B) 130 inches
(C) 126 inches
(D) 146 inches

50. A box contains 3 colors of pencils. One fourth are black, three eighths are red, and the remaining 16 are yellow. How many pencils are in the box?

(A) 19
(B) 2
(C) 43
(D) 6

STOP

If there is still time remaining, you may review your answers.

ANSWER KEY
Numerical Ability Test

1. **D**	11. **A**	21. **A**	31. **C**	41. **C**
2. **B**	12. **A**	22. **D**	32. **A**	42. **C**
3. **B**	13. **B**	23. **A**	33. **A**	43. **A**
4. **A**	14. **B**	24. **A**	34. **C**	44. **A**
5. **B**	15. **B**	25. **C**	35. **B**	45. **B**
6. **D**	16. **D**	26. **D**	36. **A**	46. **A**
7. **B**	17. **B**	27. **C**	37. **B**	47. **C**
8. **D**	18. **B**	28. **A**	38. **A**	48. **B**
9. **A**	19. **A**	29. **C**	39. **B**	49. **D**
10. **B**	20. **A**	30. **C**	40. **A**	50. **C**

NUMERICAL ABILITY TEST ANSWERS EXPLAINED

1. **(D)** 1 child : 4 slices of pizza = 16 children: x slices of pizza

$$x = 64 \text{ slices of pizza}$$
$$1 \text{ pizza}: 14 \text{ slices} = x \text{ pizza} : 64 \text{ slices}$$
$$14x = 64$$
$$x = 4.57 \text{ pizzas} = 5 \text{ pizzas}$$

2. **(B)** 1 tablet : \$2.58 = 54 tablets : x

$$x = \$139.32$$

3. **(B)** Change each fraction to a decimal to sort the numbers from least to greatest.

$$\frac{15}{45} = 0.\overline{3}$$

$$\frac{18}{75} = 0.24$$

$$\frac{45}{60} = 0.75$$

Therefore, the correct order is $\frac{18}{75}, \frac{15}{45}, \frac{45}{60}$, Choice B.

4. **(A)** Policy = \$15,000
Premium rate = \$35/\$1,000
Annual premium = x
$$\$35 : \$1,000 = x : \$15,000$$
$$1,000x = 525,000$$
$$x = \$525$$

5. **(B)** Being able to define *semiannually* is the key to solving this problem. *Semiannually* means twice a year.
Shares of stock = 800
Dividend = \$8.50/share semiannually
$$(800 \times 8.50)(2) = 13,600 = \$13,600$$

6. **(D)** $55 \text{ mph} \times 5 = 275 \text{ miles}$
$65 \text{ mph} \times 6 = 390 \text{ miles}$
$$\left(\frac{275 + 390}{11}\right) = 60.45 = 60.5 \text{ mph}$$

7. **(B)** Multiply the numbers in the parentheses, and then add.
$$(4 \times 13) + (15 \times 8) = 52 + 120 = 172$$

8. **(D)**
Least Common Multiple = 120
$$\frac{3}{5} = \frac{72}{120} \quad \frac{1}{8} = \frac{15}{120} \quad \frac{1}{6} = \frac{20}{120}$$
$$\frac{107}{120} = 89\%$$
$$100\% - 89\% = 11\%$$

9. **(A)**

circumference = 8 inches

$\pi = 3.14$

diameter = unknown	radius = unknown
$C = \pi d$	diameter = 2.5 inches
$8 = (3.14)(d)$	$r = \dfrac{1}{2}d$
$2.5 = d$	$r = \left(\dfrac{1}{2}\right)(2.5)$
	$r = 1.25$ inches

10. **(B)** Add the first two numbers together, and then subtract the third.

$17.3 + 5.75 = 23.05 - 16.02 = 7.03$

11. **(A)**

Monday:	7 A.M. – 11:20 A.M. = 4.33 hours
	12:20 P.M. – 3 P.M. = 2.67 hours
Tuesday:	3 P.M. – 8 P.M. = 5 hours
	8:30 P.M. – 11 P.M. = 2.5 hours
Wednesday:	7 A.M. – 3 P.M. = 8 hours
	3 P.M. – 11 P.M. = 8 hours

$(4.33 + 2.67 + 8) \times \$5.58 = \$83.70$

$(5 + 2.5 + 8) \times \$6.00 = \$93.00$

$\$83.70 + \$93.00 = \$176.70$

12. **(A)** $50 \times 20 = 1{,}000$ mg

13. **(B)** 1 marble : 37 = x marbles : 300

$37x = 300$

$x = 8.1 = 8$ marbles

14. **(B)** Interest = Principle × Rate × Time

Interest = $500

Rate = 8%

Time = 5 years

$P = x$

$I = PRT$

$500 = (P)(0.08)(5)$

$\$1{,}250 = P$

15. **(B)**

$\dfrac{1}{3}(\$3{,}500) = \$1{,}167$

$\dfrac{1}{5}(\$3{,}500) = \$700$

$\dfrac{1}{4}(\$3{,}500) = \$875$

$\$3{,}500 - \$1{,}167 - \$700 - \$875 = \$758$

16. **(D)** Interest = Principle × Rate × Time

$I = PRT$

$I = (750)(0.15)(2.17)$

$I = \$244.125 = \$244.13$

17. **(B)**

$\dfrac{1}{6} = 0.167 = 17\%$

17% of 89 students = 15.13 = 15 students

15% of 89 students = 13.35 = 13 students

$15 - 13 = 2$

18. **(B)** Graduate student #1 : 6 data sets/hour × 8 hours = 48 data sets

Graduate student #2 : 4.5 data sets/hour

Graduate student #1 + Graduate student #2 = 6 + 4.5 = 10.5 data sets/hour

854 data sets − 48 data sets = 806 data sets ÷ 10.5 data sets/hour = 77 hours

77 hours + 8 hours = 85 total hours

19. **(A)** Child 1 = 5 years old

Child 2 = 5 + 5 = 10 years old

Child 3 = 30 − 15 = 15 years old

Child 4 = 10 × 2 = 20 years old

Child 5 = 30 years old

20. **(A)** Jaw Lockers = \$2.50/lb

Sour Cherries = \$3.00/.5 lb = \$6.00/lb

Orange Blitzes = \$1.50/lb

Goofy Gum = \$.75/lb

$\dfrac{(\$2.50 + \$6.00 + \$1.50 + \$.75) =}{4} \dfrac{\$10.75}{4} = \$2.69$

21. **(A)** 34% of \$3,514 = (0.34)(3,514) = \$1,194.76

\$3,514 − \$1,194.76 − \$150 = \$2,169.24

22. **(D)** Subtract the number of passing graduates from the total number of graduates. The answer is the number of graduates that did not pass the licensure examination.

$950 - 843 = 107$

23. **(A)** $8 - 2 + (-10) = 6 - 10 = -4$

24. **(A)**

$\angle D = 4x$

$\angle E = 2.5x$

$\angle F = x$

$4x + 2.5x + x = 180$

$7.5x = 180$

$x = 24°$

$4x = 96°$

$2.5x = 60°$

25. **(C)** $298.60 - $157.65 = $140.95 increase

$$\frac{140.95}{157.65} = 0.894 = 89.4\%$$

26. **(D)** x = ounces of dried fruit to be added to mixture

$5 + x$ = total ounces of dried fruit in mixture

$8 + 6 + 4 + 5 + x$ = total weight of trail mix

Total ounces of dried fruit = 25% of total weight of trail mix

$5 + x = 0.25(8 + 6 + 4 + 5 + x)$

$5 + x = 0.25(23 + x)$

$20 + 4x = 1(23 + x)$

$3x = 3$

$x = 1$

27. **(C)** $\dfrac{\text{Desired} \times \text{Volume}}{\text{Available}} = \text{mL per dose}$

$$\frac{45\,\text{meq} \times 20\,\text{mL}}{30\,\text{meq}} = 30\,\text{mL} = 30\,\text{mL/dose}$$

28. **(A)** Increase = 350 mg

x = percentage of increase

What percent of 300 mg is 350 mg?

$300x = 350$

$x = 1.1666 = 1.17 = 117\%$ increase

29. **(C)** $(0.33 \times 596) + (0.20 \times 596) + (0.43 \times 596) = 197 + 119 + 256 = 572$ blankets distributed

$596 - 572 = 24$ blankets left in central supply

$$\frac{24}{596} = 4\% = 0.04 = \frac{1}{25}$$

30. **(C)** Original price = $146.25

Selling price = $1,162.50

$1,162.50 - $146.25 = $1,016.25

31. **(C)** Draw a triangle representative of the Pythagorean theorem.

Label the triangle: Horizontal line = a^2; Vertical line = b^2; Diagonal line = c^2

$a = 12$ feet (distance of guide wire from antenna)

b = unknown (height of antenna)

$c = \dfrac{80}{4} = 20$ feet (length of wire needed for one support)

$b^2 = c^2 - a^2$

$b^2 = 20^2 - 12^2$

$b^2 = 400 - 144$

$b^2 = 256$

$b = \sqrt{256} = 16$ feet

32. **(A)** $(75 \times \$.50) + (250 \times \$.25) + (150 \times \$.60) + (150 \times \$.15)$

$= \$37.50 + \$62.50 + \$90.00 + \$22.50$

$= \$212.50$

33. **(A)** $75.84 + 6.02 + 100.877 + 41.0 - 87.471 = 136.266 = 136$
Do not round numbers until the answer.

34. **(C)** $10 + 8 \times 15 + 10 \div 2 =$
Solve the problem using the order of operations. First, focus on multiplication and division.
$10 + 120 + 5 =$
Then, add the remaining numbers.
$10 + 120 + 5 = 135$

35. **(B)** 1 tablet: 125 mg = x tablets : 1,000 mg
$$125\,x = 1,000$$
$$x = 8 \text{ tablets}$$

36. **(A)** $\dfrac{1}{6} = 0.1\overline{6} = 0.167$

37. **(B)** 60 mg = 1 gr = 600 mg = x gr
$60x = 600$
$x = 10$ gr = 1 tablet

38. **(A)** $15x + 6x - 3x + 18 = 36x$
$$18x + 18 = 36x$$
$$18 = 18x$$
$$1 = x$$

39. **(B)**
$$\frac{78+84+56+96+78+85+85+95+0+73}{10} =$$
$$\frac{730}{10} = 73$$

40. **(A)** $18 + 7(2 \times 6) - (6 + 3) =$

Solve the problem using the order of operations. First, focus on any operation inside the parentheses.

$18 + 7(12) - (9) =$

Then multiply.

$18 + 84 - 9 =$

Finally, add and subtract.

$18 + 84 - 9 = 102 - 9 = 93$

41. **(C)** Set up an equation.
$5x + 14 = 54$
Solve for x.
$5x + 14 = 54$
$5x = 40$
$x = 8$

42. **(C)** Selling price – Original cost – Refurbishing cost = Profit
$\$65,000 - \$35,000 - \$20,000 = \$10,000$

43. **(A)** x = hours

  1 hour : 86 miles = x hours : 400 miles

  $$86x = 400$$

  $$x = 4.7 \text{ hours} = 4 \text{ hours } 42 \text{ minutes}$$

44. **(A)** Let percent = x. Set up an equation.

  $$(x)(15) = 8$$

  Solve for x.

  $$15x = 8$$

  $$x = 0.53 = 53\%$$

45. **(B)** Out of the choices provided, 3 is the lowest common denominator. 3 goes into 15 five times. 3 goes into 48 sixteen times. 3 goes into 63 twenty-one times.

46. **(A)** $(10 \times \$15) + (5 \times \$7.50) + (18 \times \$4) + (10 \times \$1.50) + (3 \times \$8.40)$
  $= \$150 + \$37.50 + \$72 + \$15 + \$25.20$
  $= \$299.70$

47. **(C)**
  Magazine A = $\$458 - \$13.74 = \$444.26$
  Magazine B = $\$450 - \$9.00 = \$441$
  Magazine C = $\$480 - \$24.00 = \$456$
  Magazine D = $\$440$

48. **(B)** 5(+7), 12(−3), 9(+7), 16(−3), 13(+7), 20(−3), 17

49. **(D)** All potential answers are in inches. Change the measurements in the stem of the question to inches.
  7 feet, 4 inches = $7 \times 12 = 84 + 4 = 88$ inches
  4 feet, 10 inches = $4 \times 12 = 48 + 10 = 58$ inches
  $88 + 58 = 146$ inches

50. **(C)** x = total number of pencils in box

  $\dfrac{1}{4}x$ = number of black pencils in box

  $\dfrac{3}{8}x$ = number of red pencils in box

  16 = number of yellow pencils in box
  $$0.25x + 0.375x + 16 = x$$
  $$0.625x + 16 = x$$
  $$16 = 0.375x$$
  $$42.\overline{6} = x = 43 \text{ pencils}$$

ANSWER SHEET
Verbal Ability Test

1. Ⓐ Ⓑ Ⓒ Ⓓ
2. Ⓐ Ⓑ Ⓒ Ⓓ
3. Ⓐ Ⓑ Ⓒ Ⓓ
4. Ⓐ Ⓑ Ⓒ Ⓓ
5. Ⓐ Ⓑ Ⓒ Ⓓ
6. Ⓐ Ⓑ Ⓒ Ⓓ
7. Ⓐ Ⓑ Ⓒ Ⓓ
8. Ⓐ Ⓑ Ⓒ Ⓓ
9. Ⓐ Ⓑ Ⓒ Ⓓ
10. Ⓐ Ⓑ Ⓒ Ⓓ
11. Ⓐ Ⓑ Ⓒ Ⓓ
12. Ⓐ Ⓑ Ⓒ Ⓓ
13. Ⓐ Ⓑ Ⓒ Ⓓ
14. Ⓐ Ⓑ Ⓒ Ⓓ
15. Ⓐ Ⓑ Ⓒ Ⓓ
16. Ⓐ Ⓑ Ⓒ Ⓓ
17. Ⓐ Ⓑ Ⓒ Ⓓ

18. Ⓐ Ⓑ Ⓒ Ⓓ
19. Ⓐ Ⓑ Ⓒ Ⓓ
20. Ⓐ Ⓑ Ⓒ Ⓓ
21. Ⓐ Ⓑ Ⓒ Ⓓ
22. Ⓐ Ⓑ Ⓒ Ⓓ
23. Ⓐ Ⓑ Ⓒ Ⓓ
24. Ⓐ Ⓑ Ⓒ Ⓓ
25. Ⓐ Ⓑ Ⓒ Ⓓ
26. Ⓐ Ⓑ Ⓒ Ⓓ
27. Ⓐ Ⓑ Ⓒ Ⓓ
28. Ⓐ Ⓑ Ⓒ Ⓓ
29. Ⓐ Ⓑ Ⓒ Ⓓ
30. Ⓐ Ⓑ Ⓒ Ⓓ
31. Ⓐ Ⓑ Ⓒ Ⓓ
32. Ⓐ Ⓑ Ⓒ Ⓓ
33. Ⓐ Ⓑ Ⓒ Ⓓ
34. Ⓐ Ⓑ Ⓒ Ⓓ

35. Ⓐ Ⓑ Ⓒ Ⓓ
36. Ⓐ Ⓑ Ⓒ Ⓓ
37. Ⓐ Ⓑ Ⓒ Ⓓ
38. Ⓐ Ⓑ Ⓒ Ⓓ
39. Ⓐ Ⓑ Ⓒ Ⓓ
40. Ⓐ Ⓑ Ⓒ Ⓓ
41. Ⓐ Ⓑ Ⓒ Ⓓ
42. Ⓐ Ⓑ Ⓒ Ⓓ
43. Ⓐ Ⓑ Ⓒ Ⓓ
44. Ⓐ Ⓑ Ⓒ Ⓓ
45. Ⓐ Ⓑ Ⓒ Ⓓ
46. Ⓐ Ⓑ Ⓒ Ⓓ
47. Ⓐ Ⓑ Ⓒ Ⓓ
48. Ⓐ Ⓑ Ⓒ Ⓓ
49. Ⓐ Ⓑ Ⓒ Ⓓ
50. Ⓐ Ⓑ Ⓒ Ⓓ

50 TEST ITEMS: TIME: 50 MINUTES

> **Directions:** For each of the paired words, select the answer (A, B, C, or D) that best matches the paired words. Record your answers on the Verbal Ability Answer Sheet on page 351.

1. DENTIST : TEETH :: DERMATOLOGIST :
   - (A) DISEASE
   - (B) BONES
   - (C) SKIN
   - (D) MUSCLES

2. BLANKET : MATTRESS ::
   - (A) GRASS : GROUND
   - (B) TIRE : PAVEMENT
   - (C) LEAF : TREE
   - (D) SHOE : SOCK

3. TROUT : CHORDATA :: FLATWORM :
   - (A) PLATYHELMINTH
   - (B) SQUAMATA
   - (C) ARTOIDACTYLA
   - (D) CARNIVORA

4. GOOD : SWEET ::
   - (A) BOY : GIRL
   - (B) FOOD : VEGETABLE
   - (C) NIGHT : DAY
   - (D) BAD : SOUR

5. GAINES: *BLUE BOY* ::
   - (A) LOSSES : *BASEBALL*
   - (B) INCISIVE : *AORTA*
   - (C) MICHELANGELO : *DAVID*
   - (D) CAMUS : *MONK*

6. ATROPHY : DEGENERATE :: CHICANERY :
   - (A) MEXICO
   - (B) FLIGHT
   - (C) TRICKERY
   - (D) SICKLY

7. PROPERTY : VANDAL ::
   - (A) BUILDING : POLICE
   - (B) RELIGIOUS IMAGES : ICONOCLAST
   - (C) UNDULATE : FLUCTUATE
   - (D) WRATH : ANGRY

8. CIVIL WAR : BATTLE OF SABINE PASS ::
   - (A) FRENCH REVOLUTION : BATTLE OF PARIS
   - (B) WORLD WAR I : BATTLE OF THE BULGE
   - (C) KOREAN WAR : AKITA
   - (D) WORLD WAR II : SIEGE OF DUNKIRK

9. DIMINUENDO : CRESCENDO :: ANDANTE :
   - (A) SONATA
   - (B) ALTO
   - (C) VERDI
   - (D) PRESTO

10. BEAR : FOX ::
    - (A) BOVINE : CERVINE
    - (B) PHYLUM : KINGDOM
    - (C) EOCENE : PLIOCENE
    - (D) URSINE : VULPINE

11. JOHN WAYNE : *THE COWBOYS* :: HARRISON FORD :
    - (A) *IN HARM'S WAY*
    - (B) *THE RAINMAKER*
    - (C) *INDIANA JONES*
    - (D) *THE KING AND I*

12. ABROGATE : NULLIFY ::
    - (A) DELAY : DETAIN
    - (B) MAR : HEAL
    - (C) HARDEN : INDULGE
    - (D) APPLY : NEGLECT

13. ZANY : ZEST :: ZIP :
    (A) JOIN
    (B) FLEXIBLE
    (C) ZOOM
    (D) FAST

14. NEW MEXICO : "LAND OF ENCHANTMENT" ::
    (A) TEXAS : "OIL"
    (B) ILLINOIS : "LAND OF LINCOLN"
    (C) WYOMING : "COWBOYS"
    (D) ARIZONA : "LAND OF THE GREAT CANYON"

15. BOY : GIRL ::
    (A) TALL : SHORT
    (B) STRONG : WEAK
    (C) BLUE : PINK
    (D) FOOTBALL : GOLF

16. UGLY : APPALLING :: TURN OFF :
    (A) UMBRAGE
    (B) TALENTED
    (C) DISGUST
    (D) READY

17. DIFFUSE : COMPACT ::
    (A) ASSUME : CONCLUDE
    (B) AGREE : CONCUR
    (C) COSTLY : DEAR
    (D) FEEL : DOUBT

18. 150 : 450 ::
    (A) 100 : 300
    (B) 50 : 75
    (C) 200 : 400
    (D) 375 : 475

19. FIREMAN : AX :: POLICE OFFICER :
    (A) BADGE
    (B) TASER
    (C) SIREN
    (D) RADIO

20. SISTINE CHAPEL : ROME :: NOTRE DAME :
    (A) FLORENCE
    (B) PARIS
    (C) PITTSBURGH
    (D) BERLIN

21. TURNCOAT : TRAITOR :: WAX :
    (A) WANE
    (B) SHRINK
    (C) INCREASE
    (D) ABATE

22. BOTANIST : PLANTS :: HERPETOLOGIST :
    (A) HERBS
    (B) AMPHIBIANS
    (C) FELINES
    (D) FOWL

23. IMPUDENT : INCEPTION ::
    (A) SAUCY : OUTSET
    (B) IMMODERATE : DEDUCE
    (C) NATURAL : NATIVE
    (D) REFRACTORY : COMPULSION

24. PURBLIND : DIMSIGHTED :: RESCIND :
    (A) REVOKE
    (B) LUSTFUL
    (C) DECENT
    (D) CENSURE

25. ALERT : LETHARGIC ::
    (A) LACONIC : VERBOSE
    (B) MALEFACTOR : CRIMINAL
    (C) LIMPID : LIPID
    (D) SCOURGE : WHIP

26. SCINTILLA : REATA ::
    (A) WISE : SAGE
    (B) TRACE : LARIAT
    (C) REPROVE : REPRIMAND
    (D) MATURE : VENILE

27. PULMONARY : LUNGS ::
    (A) RENAL : HEART
    (B) PALEO : LIFE
    (C) HEPATIC : LIVER
    (D) MUSCULAR : TISSUES

28. ABEYANCE : SUSTENANCE :: ASSIMILATE :

    (A) ABSORB
    (B) INTEGRATE
    (C) GENUINE
    (D) DISGORGE

29. CRYPTIC : HIDDEN ::

    (A) COULEE : GULCH
    (B) FRUSTRATE : SHORTCOME
    (C) MENTAL : VERIFY
    (D) GUILTY : CHURLISH

30. INCUBUS : NIGHTMARE :: BURDEN :

    (A) INDOLENT
    (B) PACK
    (C) CURSE
    (D) PLACID

31. DECEPTIVE : TRUE :: RICH :

    (A) FALSEHOOD
    (B) REFUTE
    (C) BLESSING
    (D) INDIGENT

32. TRIESTE : HUNGARY ::

    (A) BREST : FRANCE
    (B) VARNA : TURKEY
    (C) VENICE : DENMARK
    (D) REGA : AUSTRIA

33. NOVEMBER 22, 1963 : APRIL 5, 1865 ::

    (A) WASHINGTON : NIXON
    (B) TRUMAN : ROOSEVELT
    (C) JACKSON : JEFFERSON
    (D) KENNEDY : LINCOLN

34. $\frac{1}{2}$: 0.5 :: $\frac{7}{8}$:

    (A) 0.9
    (B) 0.875
    (C) 0.4375
    (D) 1.14

35. SAW : VERB :: BOY :

    (A) PERSONAL PRONOUN
    (B) NOUN
    (C) ADJECTIVE
    (D) CONJUNCTION

36. SUN : MERCURY ::

    (A) SUN : SATURN
    (B) SUN : EARTH
    (C) SUN : NEPTUNE
    (D) SUN : VENUS

37. INDEPENDENCE : SANTA FE TRAIL ::
    FT. BRIDGER :

    (A) OREGON TRAIL
    (B) CIMARRON CUTOFF
    (C) OLD SPANISH TRAIL
    (D) CUMBERLAND ROAD

38. FLOCK : SHEEP :: SHOAL :

    (A) GEESE
    (B) FISH
    (C) MICE
    (D) DUCKS

39. CHEYENNE : WYOMING :: DENVER :

    (A) UTAH
    (B) TEXAS
    (C) NEBRASKA
    (D) COLORADO

40. THERMOMETER : TEMPERATURE ::
    SPHYGMOMANOMETER :

    (A) HEART RATE
    (B) BLOOD PRESSURE
    (C) PULSE
    (D) RESPIRATIONS

41. X : TEN :: C :

    (A) ONE HUNDRED
    (B) TEN
    (C) ONE THOUSAND
    (D) ONE

42. DUMAS : *THE THREE MUSKETEERS* ::
    DICKENS :

    (A) *OLIVER TWIST*
    (B) *SISTER CARRIE*
    (C) *AS I LAY DYING*
    (D) *MADAME BOVARY*

43. CRAZY HORSE : SIOUX :: QUANAH PARKER :

   (A) MOHAWK

   (B) COMANCHE

   (C) APACHE

   (D) CROW

44. DECEMBER 25 : APRIL 1 ::

   (A) ARBOR DAY : MEMORIAL DAY

   (B) COLUMBUS DAY : LABOR DAY

   (C) CHRISTMAS DAY : APRIL FOOL'S DAY

   (D) PRESIDENT'S DAY : VALENTINE'S DAY

45. STERILE : FERTILE :: UNFRUITFUL :

   (A) STAID

   (B) TERSE

   (C) SALUBRIOUS

   (D) FECUND

46. DEONTOLOGY : ETHICS :: HISTOLOGY :

   (A) FOSSILS

   (B) LIVING TISSUES

   (C) REVERED PERSONS

   (D) ANIMALS

47. PEARY : AMERICAN :: AMUNDSON :

   (A) SPANISH

   (B) ENGLISH

   (C) NORWEGIAN

   (D) FRENCH

48. BISMARCK : GERMANY ::

   (A) WHITNEY : AMERICA

   (B) GARIBALDI : ENGLAND

   (C) PIZARRO : ITALY

   (D) O'HIGGINS : CHILE

49. CUBISM : FRANCE ::

   (A) FUTURISM : ITALY

   (B) ENGRAVING : AMERICA

   (C) SURREALISM : CHINA

   (D) FAUVISM : BRAZIL

50. WILDER : *OUR TOWN* :: WILLIAMS :

   (A) *LEAVES OF GRASS*

   (B) *CAT ON A HOT TIN ROOF*

   (C) *THE COLOR PURPLE*

   (D) *THE HOBBIT*

If there is still time remaining, you may review your answers.

ANSWER KEY
Verbal Ability Test

1. **C**	11. **C**	21. **C**	31. **D**	41. **A**
2. **A**	12. **A**	22. **B**	32. **A**	42. **A**
3. **A**	13. **C**	23. **A**	33. **D**	43. **B**
4. **D**	14. **B**	24. **A**	34. **B**	44. **C**
5. **C**	15. **C**	25. **A**	35. **B**	45. **D**
6. **C**	16. **C**	26. **B**	36. **D**	46. **B**
7. **B**	17. **D**	27. **C**	37. **A**	47. **C**
8. **D**	18. **A**	28. **D**	38. **B**	48. **D**
9. **D**	19. **B**	29. **A**	39. **D**	49. **A**
10. **D**	20. **B**	30. **B**	40. **B**	50. **B**

VERBAL ABILITY TEST ANSWERS EXPLAINED

1. **(C)** A dentist specializes in the care of teeth. A dermatologist specializes in the care of skin.

2. **(A)** A blanket covers a bed. Grass covers the ground.

3. **(A)** Trout belong to the phylum Chordata. Flatworms belong to the phylum Platyhelminth.

4. **(D)** Good and bad are antonyms, as are sweet and sour.

5. **(C)** Gaines painted the *Blue Boy*. Michelangelo sculpted *David*.

6. **(C)** Atrophy and degenerate are synonyms, as are chicanery and trickery.

7. **(B)** A vandal destroys property. An iconoclast destroys religious images.

8. **(D)** The Battle of Sabine Pass was fought in Texas during the Civil War. The Siege of Dunkirk was fought in France during World War II.

9. **(D)** Diminuendo and crescendo are antonyms, as are andante and presto. All are musical terms.

10. **(D)** The adjective form of bear is ursine. The adjective form of fox is vulpine.

11. **(C)** The actor, John Wayne, starred in *The Cowboys*. The actor, Harrison Ford, starred in *Indiana Jones*.

12. **(A)** Abrogate and nullify are synonyms, as are delay and detain.

13. **(C)** All of the words begin with the letter *Z*.

14. **(B)** "Land of Enchantment" is inscribed on New Mexico license plates. "Land of Lincoln" is inscribed on Illinois license plates.

15. **(C)** Blue is typically considered a boy's color, whereas pink is typically considered a girl's color.

16. **(C)** Ugly and appalling are synonyms, as are turn off and disgust.

17. **(D)** Diffuse and compact are antonyms, as are feel and doubt.

18. **(A)** Four hundred fifty is three times greater than one hundred fifty. Three hundred is three times greater than one hundred.

19. **(B)** An ax is a hand tool for a fireman. A taser is a hand tool for a police officer.

20. **(B)** The Sistine Chapel is located in Rome. Notre Dame is located in Paris.

21. **(C)** Turncoat and traitor are synonyms, as are wax and increase.

22. **(B)** A botanist works with plants. A herpetologist works with amphibians.

23. **(A)** Impudent and saucy are synonyms, as are inception and outset.

24. **(A)** Purblind and dimsighted are synonyms, as are rescind and revoke.

25. **(A)** Alert and lethargic are antonyms, as are laconic and verbose.

26. **(B)** Scintilla and trace are synonyms, as are reata and lariat.

27. **(C)** The term pulmonary refers to the lungs. The term hepatic refers to the liver.

28. **(D)** Abeyance and sustenance are antonyms, as are assimilate and disgorge.

29. **(A)** Cryptic and hidden are synonyms, as are coulee and gulch.

30. **(B)** Incubus and nightmare are synonyms, as are burden and pack.

31. **(D)** Deceptive and true are antonyms, as are rich and indigent.

32. **(A)** The city of Trieste is in Hungary. The city of Brest is in France.

33. **(D)** President Kennedy was assassinated on November 22, 1963. President Lincoln was assassinated on April 5, 1865.

34. **(B)** One half is written both as a fraction and as a decimal. Seven-eighths is also written as a fraction and as a decimal.

35. **(B)** The word *saw* is a verb. The word *boy* is a noun.

36. **(D)** Mercury is the planet closest to the sun. Venus is the only other planet closer to the sun than Earth.

37. **(A)** The Santa Fe Trail began in Independence, Missouri. The Oregon Trail began at Ft. Bridger.

38. **(B)** A group of sheep is called a flock of sheep. A group of fish is called a shoal of fish.

39. **(D)** Cheyenne is the capital of the state of Wyoming. Denver is the capital of the state of Colorado.

40. **(B)** A thermometer is used to determine temperature. A sphygmomanometer is used to determine blood pressure.

41. **(A)** The number ten in Roman numerals is X. One hundred in Roman numerals is C.

42. **(A)** Dumas wrote the literary piece *The Three Musketeers*. Dickens wrote *Oliver Twist*.

43. **(B)** Crazy Horse was a Sioux chief. Quanah Parker was a Comanche chief.

44. **(C)** Christmas day is on December 25. April Fool's day is on April 1.

45. **(D)** Sterile and fertile are antonyms, as are unfruitful and fecund. Sterile and unfruitful are synonyms, as are fertile and fecund.

46. **(B)** Deontology is the study of ethics. Histology is the study of living tissues.

47. **(C)** Peary was an American. He was the first to reach the North Pole. Amundsen was a Norwegian. He was the first to reach the South Pole.

48. **(D)** Bismarck is considered the unifier of Germany. O'Higgins is considered the unifier of Chile.

49. **(A)** The art style, cubism, developed in France. The art style, futurism, developed in Italy.

50. **(B)** Thornton Wilder wrote *Our Town*. Tennessee Williams wrote *Cat on a Hot Tin Roof*.

ANSWER SHEET
Reading Comprehension Test

1. Ⓐ Ⓑ Ⓒ Ⓓ
2. Ⓐ Ⓑ Ⓒ Ⓓ
3. Ⓐ Ⓑ Ⓒ Ⓓ
4. Ⓐ Ⓑ Ⓒ Ⓓ

5. Ⓐ Ⓑ Ⓒ Ⓓ
6. Ⓐ Ⓑ Ⓒ Ⓓ
7. Ⓐ Ⓑ Ⓒ Ⓓ
8. Ⓐ Ⓑ Ⓒ Ⓓ

9. Ⓐ Ⓑ Ⓒ Ⓓ
10. Ⓐ Ⓑ Ⓒ Ⓓ

10 TEST ITEMS: TIME: 15 MINUTES

Read the following selection. Then, select the choice (A, B, C, or D) that best answers the question. Record your answers on the Reading Comprehension Answer Sheet on page 361.

Selection: Coming of Age in Samoa by Margaret Mead, 1928.

By the time a child is six or seven a girl has all the essential avoidances well enough by heart to be trusted with the care of a younger
Line child. She also develops a number of simple
(5) techniques. She learns to weave firm square balls, to make pinwheels of palm leaves…, to climb a coconut tree by walking with flexible little feet, to break open a coconut…, to play a number of group games and sing the songs
(10) which go with them, to tidy the house… and to exercise tact in begging slight favours from relatives.

But in the case of the little girls all of these tasks are merely supplementary to the main
(15) business of baby tending. Very small boys also take care of the younger children, but at eight or nine years of age they are usually relieved of the duty. Whatever rough edges have not been smoothed off by this
(20) responsibility for younger children are worn off by their contact with older boys. For little boys are admitted to interesting and important activities only as long as their behavior is circumspect and helpful. Where
(25) small girls are abruptly pushed aside, small boys will be patiently tolerated and they become adept at making themselves useful. The four or five little boys who all wish to assist at the important business of helping a
(30) grown youth lasso reef eels, organize themselves into a highly working team; one boy holds the bait, another holds an extra lasso, others poke eagerly about in holes in

the reef looking for prey, while still another
(35) tucks the captured eels into his *lavalava*. The small girls, burdened with heavy babies or the care of little staggerers who are too small to adventure on the reef, discouraged by the hostility of the small boys and the scorn of
(40) the older ones, have little opportunity for learning the more adventurous forms of work and play. So while the little boys first undergo the chastening effects of baby-tending and then have many opportunities to learn
(45) effective cooperation under the supervision of older boys, the girls' education is less comprehensive. They have a high standard of individual responsibility, but the community provides them with no lessons in cooperation
(50) with one another. This is particularly apparent in the activities of young people; the boys organize quickly; the girls waste hours in bickering, innocent of any technique for quick and efficient
(55) cooperation.

1. In the above selection by Margaret Mead, she presents

   (A) facts and interpretations of her observations.
   (B) facts based on her observations.
   (C) growing up in Samoa almost 90 years ago.
   (D) misconceptions of Samoan parenting.

2. Based on lines 15–21, little boys are castigated for caring for younger children because

   (A) caring for children requires little understanding of children.
   (B) once boys reach a certain age, childcare is considered a female role.
   (C) little boys do not have the developmental skills to interact with older children.
   (D) Not enough information is given to determine an answer.

3. What is the most important point in the first paragraph (lines 1–12)?

   (A) Only trusted girls, 7 or 8 years old, are allowed to care for smaller children.
   (B) Small girls are taught skills for homemaking as adults.
   (C) Learning life skills, such as opening a coconut, is extremely important for small girls.
   (D) The girls' predominant task is caring for children.

4. What is the most precise definition of *supplementary* in line 14?

   (A) primary
   (B) fundamental
   (C) extra
   (D) critical

5. What is meant when the author says that the girls' education is "less comprehensive" in lines 46–47?

   (A) The girls' education is not all encompassing like the boys' education is.
   (B) The girls do not want as much education as the boys do.
   (C) The girls have no levels of responsibility whatsoever.
   (D) It takes the girls until they are 16 or 17 to complete their education, whereas the boys continue their education well into their 20s.

6. Lines 21–24 and 28–35 suggest that the interactions between the smaller boys and the older boys are meant to be

   (A) activities filled with excitement and adventure.
   (B) a bonding experience for smaller boys.
   (C) a fairly rigid learning experience.
   (D) the beginning of the journey to manhood.

7. Line 25 states that "girls are abruptly pushed aside." What does this statement suggest?

   (A) Females, especially when pregnant, are more vulnerable to injuries sustained by males.
   (B) Females are not as smart as males and would take too long to teach.
   (C) Females are not strong enough to learn or perform male roles.
   (D) There may be a taboo against females learning traditional male roles.

8. A <u>synonym</u> for *organize* in line 30 is

   (A) club.
   (B) disarrange.
   (C) establish.
   (D) systemize.

9. One reason that the smaller boys interact with the older boys is to introduce and reinforce the concept of

   (A) group play.
   (B) male domination in the society.
   (C) socialization of small girls and boys with older girls and boys.
   (D) teamwork.

10. *Bickering* in line 53 is an <u>antonym</u> for

   (A) altercating.
   (B) making peace.
   (C) duking it out.
   (D) chatting.

If there is still time remaining, you may review your answers.

ANSWER KEY
Reading Comprehension Test

1. **B**	3. **D**	5. **A**	7. **D**	9. **D**
2. **B**	4. **C**	6. **C**	8. **C**	10. **B**

READING COMPREHENSION TEST ANSWERS EXPLAINED

1. **(B)** Margaret Mead was an American cultural anthropologist. When studying the cultures of other groups, she wrote about what she observed. She did not attempt to explain or interpret what she observed. The selection does not address growing up in Samoa or Samoan parenting.

2. **(B)** The only logical answer is that taking care of children is a traditional role for females. The remaining answers are not addressed in the selection, and more than enough information is presented to determine an answer.

3. **(D)** Lines 1–12 discuss the role of a young girl, 6 or 7 years of age. She is old enough and knows enough to care for younger children and to perform simple tasks. The first paragraph does not address trust as a determining issue, homemaking skills, or the importance of life skills.

4. **(C)** In this sentence, *supplementary* means extra. The skills that girls develop are all considered just an added bonus to their primary role in this community, which is baby tending.

5. **(A)** By saying that the girls' education is "less comprehensive," the author means that the girls do not receive the same thorough level of education that the boys do. There is no evidence in the selection that suggests that girls do not want education. Lines 47 and 48 state specifically that the girls do still have a "high standard of individual responsibility" despite their lack of a full education. Although the boys continue to receive education for a longer period of time than the girls do, these ages are never mentioned in this selection.

6. **(C)** At first glance, all of the choices seem plausible. However, upon critical review of the information in the passage, only choice C stands out. The smaller boys are chastised by the older boys, and the smaller boys are only allowed in activities if their behavior is deemed appropriate.

7. **(D)** Based on information presented in the selection, young girls are relegated to the performance of simple tasks and child tending. While young boys eventually leave these tasks behind, their role changes to a "males only" role. Since girls are not included, there is a strong possibility that females learn that male roles are taboo and off limits to them. The remaining responses are unjustified assumptions.

8. **(C)** In this context, *organize* means to establish. The boys are establishing themselves as a "highly working team." They may be considered a club, but *organize* does not mean *club*. *Disarrange* is not a synonym of *organize*. While *systemize* is a synonym of *organize*, that is not the meaning of *organize* in this sentence.

9. **(D)** The selection provides examples of young boys working together and having the opportunity to learn cooperation when working with older youths. This teaches teamwork. The presented information does not mention interacting with older boys as play. Male dominance is not mentioned in this context, and while the male interaction is a form of socialization, nothing is mentioned regarding small girls socializing with older girls.

10. **(B)** In this sentence, *bickering* means fighting. Remember to pay attention to what the question is asking for. If you chose synonyms of *bickering*, such as *altercating* and *duking it out*, you did not read the question carefully. The antonym of *bickering* is *making peace*.

ANSWER SHEET
Science Test

1. Ⓐ Ⓑ Ⓒ Ⓓ
2. Ⓐ Ⓑ Ⓒ Ⓓ
3. Ⓐ Ⓑ Ⓒ Ⓓ
4. Ⓐ Ⓑ Ⓒ Ⓓ
5. Ⓐ Ⓑ Ⓒ Ⓓ
6. Ⓐ Ⓑ Ⓒ Ⓓ
7. Ⓐ Ⓑ Ⓒ Ⓓ
8. Ⓐ Ⓑ Ⓒ Ⓓ
9. Ⓐ Ⓑ Ⓒ Ⓓ
10. Ⓐ Ⓑ Ⓒ Ⓓ
11. Ⓐ Ⓑ Ⓒ Ⓓ
12. Ⓐ Ⓑ Ⓒ Ⓓ
13. Ⓐ Ⓑ Ⓒ Ⓓ
14. Ⓐ Ⓑ Ⓒ Ⓓ
15. Ⓐ Ⓑ Ⓒ Ⓓ
16. Ⓐ Ⓑ Ⓒ Ⓓ
17. Ⓐ Ⓑ Ⓒ Ⓓ
18. Ⓐ Ⓑ Ⓒ Ⓓ

19. Ⓐ Ⓑ Ⓒ Ⓓ
20. Ⓐ Ⓑ Ⓒ Ⓓ
21. Ⓐ Ⓑ Ⓒ Ⓓ
22. Ⓐ Ⓑ Ⓒ Ⓓ
23. Ⓐ Ⓑ Ⓒ Ⓓ
24. Ⓐ Ⓑ Ⓒ Ⓓ
25. Ⓐ Ⓑ Ⓒ Ⓓ
26. Ⓐ Ⓑ Ⓒ Ⓓ
27. Ⓐ Ⓑ Ⓒ Ⓓ
28. Ⓐ Ⓑ Ⓒ Ⓓ
29. Ⓐ Ⓑ Ⓒ Ⓓ
30. Ⓐ Ⓑ Ⓒ Ⓓ
31. Ⓐ Ⓑ Ⓒ Ⓓ
32. Ⓐ Ⓑ Ⓒ Ⓓ
33. Ⓐ Ⓑ Ⓒ Ⓓ
34. Ⓐ Ⓑ Ⓒ Ⓓ
35. Ⓐ Ⓑ Ⓒ Ⓓ
36. Ⓐ Ⓑ Ⓒ Ⓓ

37. Ⓐ Ⓑ Ⓒ Ⓓ
38. Ⓐ Ⓑ Ⓒ Ⓓ
39. Ⓐ Ⓑ Ⓒ Ⓓ
40. Ⓐ Ⓑ Ⓒ Ⓓ
41. Ⓐ Ⓑ Ⓒ Ⓓ
42. Ⓐ Ⓑ Ⓒ Ⓓ
43. Ⓐ Ⓑ Ⓒ Ⓓ
44. Ⓐ Ⓑ Ⓒ Ⓓ
45. Ⓐ Ⓑ Ⓒ Ⓓ
46. Ⓐ Ⓑ Ⓒ Ⓓ
47. Ⓐ Ⓑ Ⓒ Ⓓ
48. Ⓐ Ⓑ Ⓒ Ⓓ
49. Ⓐ Ⓑ Ⓒ Ⓓ
50. Ⓐ Ⓑ Ⓒ Ⓓ
51. Ⓐ Ⓑ Ⓒ Ⓓ
52. Ⓐ Ⓑ Ⓒ Ⓓ
53. Ⓐ Ⓑ Ⓒ Ⓓ

53 TEST ITEMS: TIME: 53 MINUTES

Select the choice (A, B, C, or D) that best answers each question. Record your answers on the Science Test Answer Sheet on page 367.

1. The kidneys are located
   (A) in the chest between the lungs, behind the sternum, and above the diaphragm.
   (B) in the right hypochondriac region above the right lumbar region.
   (C) posterior abdomen behind the peritoneum on either side of the vertebral column between the 12th thoracic vertebrae and the 3rd lumbar vertebrae.
   (D) under the ribcage and superior to the stomach in the left upper quadrant of the abdomen.

2. Which component of the upper respiratory system is responsible for maintaining middle ear pressure?
   (A) larynx via the upper airways
   (B) Eustachian tube via the pharynx
   (C) nose via the nasopharynx
   (D) sinuses via the trachea

3. Red blood cells have a life span of approximately
   (A) 30 days.
   (B) 60 days.
   (C) 90 days.
   (D) 120 days.

4. All of the following are essential physiologic roles of electrolytes EXCEPT
   (A) altering tissue permeability.
   (B) influencing blood clotting time.
   (C) maintaining electroneutrality in fluid compartments.
   (D) regulating nerve impulse transmission.

5. Calcitonin
   (A) assists in the conversion of amino acids into glucose.
   (B) inhibits calcium from the parathyroid gland from entering the intestines.
   (C) decreases the release of calcium into the blood.
   (D) stimulates the breakdown of the bone matrix.

6. Select the correct conduction system for the heart.
   (A) SA node ⇒ AV node ⇑ Bundle of Purkinje (splits into left and right apex) ⇓ Bundle fibers
   (B) SA node ⇒ AV node ⇒ Bundle of His (splits into left and right bundle) ⇒ Purkinje fibers
   (C) AV node ⇒ SA node ⇒ Bundle of His (splits into left and right bundle) ⇒ Ventricular fibers ⇒ SA node
   (D) SA node ⇒ AV node ⇒ Bundle of His (splits into left and right bundle) ⇔ Purkinje fibers

7. The left coronary artery has the following branches:
   (A) great cardiac and small cardiac
   (B) left anterior descending and circumflex
   (C) posterior interventricular and marginal
   (D) small cardiac and middle cardiac

8. The liver occupies

    (A) most of the left lower quadrant and lies above the diaphragm.
    (B) most of the right lower quadrant and lies alongside of the diaphragm.
    (C) most of the left upper quadrant and lies behind the diaphragm.
    (D) most of the right upper quadrant and lies under the diaphragm.

9. The _____ represents the depolarization of the atria. During this wave, the muscles of the atria are contracting.

    (A) P wave
    (B) Q_1 wave
    (C) QRS complex
    (D) T wave

10. Which three of the following factors regulate heart rate?

    1. Autonomic nervous system
    2. Other factors
    3. Cardiac output
    4. Preload
    5. Chemicals
    6. Stroke volume
    7. Diastasis

    (A) 1, 2, 3
    (B) 1, 3, 6
    (C) 2, 4, 7
    (D) 5, 6, 7

11. All of the following are mechanisms of a nonspecific first line of body defenses EXCEPT

    (A) antibodies.
    (B) antimicrobial proteins.
    (C) cilia.
    (D) gastric juices.

12. Endocrine glands are classified as _____ or _____.

    (A) endocrine, exocrine
    (B) fat soluble, water soluble
    (C) sensory, motor
    (D) releasing, inhibiting

13. Ideal plasma pH is

    (A) 7.00–7.35
    (B) 7.35–7.45
    (C) 7.40–7.50
    (D) All of the above.

14. Platelets may also be referred to as

    (A) thrombin.
    (B) thrombocytes.
    (C) thromboplastin.
    (D) thrombusi.

15. Steroid and thyroid gland hormones that diffuse through cell membranes of target cells are known as _____ hormones.

    (A) lipid-soluble
    (B) inhibiting
    (C) releasing
    (D) water-soluble

16. All of the following are secreted by the pancreas EXCEPT

    (A) cholecystokinin.
    (B) glucagon.
    (C) insulin.
    (D) trypsin.

17. The human body cannot sustain life if pH is

    (A) <6.50 or >7.50
    (B) <6.80 or >7.80
    (C) <7.35 or >7.45
    (D) <8.00 or >8.50

18. A normal human pregnancy ranges from

    (A) 32 to 36 weeks
    (B) 38 to 42 weeks
    (C) 43 to 47 weeks
    (D) The number of weeks depends on when conception took place.

19. Neurotransmitters can be described as

   (A) activators of the reticular activation system.
   (B) chemical messengers.
   (C) inhibitors of the reflex arc.
   (D) responsible for integrating sensory information.

20. All of the following are used to supplement the immune response EXCEPT

   (A) antibiotics.
   (B) inborn immunity.
   (C) passive immunity.
   (D) vaccines.

21. Buffer systems control _____ ion concentrations.

   (A) bicarbonate
   (B) carbonic
   (C) hydrogen
   (D) plasma

22. What controls the autonomic nervous system?

   (A) hypothalamus
   (B) limbic system
   (C) pituitary
   (D) thalamus

23. Chemical digestion begins in the

   (A) duodenum.
   (B) esophagus.
   (C) mouth.
   (D) stomach.

24. Which one of the following is a *true* statement regarding the reflex arc in humans?

   (A) It is voluntary and nearly instantaneous movement in response to a specific stimulus.
   (B) Most sensory neurons do not pass directly into the brain, but synapse in the spinal cord.
   (C) The patellar reflex is polysynaptic, as opposed to monosynaptic.
   (D) The reflex arc types are autonomic and sensory.

25. One constituent of plasma is/are

   (A) albumin.
   (B) leukocytes.
   (C) monocytes.
   (D) platelets.

26. All of the following are pancreatic enzymes EXCEPT

   (A) chymotrypsin.
   (B) lipase.
   (C) somatotropin.
   (D) trypsin.

27. The appendix is part of the

   (A) accessory organs.
   (B) biliary system.
   (C) colon.
   (D) duodenum.

28. The _____ is the only muscle in the body under voluntary control.

   (A) endomysial muscle
   (B) perimysied muscle
   (C) smooth muscle
   (D) striated muscle

29. Simply put, the primary purpose of the hematological system is

   (A) erythropoesis.
   (B) formation of blood cells.
   (C) pH maintenance.
   (D) transportation.

30. What are the final branches of the bronchial tree called?

   (A) alveolar ducts
   (B) alveolar pores
   (C) alveolar sacs
   (D) alveolus

31. Which of the following is an example of a specific defense of the immune system?

   (A) B-cells
   (B) inflammatory response
   (C) phagocytes
   (D) vasodilation

32. Select the best definition for the glomeruli.

   (A) a dense ball of capillaries that branches from the afferent arteriole and enters the nephron
   (B) a double-walled, cup-shaped structure around the convex side of each nephron
   (C) the highly vascularized inner layer of the kidney
   (D) the thin membranous sheath that covers the inner surface of each kidney

33. The function of the sebum is to

   (A) discharge a liquid in reaction to stress or sexual excitement.
   (B) hinder the growth of bacteria and help constrain drying of the hair.
   (C) prevent foreign bodies from entering the internal ear canal.
   (D) promote evaporation to cool the skin.

34. The ejaculatory ducts connect the ductus deferens to the

   (A) external urethral orifice.
   (B) penis.
   (C) spermatic cord.
   (D) urethra.

35. The _____ response involves B-cells that identify antigens or pathogens circulating in the lymph or blood.

   (A) B-lymphocyte
   (B) humoral
   (C) inflammatory
   (D) cell-mediated

36. The human musculoskeletal system provides/supports/protects for all of the following EXCEPT

   (A) internal framework for muscle attachment.
   (B) movement through relaxation.
   (C) organs from injury.
   (D) leverage and movement.

37. What occurs when there are no nerve impulses to stimulate contraction?

   (A) muscle fatigue
   (B) muscle tone
   (C) muscle synergy
   (D) muscle relaxation

38. The eleventh cranial nerve is a _____ whose function is _____.

   (A) motor nerve, head and shoulder movement
   (B) motor nerve, eyelid and eyeball movement
   (C) sensory nerve, equilibrium and hearing
   (D) sensory nerve, facial expression and salivation

39. All of the following are types of muscles EXCEPT

   (A) cardiac.
   (B) coarse.
   (C) skeletal.
   (D) smooth.

40. What keeps the trachea from collapsing during inspiration?

   (A) hyaline cartilage
   (B) lower vocal folds
   (C) primary bronchi
   (D) windpipe

41. Antagonists are skeletal muscles that cause movement opposite to that of the _____.

   (A) parallel fascicles
   (B) prime mover
   (C) synergist
   (D) multipolar neurons

42. Keratin, found in the epidermis, is best defined as a protein that

   (A) defends cells from ultraviolet radiation.
   (B) interacts with leukocytes during an autoimmune response.
   (C) serves as a sensory function.
   (D) toughens and makes the skin impervious to water.

43. The communication network of _____ allows the human organism to interact with the external and internal environment.

   (A) axons
   (B) motor dendrites
   (C) neurotransmitters
   (D) sensory neurons

44. The reproductive system can be described as

   (A) a delectation system.
   (B) a gestational system.
   (C) systems that are separate but dependent.
   (D) systems that are separate but symbiotic.

45. The uterus is held in place by all of the following ligaments EXCEPT the

   (A) broad.
   (B) cardinal.
   (C) perimetrial.
   (D) round.

46. The function of the respiratory system is _____.

   (A) delivery of air to the lungs
   (B) external respiration
   (C) gas transport
   (D) pulmonary ventilation

47. Skin is regarded as an organ because it comprises

   (A) accessory organs such as sebaceous and sudoriferous glands.
   (B) differing layer of tissues. The entire body has four layers and the soles of the feet have five layers.
   (C) stratified squamous epithelium, such as Langerhans and Merkel cells.
   (D) two tissues, the connective and epithelial.

48. Urine formation, occurring in the nephrons, involves all of the following processes EXCEPT

   (A) filtration.
   (B) homeostasis.
   (C) reabsorption.
   (D) secretion.

49. In order for normal urination to occur, all parts of the urinary tract need to work together in the correct order.

   (A) False
   (B) False, providing urinary output is unchallenged
   (C) True
   (D) True, providing the efferent arteriole carries blood toward the glomeruli

50. Basic biological concepts include all of the following EXCEPT

   (A) adaptation.
   (B) homeostasis.
   (C) metabolism.
   (D) reproduction.

51. An object that maintains shape, occupies volume, has an identifying density, cannot be forced into a smaller space, and does not increase under pressure satisfies the definition of a

   (A) colloid.
   (B) gas.
   (C) liquid.
   (D) solid.

52. _____ is a group of different kinds of tissues working together to perform a particular activity.

(A) A cell
(B) An organ
(C) An organism
(D) An organ system

53. Select the correct statement.

(A) The skin is inferior to the muscle.
(B) The spleen and descending colon are ipsilateral.
(C) Bones are superficial to the muscle.
(D) The heart is proximal to the lungs.

STOP

If there is still time remaining, you may review your answers.

ANSWER KEY
Science Test

1. **C**	12. **A**	23. **C**	34. **D**	45. **C**
2. **B**	13. **B**	24. **B**	35. **B**	46. **A**
3. **D**	14. **B**	25. **A**	36. **B**	47. **D**
4. **A**	15. **A**	26. **C**	37. **D**	48. **B**
5. **C**	16. **A**	27. **C**	38. **A**	49. **C**
6. **B**	17. **B**	28. **D**	39. **B**	50. **D**
7. **B**	18. **B**	29. **D**	40. **A**	51. **D**
8. **D**	19. **B**	30. **A**	41. **B**	52. **B**
9. **A**	20. **B**	31. **A**	42. **D**	53. **B**
10. **A**	21. **C**	32. **A**	43. **D**	
11. **A**	22. **A**	33. **B**	44. **D**	

SCIENCE TEST—ANSWERS EXPLAINED

1. **(C)** Choice C describes the correct location of the kidneys.

2. **(B)** The middle ear, also known as the tympanic cavity, is an air filled space. The Eustachian tube maintains pressure in the middle ear.

3. **(D)** Review erythrocytes (RBCs) on page 257.

4. **(A)** Most electrolytes have more than one physiologic role in the body. Several electrolytes may work together to mediate chemical events. The physiologic roles of electrolytes include: changing cell membrane permeability, influencing blood clotting time, upholding electroneutrality in fluid compartments, facilitating enzyme reactions, regulating muscle contraction and relaxation, and regulating nerve impulse transmission. Electrolytes do not alter tissue permeability.

5. **(C)** Calcitonin, a hormone, is released by the thyroid to decrease the level of calcium in the blood.

6. **(B)** Review impulse conduction in the heart on page 212 if you missed this question.

7. **(B)** Review blood supply to the heart on page 212.

8. **(D)** Choice D provides the correct location of the liver.

9. **(A)** The cardiac cycle (PQRST) is seen as wave patterns on an EKG. The P wave in the SA node causes the atria to contract. The R wave in the AV node of the right atrium causes the ventricles to contract (QRS wave), and the T wave represents the repolarization of the cardiac muscle.

10. **(A)** The sympathetic or parasympathetic systems influence the heart by increasing or decreasing the heart rate. Other factors that influence heart rate are activity level, age, body temperature, and various pathologies.

11. **(A)** Antibodies are immunoglobulins, specialized immune proteins, produced when an antigen is introduced into the body. They have the ability to combine with the antigen that triggered its production.

12. **(A)** Glands are classified as endocrine or exocrine. Endocrine glands, or ductless glands, release hormones directly into the blood stream. Exocrine glands, or ducted glands, release enzymes and other products into ducts.

13. **(B)** The ideal plasma pH is 7.4, and exists within a range of 7.35–7.45.

14. **(B)** Review platelets on page 258 if you missed this question.

15. **(A)** Water-soluble and lipid-soluble hormones are contained within the endocrine system. They differ in how they bind to receptors in or on target cells. Water-soluble hormones bind or form a chemical bond with receptors on the exterior of target cells and do not easily pass through the plasma membrane that surrounds target cells. Lipid-soluble hormones pass through the plasma membrane and bind to receptors in the cytoplasm or nucleus of the cell.

16. **(A)** Cholecystokinin is an intestinal hormone. It stimulates contraction of the gallbladder and the release of pancreatic juice.

17. **(B)** The human body exists within a narrow pH band. A pH of less than 6.80 or greater than 7.80 cannot sustain life.

18. **(B)** Human gestation begins at conception when the sperm from the man fertilizes the ovum of the woman. The gestation period continues until the child is born. The "normal" gestation period is around 40 weeks, but may range from 37 or 38 to 42 weeks and still be considered a normal pregnancy.

19. **(B)** A neurotransmitter is a chemical messenger that transports, boosts, and regulates signals between neurons and other cells in the body. In the majority of instances, a neurotransmitter is discharged from the axon terminal after an action potential has arrived at the synapse. The neurotransmitter then transverses the synaptic gap to reach the receptor site of the other cell or neuron. Once the site is reached, the neurotransmitter connects to the receptor site and is reabsorbed by the neuron in a process known as reuptake.

20. **(B)** Inborn immunity is inherited. Supplements add to, complement, or enhance something. In terms of supplementing immunity, these are antibiotics (bacteriostatic or bacteriocidal preparations), passive immunity (obtained when antibodies are transferred from an individual who has had a disease, or from breast milk), and vaccines (substances that stimulate the production of memory cells; may require a booster).

21. **(C)** Acid-base balance is associated with the hydrogen concentration in body fluids. A buffer is a solution that thwarts substantial changes in pH when amounts of acids or bases are added. The phosphate carbonic acid-sodium bicarbonate, and protein are buffer systems in the body.

22. **(A)** The autonomic nervous system is regulated by the hypothalamus.

23. **(C)** Review the digestive process (oral cavity) on page 245.

24. **(B)** Reflex arcs are involuntary, somatic, and the patellar reflex is monosynaptic. A reflex arc is a neural pathway that regulates an action reflex. In humans, most sensory neurons do not pass promptly into the brain, but synapse in the spinal cord. This feature allows reflex actions to occur relatively fast by activating spinal motor neurons without the delay of steering signals through the brain, even though the brain will receive sensory input while the reflex action occurs. There are two types of reflex arcs: the autonomic reflex arc (affecting inner organs) and the somatic reflex arc (affecting muscles).

25. **(A)** Review the constituents of plasma in Figure 6.7. Composition of Whole Blood on page 256.

26. **(C)** Somatotropin, produced by the anterior pituitary, is a growth hormone.

27. **(C)** The appendix is attached to the cecum, a bag-like structure of the colon, located at the connection of the small and large intestine.

28. **(D)** The striated muscle may be referred to as voluntary muscle because contractions of this muscle can be deliberately controlled.

29. **(D)** Review the Overview of the Hematologic System on page 255 if you missed this question.

30. **(A)** The alveolar ducts are the final branches of the bronchial tree.

31. **(A)** B-cells, or lymphocytes, are lymphocytes developed in the bone marrow. Antigen receptors of the B-cells bond freely to antigens circulating in the vascular or lymph system. Inflammatory responses, phagocytes, and vasodilation are the second line of (nonspecific) defenses that arbitrarily confront foreign invaders inside the body.

32. **(A)** The key phrase is "dense ball of capillaries." Choice A is the correct definition of glomeruli.

33. **(B)** Sebum, secreted from sebaceous glands, serves to hinder the growth of bacteria and help constrain drying of the hair. It also has antibacterial properties.

34. **(D)** Review the ejaculatory ducts on pages 315–316 if you had difficulty answering this question.

35. **(B)** The humoral response (antibody-mediated response) engages cells that identify antigens (pathogens) circulating the blood or lymph.

36. **(B)** Skeletal muscles move in response to muscles that work like levers. This allows a variety of movements such as bending, running, sitting, and stooping. Skeletal muscles will not contract unless stimulated by neurons whereas smooth and cardiac muscles will. A muscle relaxes where there are no nerve impulses to stimulate it to contract.

37. **(D)** Muscles respond to stimuli. When no stimuli are present, the muscles are in a state of rest or relaxation.

38. **(A)** Review the eleventh cranial nerve on page 300.

39. **(B)** There are no muscles that are considered coarse muscles.

40. **(A)** The hyaline cartilage is composed of approximately 20 rigid, C-shaped rings embedded in the submucosa of the trachea that prevent the trachea from collapsing during inspiration.

41. **(B)** Several muscles influence any particular body movement. The prime mover is the muscle most responsible for the movement. The antagonist is the muscle or muscles that move opposite to the prime mover.

42. **(D)** Choice D provides the best definition of keratin.

43. **(D)** Nerves of the peripheral nervous system are classified by the direction of nerve spread. Sensory (afferent) neurons transmit impulses from the skin and other sensory organs toward the central nervous system. Motor (efferent) neurons transmit impulses away from the central nervous system to effectors (muscles or glands).

44. **(D)** Symbiotic relationships are interdependent, reciprocal, and suggest a mutually beneficial relationship. Male and female relationships are, for the most part, symbiotic for many reasons. This is particularly true in terms of reproduction.

45. **(C)** The perimetrial ligament does not exist. There is the perimetrium which is the outer layer of the uterus, but it does not need a ligament. When weighing answer choices, beware of selecting terms you have never heard of or seen before.

46. **(A)** External respiration and gas transport are processes of respiration. Pulmonary ventilation is the process of inspiration and expiration, or breathing.

47. **(D)** Review the Overview of the Integumentary System on page 277 if you missed this question.

48. **(B)** Filtration, reabsorption, and secretion all take place within the nephron. Homeostasis does not.

49. **(C)** The key to answering this question correctly is recognizing the word "normal" in the question stem.

50. **(D)** Adaptation, homeostasis, and metabolism are necessary for an individual or species to survive and are characteristics of all living things. Reproduction is a method by which new individuals are produced. A species will become extinct if it loses its reproductive potential.

51. **(D)** The question stem is the definition of a solid.

52. **(B)** A cell is the smallest unit of life, and may be specialized, but it is not considered an organ. An organism is a system having the physiognomic of living things. An organ system is two or more organs working in tandem to perform a function.

53. **(B)** Review Table 3.4. Anatomical Directional Terms on page 47 if you had difficulty answering this question.

References

American Heritage Dictionary. Boston: Houghton Miffin Co., 2014.

Arco Educational Board. *Vocabulary, Spelling, and Grammar: Self Taught To Increase Your Personal Effectiveness*. New York: Arco Publishing, Inc., 1982.

Bobrow, J. *Math Review for Standardized Tests*. Lincoln, NE: Cliffs Notes, 1985.

Chen, L. *Painless Chemistry*. Hauppauge, NY: Barron's Educational Series, Inc., 2011.

Dickinson, E. "I Heard a Fly Buzz When I Died," in *The Norton Anthology of Poetry (Shorter Edition)*, edited by A.M. Eastman (Coordinating Editor). New York: W.W. Norton & Company, Inc., 1970.

Edwards, G. I., & C. Pfirrman. *E–Z Biology*. Hauppauge, NY: Barron's Educational Series, Inc., 2009.

Fluids and Electrolytes Made Incredibly Easy. Springhouse, PA: Springhouse, 1997.

Frost, R. "Stopping By Woods on a Snowy Evening," in *The Norton Anthology of Poetry (Shorter Edition)*, edited by A.M. Eastman (Coordinating Editor). New York: W.W. Norton & Company, Inc., 1970.

Hargrove-Huttel, R. *Review Series: Medical-Surgical Nursing, 4th Edition*. Philadelphia: Lippincott Williams & Wilkins, 2005.

Hogan, A., & D. Wane. *Fluids, Electrolytes, and Acid-Base Balance: Reviews and Rationales*. Upper Saddle River, NJ: Pearson Education, Inc., 2003.

http://breastfeeding-problems.com/breastfeeding-with-small-breasts.html

http://courses.cvcc.vccs.edu/wisemand/discussion of the pyramids.htm

http://medical-dictionary.thefreedictionary.com

http://ptdirect.com/training-design/anatomy-and-physiology/joints-joint-action-examples of movement

http://study.com/academy/lesson/what-is-collagen-definition-types-and-diseases.html

http://umm.edu/health/medical/altmed/supplement/calcium#ixzz3icQ2daXA

http://www.boundless.com/textbooks/boundless-biology-textbook

http://www.emedicinehealth.com/electrolytes/

http://www.md-health.com/Lobes-Of-The-Brain.html

http://www.medicalnewstoday.com/articles/153188.php

http://www.medicinenet.com

http://www.newhealthguide.org/Gestation-Period-for-Humans.html

http://www.nlm.nih.gov/medlineplus

http://www.wiley.com/legacy/products/subject/life/elgert/CH04.pdf

http://www.yourhormones.Info/Hormones/Prolactin.aspx

Hensyl, W. R. *Steadman's Medical Dictionary, 25th Edition.* Baltimore, Lippincott Williams & Wilkins, 1990.

Jones, D. (2012). *Painless Reading Comprehension.* Hauppauge, NY: Barron's Educational Series, Inc., 2012.

Krumhardt, B., & I.E., Alcamo. *E–Z Anatomy and Physiology.* Hauppauge, NY: Barron's Educational Series, Inc., 2010.

Mead, M. *Coming of Age in Samoa: A Psychological Study of Primitive Youth for Western Civilisation [sic], Non-copyright Edition.* New York: William Morrow & Company, 1928.

Pack, P. E. *Anatomy and Physiology.* Lincoln, NE: Cliffs Notes, 1997.

Phillips, L. D. *Manual of IV Therapeutics.* Philadelphia: F.A. Davis, 2005.

Index

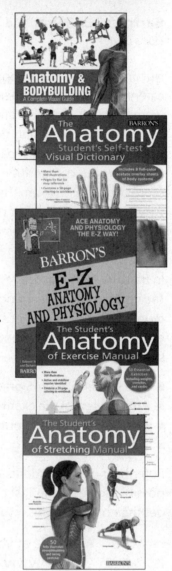

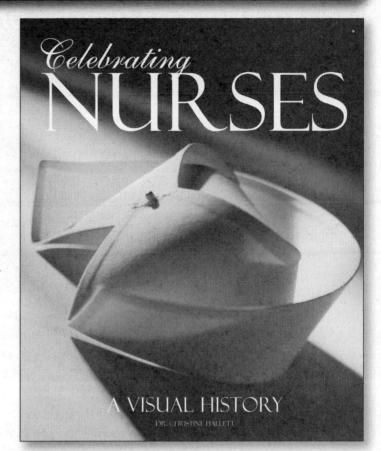
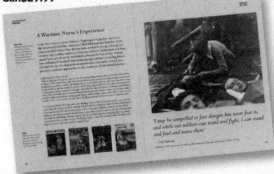
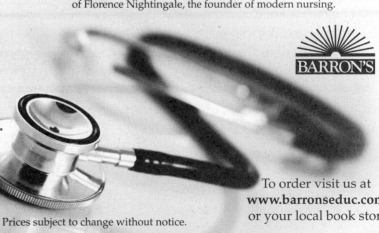

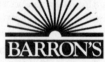
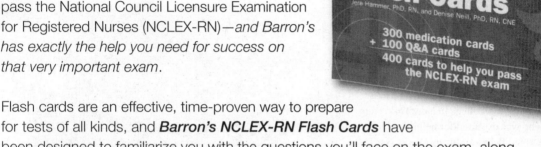
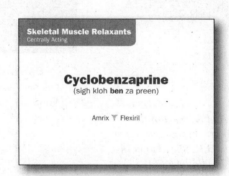